THE HANDBOOK OF COMPLEMENTARY MEDICINE

Second Edition

THE HANDBOOK OF COMPLEMENTARY MEDI-CINE in its first edition, was acknowledged to be the most authoritative and complete guide to alternative medicine in the UK. Growing out of a two-year research project it covered all aspects of complementary medicine – ranging from why people turned to complementary practitioners in the first place to providing a detailed guide to some 250 organisations in the field.

This new updated edition reflects the dramatic increase in public interest in complementary medicine over the last few years. This has been fuelled in no small part by the Royal Family's support and interest in such therapies.

This is an invaluable reference guide for both the professional and the layman. Written with great clarity it is a valuable guide to what is fast becoming the second health service in the country.

The Handbook of Complementary Medicine

Second Edition

Stephen Fulder

With a Foreword by John Thompson,
Professor of Pharmacology,
University of Newcastle upon Tyne

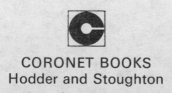

CORONET BOOKS
Hodder and Stoughton

Copyright © 1988 by
Stephen Fulder

First published in Great
Britain in paperback by
Coronet Books 1984

First revised and updated
hardback edition by Oxford
University Press 1988

Coronet revised and updated
edition 1989

British Library C.I.P.

Fulder, Stephen
    The handbook of
complementary
medicine.—
    2nd ed.
    1. Alternative medicine
    I. Title
    615.5

ISBN 0-340-49484-0

Printed and bound in Great
Britain for Hodder and
Stoughton Paperbacks, a
division of Hodder and
Stoughton Ltd., Mill Road,
Dunton Green, Sevenoaks,
Kent TN13 2YA (Editorial
Office: 47 Bedford Square,
London WC1B 3DP) by
Richard Clay Ltd., Bungay,
Suffolk.

Foreword

John W. Thompson M.B., Ph.D., F.R.C.P.

*Professor of Pharmacology, University of
Newcastle upon Tyne and Consultant Clinical
Pharmacologist and Consultant in Charge,
Pain Relief Clinic, Royal Victoria Infirmary,
Newcastle upon Tyne*

Be ye doers of the word, and not hearers only.
James i: 22

What *is* complementary (or alternative) medicine; and how does it
relate to orthodox or conventional medicine? The fact that you are
reading this foreword may indicate that you are one of a large and
growing number of people who wish to find out more about this
fascinating and important subject. Without this book you would
have found it extremely difficult to collect this information;
although many books and papers on this subject exist, each deals
with only a small area and has usually been written by a specialist.
What has been lacking is a comprehensive and critical account of the
entire field of complementary medicine. But such a review could
only be undertaken by someone who possesses a rare combination of
skills. Ideally, the author needs to have a trained and experienced
scientific mind; a wide and deep knowledge of complementary
medicine; an accurate and lucid style of writing and an objectivity of
outlook that would only be possible in someone who does not
practise complementary or conventional medicine. Fortunately such
a person exists in the form of Dr. Stephen Fulder who has degrees in
biochemistry, chemical pharmacology, and genetics and has held
important posts at the National Institute for Medical Research and
also Chelsea College, London, before setting up his own Con-
sultancy and Research Organization on Biomedicine (CAROB). In
writing a review of this whole field, Dr. Fulder has been constantly

aware of the important fact that if complementary medicine has anything important to offer—and it certainly seems that it has—then wherever possible it must be investigated and tested fully by means of controlled laboratory experiments and rigorous clinical trials in just the same way as is required for orthodox or conventional medicine. Even if some form of treatment is not based on currently accepted theories of biomedical science, it should still be possible for it to be tested using present-day scientific methods; and the author has painstakingly sifted through the evidence available. Conventional medicine does not hold all the answers to the problems of disease and that is why it so important to find out what positive contributions can be made by complementary medicine. The best of both systems then need to be brought to work together for the greater benefit of the human race.

Dr. Fulder is to be congratulated on tackling a marathon task and to have produced a fascinating, stimulating, and critical account of complementary medicine. Certainly no-one having read this book can fail to be anything but better informed and more critically orientated towards a subject that should be the concern of all of us.

Preface

Alternative approaches to traditional medicine currently command great interest. Although many books containing information on individual therapies have been published, no thorough examination of the present state of these alternatives has yet been written. There is no comprehensive review of the organizations and training establishments involved with alternative therapies. Nor is there a summary of the rationale and practice of the therapies which is written with the sceptical conventional medical practitioner as much in mind as the devotees and practitioners of the therapies themselves. For these reasons I have attempted to rectify the situation with the publication of this book which I hope will fulfil both professional and lay requirements.

Lack of data has been the principal reason that a book like this has not previously been published. Indeed, inadequate information concerning the extent of public use of the therapies and the practices of therapists has made it difficult for society to appreciate their role. To remedy this the Threshold Foundation (see Chapter 3) provided a generous grant to Robin Monro and myself to gather and compile all available information on the state of the therapies today. Where necessary we had to carry out primary research by means of questionnaires. The project took a hectic fifteen months to complete.[1] We collected documents, papers, and reports on scientific, social, and legal aspects, keyworded for accessibility. We prepared a comprehensive classified directory of organizations and their activities, with some 500 entries, up-to-date scientific bibliographies, files of practitioners, book titles, press cuttings, and so on. The material is available at the Research Council for Complementary Medicine, Suite 1, 19a, Cavendish Square, London W1M 9AD, and the library of the British School of Osteopathy. The collection of this material has made this book possible.

Both Robin Monro and myself are scientists, not practitioners, and we hope this background has provided us with a useful degree of objectivity. I have attempted to present the activities of therapists as fairly as possible, disregarding the prejudices still to be found on both sides of the medical divide. No judgements are intended regarding the relative qualities of the therapies. These valuations must be made at a later date. However, I must state at the outset my conviction that complementary medicine has a vital role to play in our future; because of its emphasis on safe and subtle treatment methods and self-care, it will be able to contain many chronic and insidious diseases which conventional medicine has failed to cure. I believe in a pluralistic health system and these views are expressed and supported in this book.

In order to keep this book in manageable proportions some boundaries have had to be drawn. First, the book encompasses therapies that treat the body and the whole being but I have had to exclude all the purely psychological and psychotherapeutic therapies: encounter, psychosynthesis, meditation, Gestalt, bioenergetics, and the other 140 psychotherapies listed by President Carter's commission on mental health. However, since mental and physical health are interconnected, psychological therapies that are more psychosomatic, such as hypnotherapy, autogenics, and biofeedback, are included. I have also distinguished between healing and general inner development, regretfully omitting such disciplines as yoga, T'ai-Chi, martial arts, or sports. These are primarily designed for the healthy, and although they can also be invaluable in treating the sick, they are rarely tailored specifically to the diagnosed condition of each individual.

Every effort has been made to be accurate and as up to date as possible. Entries for the organizational directory were sent to each establishment for checking; the material is therefore dependent on their willingness to supply accurate information. I hope that organizations will approach the author through the publishers with further information to maintain the accuracy of this handbook.

July 1987 S.F.

Note on terminology

Where the word *medicine* is used, it is distinguished by the adjectives *conventional* or *complementary*. Where practitioners are referred to, *doctor* or *physician* are used exclusively in connection with conventional medicine and *therapist* in connection with complementary medicine. *Practitioner* on its own is used interchangeably with its meaning defined by its context.

Notes

1. Fulder, S.J. and Monro, R. (1981). *The status of complementary medicine in the United Kingdom.* Threshold Foundation, London.

   Fulder, S.J. and Monro, R. (1985). Complementary medicine in the United Kingdom: patients, practitioners, and consultations. *Lancet*, **2**, 542–5. The survey data is referred to frequently in this book. We carried out two primary projects from October 1980 to April 1981. The first was a poll which sought information from all the organizations representing therapists (including healers) on membership, practising membership, change in numbers of members over time, numbers of doctor members, estimates as to total number of practising therapists in the UK in that therapy, and then premises, book lists, opinions and attitudes, educational standards, etc. Response was virtually 100 per cent. The second was a questionnaire submitted to therapists whose names were obtained from registers, yellow pages, local periodicals, health shops and centres, other therapists, etc. Probably all the therapists practising in Oxfordshire and Cambridge were identified and by means of follow-up interviews 80–90 per cent completed questionnaires. In Cardiff, Exeter, Sheffield, Hereford, and Cumbria detection of therapists was less complete and since postal questionnaires were self-administered, only a third were completed. Only professional therapists who let it be known that they were able to treat members of the public, normally for a fee, were interviewed. A total of 137 questionnaires were received.

Acknowledgements

I should like to acknowledge Robin Monro, my friend and partner in the Threshold Project for his extensive and careful work; Ruth West, William Cash, Mr A.J. de Wit of the Dutch Commission on Alternative Medicine, Herta Larive, and the many others who have supplied information to us; John Blackwood for his careful reading of the manuscript; Clare Wright whose steady and intelligent assistance is greatly appreciated and whose considerable understanding of therapy has helped me through more than one boggy patch; and my wife Rachel, for her forbearance and intuition.

I am greatly indebted to the following leading practitioners with whom the chapters indicated have been written, and without whom this book would have been impossible: Peter Bartlett LCSP (Applied Kinesiology); Robert Davidson R.S. Hom., MCH, (Homeopathy); Colin Dove MRO (Osteopathy); Jonathan Drake MD (Alexander Technique); Michael Endacott (Healing); Michael Evans MD (Anthroposophical Medicine); Nicola Hall (Reflexology); Simon Mills MNIMH (Herbalism); Roger Newman-Turner ND, DO, B.Ac. (Naturopathy and Nutrition Therapy); Iris Oliver (Remedial Massage); David Tansley DC (Radionics); Lorraine Taylor, SRN, B.Ac. (Acupuncture and Oriental Medicine).

I am most grateful to the Threshold Foundation for supporting the national survey which generated a good deal of the data and material on which this book is based, and to Harold Wicks, past General Secretary of the Research Council for Complementary Medicine, for his tireless support.

Contents

Glossary and classification of therapies

Medical systems

Complementary medicine
  Alternative medicine
  Fringe medicine
  Unconventional
    medicine
  Unorthodox medicine
  Natural medicine

The aggregate of diagnostic and therapeutic practices and systems which are separate from and in contrast to conventional scientific medicine.

Conventional medicine
  Scientific medicine
  Orthodox medicine
  Technical medicine
  Modern medicine

The aggregate of diagnostic and therapeutic concepts and practices which attempt to adhere to modern scientific principles.

Far Eastern medicine
  Oriental medicine
    Chinese, Korean,
    Japanese, Tibetan,
    etc.

The aggregate of unique diagnostic and therapeutic practices developed in Far Eastern countries, in particular acupuncture, constitutional medicine, herbalism, movement, massage, and dietary control.

Folk medicine

The aggregate of practices, remedies, and recipes which form a largely unwritten and unsystematic body of knowledge among the lay population.

Holistic medicine

The combined use of conventional medicine, complementary medicine, psychotherapy, and health education by medical and other practitioners and

---

Main therapeutic specialties are in **bold** type, therapeutic subspecialties are in *italics*. Synonyms are in roman type.

	instructors, often within a General Practice setting.
Indian medicine	The unique traditional medicine and remedies of the Indian sub-continent.
Ayurvedic medicine	The aggregate of diagnostic and therapeutic practices, based on the Vedic texts, incorporating a complete life instruction and branches on constitutional medicine, surgery, remedies, longevity practices, etc.
Unani medicine	Ayurvedic medicine joined with ancient Arabic medicine.
Siddha medicine	Ayurvedic medicine joined with the indigenous medicines of the Dravidian people of Southern India.
Traditional medicine Primitive medicine Indigenous medicine	The aggregate of indigenous diagnostic and the therapeutic practices, which may or may not be formal and systematic, which have developed to form an integral part of a culture.

Therapies in complementary medicine

Acupuncture	Techniques whereby needles are inserted into specific sites on the body surface to improve the flow of energy around the body, thus preventing and treating disease and disability.
Acupressure Shiatzu	Techniques whereby finger massage is applied to these same points, combined, in shiatzu, with general massage.
Electro-acupuncture	Adaption of acupuncture in which small electrical currents are applied to

needles inserted into the acupuncture points.

Ear acupuncture
  Auricular therapy

Acupuncture solely applied to points in and around the ear in order to affect other parts of the body.

Moxibustion

The burning of rolled cones of dried *Artemisia* (mugwort) over acupuncture points in order to affect the flow of energy at those points to prevent and treat diseases and disabilities.

Anthroposophical medicine

A therapeutic system based on the 'anthroposophical' teachings of Rudolf Steiner in which physical health is achieved through harmony between the various co-existent aspects of man and the environment. Creativity, self-observation, and special (including homeopathic) remedies are used.

Eurythmy

The use of rhythmical movements to heal and reintegrate healthy, sick, or disabled people.

Speech therapy

The similar use of sound, speech, and breath.

Art therapy

The similar use of art, colour, and form.

Breathing therapies

Use of breath for therapeutic purposes.

Pranayama

Indian yogic methods of breath control often used for therapeutic purposes.

Diagnosis

Iridology

Diagnosis by observation of the marks, patterns, and colours of the iris, which are reflections of body diseases and experiences.

Auric diagnosis

Psychic diagnosis by analysis of the colours and changes of the aura perceived by sensitives.

Kirlian photography

Diagnostic method which photographs the corona discharge of 'bioenergy' around the body.

Electrical therapies

Use of electromagnetic energy directly for therapeutic purposes.

Magnetic field therapy

Use of a magnetic field to aid repair, regeneration, and healing of tissues.

Diathermy

Special equipment sending pulses of electromagnetic energy deep into tissues to warm them and heal them.

Ion generators

Equipment to generate and emit negatively charged ion particles in order to aid mood and concentration.

Healing
  Faith healing
  Spiritual healing
  Magnetic healing
  Mental healing
  Laying on of hands

The direct transmission of psychic energy for therapeutic purposes.

Absent healing

Healing which is given by healer to a patient who is at a distance.

Prayer healing

Healing which is focused, transmitted, and effected by means of prayer.

Spirit healing
  Exorcism

Use of discarnate entities in healing.

Auric healing	Healing directed towards the subtle or etheric aura of the body to cure its susceptibilities and prevent their manifestation in the body as diseases.
Homeopathy	A therapeutic system developed by Samuel Hahnemann, which treats the symptoms of a patient with microscopic doses of those remedies which create similar symptoms in the healthy.
Biochemic remedies	Small amounts of salts used on homeopathic principles.
Bach flower remedies	Extracts of flowers diluted according to homeopathic principles which are applied to cure subtle emotional roots of disease.
Hydrotherapy Balneology	The use of mineral water, thermal springs, mud, pools, and bathing in therapy.
Spas	Health resorts primarily devoted to hydrotherapy
Manipulative therapies	Treatment by means of manual force or touch or pressure applied to the body.
Chiropractic	A technique in which movement is restored, especially between the vertebrae, by means of massage and short sharp thrusts. This is intended to restore circulation and enervation of connected organs.
Osteopathy	A technique in which movement and function of the musculoskeletal system is restored by means of leverage and repeated manual articulation.

Cranial osteopathy	Pressure applied to the bones of the cranium to affect musculature and body fluids for the treatment of specific conditions.
Manipulation	Leverage and articulation of the body used pragmatically, usually by medical doctors, without connection to the techniques of osteopathy and chiropractic.
Bonesetting	The restoration of alignment and integrity of limbs after injury.
Massage	Any technique in which pressure and touch are applied to the body to stimulate the circulation and relax the tissues.
Kinesiology	A technique in which muscular strength and balance at distant points is used to determine the site and nature of a local impairment.
Reflexology Reflex zone therapy	Massage of areas of the feet to treat organ systems with which they are in developmental relationship.
Polarity therapy	Combination of massage and the teaching of awareness of the body and its dimensions and interrelations.
Rolfing	A deep massage technique to make structural alterations in the musculature, to liberate tensions, and to awaken protected, underused areas.
Postural integration	A massage and instructural process which realigns the body, liberating tensions and inhibitions.
Naturopathy Nature cure	Systems which use predominantly the body's own self-healing capacities in a

	Hippocratic manner, eschewing most external remedies.
Hygienic systems	Strict nature cure, relying on fasting and purifications, without any recourse to remedies.
Nutritional therapy	Treatment by dietary control and the use of food supplements and components as medicines.
Clinical ecology	Treatment by the detection and elimination of allergenic and irritant foods from the diet.
Dietetics	Planning appropriate diets according to the nutritional principles laid down by conventional medicine.
Monodiets	Diet restricted to one item for a specific period, such as a grape juice diet.
Fasting	A common component of naturopathy in which little or no food is taken for a specific period.
Vegetarianism	A way of life which excludes the consumption of birds, animals, or fish.
Veganism	A way of life which excludes the consumption of all bird, animal or fish products including eggs and milk products.
Macrobiotics	Diets according to the principles established in Zen monasteries in which the grain-, vegetable-, animal-, salt-, heat- or cold-producing and *yin* or *yang* qualities of food are balanced appropriately.

Postural therapies   Treatment of posture by reconditioning mental and physical attitudes to self and habitual patterns of movement.

Alexander Technique   A technique developed by F.M. Alexander for postural improvement by means of constant self-awareness.

Feldenkrais Technique   A technique developed by M. Feldenkrais for restoration of postural balance, relaxation, and ease of movement by learning natural, pleasurable, and harmonious movement.

Psionic medicine   Use of pendulum and instruments
  Medical Dowsing   focusing psychic power to diagnose
  Radiesthesia   and select appropriate treatments (usually homeopathic), which attack long-term predispositions to diseases, rooted in the subtle body of the patient.

Radionics   Use of equipment on radiesthetic principles expressing diagnosis and the required remedy in quantitative terms.

Psychosomatic therapies   Procedures and therapies which create mental states and behaviour patterns beneficial to general health and recovery from disease.

Autogenic Training   A technique of implanting positive
  Autosuggestion   suggestions into the subconscious by repeated self-instructions, particularly in relation to relaxation and stress diseases.

Hypnotherapy   The use of hypnotic suggestion to
  Hypnosis   treat illness and destructive behavioural patterns.

Bioenergetics
  Biodynamics
  Reichian therapeutics

Behavioural and psychological encounters with a therapist resulting in an often explosive release of psychological blocks, body tensions, and inhibitions, leading to improved general health and well-being.

Biofeedback

The use of equipment to self-monitor physiological signals from the mind or body and thus to bring involuntary processes under voluntary control.

Relaxation techniques

Techniques for calming the mind and body and releasing muscle tensions so as to induce deep relaxation.

Meditation
  Visualisation

Techniques for calming, concentrating, and purifying the mind by persistent focusing, leading to self-transcendence.

Remedies
  Home remedies
  Natural medicines

Materials in the natural world, excluding drugs, taken with therapeutic intent. Can even be foods.

Herbs

Plant materials so taken.

Health remedies
  Health products

Remedies or food supplements which are taken for preventive and health promoting purposes.

Mineral remedies

Salts and inorganic materials taken as remedies.

Organic remedies

Tissues, enzymes, extracts, and biological materials, processed or unprocessed, taken as remedies.

Cell therapy

Techniques pioneered by Paul Niehans in which cells from the homologous organ of foetal animals are injected to cure a diseased organ in man.

Herbalism

Therapeutic systems based exclusively

Phytotherapy	on the curative power of herbal and mineral remedies.
Sense therapies	Use of specific patterns of sense impressions to heal imbalances and assist in cure.
Aroma therapies	Use of oils, vapours, and essences for therapeutic purposes.
Colour therapy	Use of specific coloured environments, clothes, and lights for therapeutic purposes.
Sound therapy	Use of patterns of sound for therapeutic purposes.

PART 1

General survey

1

The background

Introducing complementary medicine

It would be unrealistic to attempt an exact definition of those therapies which are found outside mainstream conventional medicine. For they are a diverse assortment, both ancient (e.g. acupuncture) and modern (biofeedback). Some provide more fundamental curative treatment (naturopathy), while others can, at times, be highly symptomatic (medical homeopathy). Some shun any artificial aid (nature cure) while others use extensive medicinal intervention (herbalism). Useful working definitions therefore usually focus on the one aspect that is common to all: the fact that they are separate from conventional scientific medicine. Even here there are no sharp dividing lines: the philosophies of radionics or healing are utterly at odds with conventional medical principles but the bases of osteopathy or herbalism are quasi-scientific and could be incorporated into conventional medicine without stretching its scientific model to breaking point.

After extensive discussions, the author and many others who are working in this area concluded that *complementary medicine* is the most accurate and reasonable umbrella description of the therapies. It sees them as partners to, though different in nature from, scientific medicine. 'Alternative medicine' is an unsatisfactory description, for the therapies could never entirely replace conventional medicine. 'Fringe', 'unorthodox', or 'unconventional' are based on an out-of-date view of the therapies and place them in a rather alienated and embattled light.

Despite their diversity, a common bond unites the therapies.[1] They all attempt, in varying degrees, to recruit the self-healing capacities of the body. They amplify natural recuperative processes and augment the energy upon which the patient's health depends, helping him to adapt harmoniously to his surroundings. Symptoms are sometimes treated at the outset, as in osteopathy or chiropractic, or are left to clear up by themselves as the individual progresses towards health, as in traditional acupuncture. In all cases, however, the symptoms are used as guides to the origin of the patient's upset or imbalance.

Several distinctive practical attitudes arise from this emphasis on self-healing. Firstly, symptoms may only be assessed in relation to a particular personality. For this reason therapists attempt to gain a full constitutional and biographical picture of a patient. Treatment seeks to realign and restore imbalances, defects and destructive patterns by determining why they arose in this particular individual. The patient is very rarely assessed against a statistical norm. 'Normal' instead means the potential capacity for health of the individual consulting the therapist.

Secondly, since it is the individual who is treated as well as his symptoms, there are no special reasons to erect or maintain barriers between mind, body, and spirit. Lifestyle, attitudes, caste of mind, vital energy, posture, and bearing are considered relevant in most of the therapies. Even in the manipulative therapies (osteopathy and chiropractic), efforts will be made to identify the sources of tensions and stresses within the body and make the patient aware of them.

Thirdly, complementary medicine uses a broad definition of health. This goes beyond the mere absence of symptoms to include a state of complete physical and mental well-being (the definition of health used by the World Health Organization). Poor vitality and low resistance are conventionally regarded as states of health rather than illness; only complementary therapists take them seriously. Most practitioners will continue to work with a patient after all his symptoms have disappeared, in an effort to improve his health and well-being. Therefore, a good deal of complementary medicine is preventive.

Fourthly, complementary medicine is most at home treating chronic, psychogenic, and organic diseases for which the resistance and health of the patient is a key to recovery. It is least comfortable with acute and epidemic diseases and injuries although here it can have an adjunctive role to play. This is in contrast to conventional medicine.

Fifthly, since the goal of complementary medicine is self-healing, the therapies are generally harmless when practised competently, and remedies are non-toxic. The therapies have not always been so harmless but certain more toxic and powerful procedures, such as the use of the apothecary's mineral remedies, have been abandoned over the last hundred years. There are certain risks with all therapies and these are described in the relevant chapters but they are very small compared to those of conventional medicine.

This emphasis on self-healing means that the patient must do what he can to help himself. All therapies are partly instructional and some, such as the Alexander or relaxation techniques, are almost entirely so. Virtually all therapists will have something to say about diet and exercise, believing that many current chronic diseases are caused or exacerbated by improper eating habits and superfluous, impure, and unhealthy foods. The patient is encouraged to discover why he is sick and to work for his own cure, with the therapist as a partner whose function is partly catalytic. With most therapies, in particular the Alexander technique, acupuncture, anthroposophy, hypnotherapy, the 'psychosomatic' therapies, and naturopathy, the patient is encouraged to use the changes that happen to him during treatment as a journey of self-discovery.

It is clearly hard to draw boundaries around complementary medicine. A naturopathic diet, for example, may be no different from the usual eating habits of those inclined towards natural unre-fined foods. It may be impossible and usually fruitless to distinguish what is therapy and what is not. Anthroposophical methods work through reappraisal of the self so that treatment and self-develop-ment become identical. Laying on of hands, radionics, and perhaps even homeopathy act through subtle channels that we know very little about, but at least demonstrate the connection between healing and spiritual sustenance.

These principles are strikingly different from the fundamental tenets of conventional medicine.[2] We will examine how the diver-gence in approach came about later in the chapter (p. 12).

The art of diagnosis

Diagnosis in complementary medicine is radically different from that in conventional medicine. The methods invariably consist of very sensitive observation of areas and functions of the body, and detailed questions concerning the patient's feelings, habits, and life-style. Diagnosis is not invasive, nor is it intrusive. Just as the conven-tional medical requirement to probe, cut, biopsy, and X-ray the interior of the body is a necessary product of the anatomical character of conventional pathology, so observational diagnosis is a corollary of the character of complementary pathology.

The diagnostic skills of Oriental medicine are typical of complementary medicine. They are the result of thousands of years of development and refinement, and they contain most of the procedures used by other therapies. The key to Oriental diagnosis is the concept that inner states are projected on to the surface of the body as a film is projected on to a screen. Oriental pathology is highly complex and systematic, classifying diseases by means of qualities of body function (such as hot/cold, watery/dry) and qualities of the various body energies (such as scattered, stuck, and withdrawn). There are no anatomical boundaries to restrict these qualities, which can only be read by a sensitive and trained practitioner. The colour and texture of the tongue and skin, the timbre of the voice, the distribution of hot or cold patches, the responses and actions, the smell or appearance of urine and body secretions, and above all, the textures of the 12 pulses (read like waves on an oscilloscope) are all used as messages. Through them the practitioner gains a type of continuous log of the patient's condition and prognosis, and the alterations produced by treatment or other events. The traditional acupuncturist today will use these methods.

Although the conventional physician will also examine the same parts of the body—the pulse, tongue, skin, and urine—he is looking for very different things and translating his perceptions into a different language. For example he will count pulses rather than feel their 'shape' and texture.

Nonetheless, since much of the sensitivity to a patient's condition comes with experience and an open mind, one can find GPs so well versed in their diagnosis that they can tell the condition of some patients as soon as they walk into the surgery.

Other therapies diagnose in a similar manner, although interpretations are again different. Body therapists, including many masseurs, read the postures, actions, balances, and breaths of the body as a language expressing a person's psychophysical make-up. They read character and emotional tone from the patterns of tensions and alignments. Physical therapists, chiropractors, and osteopaths read posture with equal sensitivity, although here it is dimensions, stresses, pressures, and flexions which are invoked to explain the patient's condition. Many naturopaths use a diagnostic technique called iridology, the basic premise of which is that all the parts of the body are specifically reflected in areas of the iris of the eye. An examination of the spots, marks, blemishes, fibres, patterns, and colours of the iris suggests an historical record of the patient's condition.[3]

All the diagnostic methods described so far use the normal senses as tools. The use of paranormal senses is also common in complementary medicine. (Paranormal senses may also, of course, be part of the unconscious intuition which any physician will have about his patients.) The use of paranormal faculties in diagnosis today is not usually expressed in such mystical or sacramental terms as it was before the era of quantum physics. Therapists tend now to regard such faculties as some kind of physical phenomenon, although below the threshold of normal perception and beyond the threshold of current scientific explanation. Dowsing, for example, has long been used and virtually accepted as a specially developed sense on the physical plane; water diviners use a stick which is believed to augment their minute body response to the signals that they pick up. The pendulum as the corresponding amplifier is the basis of diagnosis in psionic medicine and radionics. Psychic diagnosis also often involves visualization of the 'aura' around individuals, or patches of light or shade on their bodies.[4]

Whereas the scientific verification of complementary treatments is fraught with complications and fundamental incongruities, (see p. 20), diagnosis should be more easily testable. Indeed, diagnosis of distant pain sites from observation of the ear alone by acupuncturists has been confirmed in a controlled experiment at the University of California. In a further study there, 4 patients who had lung cancer were correctly picked out from 30 individuals, by measuring the electrical activity of the lung acupuncture points on the hand. The testers saw no other part of the body.[5] Clairvoyant diagnosis near silent patients and even from photographs has been found to be up to 80 per cent accurate, depending on the clairvoyant and the conditions under which he can operate.[6] There are machines available which can detect acupuncture points or measure several pulses on each wrist and record them on a continuous trace. Kirlian photography, when executed properly, can photograph some kind of bioenergetic corona discharge around the human body, the patterns of which are very sensitive to disease, mood, vitality, drug consumption, and the psychophysical state of the individual.[7]

Holistic medicine—the new Hippocratism

Holistic medicine is a movement evolving within the medical profession in response to the need to find new methods of dealing with stress-related and degenerative health problems. It is also a reaction against increasing specialization within medicine. Holistic medicine integrates a variety of potential psychological and physical treatments with preventive instruction. It attempts to give a global treatment to each patient with as much emphasis on psychological and preventive care as on the treatment of pathologies. This is how it is defined by the American Holistic Medical Association: 'Holistic Medicine is a system of health care which emphasises personal responsibility, and fosters a co-operative relationship among all those involved, leading toward optimal attunement of body, mind, emotions and spirit.[8]

In practice, holistic medicine uses both conventional and complementary methods simultaneously in treatment. The complementary approach is as we have just described it, although there is a more strongly psychotherapeutic approach, including group therapy, sexual guidance, and analysis of important events in the patient's life; and there is an attempt to provide a continuous preventive guide throughout life.[8] For example:

Holistic practitioners are as interested in the colouring of the mood that preceded an attack of chest pain and the meaning it had for the patient as in the dimensions of the electro-cardiographic change that followed it. Their therapeutic approach may include a meditative technique; dietary changes and exercises to improve cardiovascular functioning; psychotherapy to mitigate the depression and rage that predispose an individual to myocardial infarction (heart attack); or pastoral counselling to help someone confront the despair that can be as lethal as any anatomic pathology.[9]

Holistic practitioners examine minutely the patient's lifestyle, often by means of extensive questionnaires on life habits, attitudes, relationships, and psychological traits, as well as bodily symptoms. In this way they attempt to spot susceptibilities and preconditions for disease. They can then guide the client through his disease towards the discovery of the manner in which his personality and habits influence his physical and psychological health.[10]

Holistic medicine is in consequence concerned with the long-term development of each individual rather than the short-term response to each incident of disease. It also brings the family into the process of healing an individual since the family is critical in creating a positive or negative ambience, and may have been involved in the emotional roots of a disease in the first place. In the same way since health-promoting or health-destroying concepts and habits are rooted in society, a holistic health centre tries to involve the local community.

The medical background

Since childhood Dennis has had diabetes, with the full range of pathologies, including, until recently, steadily declining kidney function. According to conventional medicine the failing kidney is an irreversible condition. At Dennis's clinic the doctors recorded his downward progress, helplessly witnessing his deterioration and movement towards inevitable kidney transplantation. 1981 saw a dramatic turnaround in Dennis's fortunes. He went to a traditional acupuncturist. His kidneys began to improve. The clinic found this phenomenon inexplicable; the doctors refused to consider the possibility that acupuncture might be responsible for the improvement. Dennis's health has continued to improve through the use of acupuncture and herbal and dietary treatments although he must also continue to take insulin. However, it appears that the more subtle methods of unconventional medicine are achieving that which is beyond the grasp of conventional medicine: enabling the body to adapt to its disturbed glands. Conventional medicine (insulin) is keeping Dennis alive, but complementary medicine (acupunture, herbal, and dietary treatments) is helping him live.

Dennis's case demonstrates the potential of pluralistic medicine. This takes a middle way between the professional territorialism of conventional medicine that can look on all other healing methods as humbug, and the equally short-sighted exponents of a Luddite natural medicine that can view all technical intervention as dangerous symptomatic meddling.

Dennis's case also illustrates the fact that both conventional and complementary medicine have a part to play in treatment. One cannot blame his doctors for being unfamiliar with acupuncture. However, have they failed to appreciate the limitations of their own system, by accepting his decline rather than acknowledging that there might be others who could do better? Similarly, the significant number of doctors who consider that their main option for the treatment of bad backs is to give codeine for the pain do not understand that technical medicine may not be able to treat the underlying condition and alternatives could usefully be sought.[11]

Doctors are becoming uncomfortably aware that modern scientific medicine has, like all other medical systems, areas of excellence and areas of failure. Its tremendous successes—the control of acute infection, vaccinations against diphtheria, smallpox, or typhoid; skills in surgery, dentistry, anaesthetics, prosthetics, and immunology, and the feat of keeping perinatal mortality down to less than 2 children lost per 100 births[12]—must be given due credit. Yet the statistics in Table 1.1 show that while the cost of health care and the resources ploughed into it are rising steadily, lifespan remains unchanged, and according to the World Health Organization (WHO) there has been a 50 per cent increase in chronic illness in the UK since 1972.

The dominance of technical medicine in the last hundred years has resulted in a change in the kinds of diseases with which society today is particularly afflicted. Today's major diseases are the cardiovascular, neoplastic, arthritic, and cerebral degenerations. Fifteen per cent of Americans suffer from high blood pressure. These diseases are insidious, they build up slowly and invisibly from an early age, they are largely the result of behaviour and environment and they are therefore preventable. They are also virtually irreversible. Modern medicine has found itself unable to cure these conditions by using its disease-attacking principles.[13] For example, the 5 year cure rate for all cancers put together has changed little in the last 20 years.[14]

Conventional medicine's treatment of blood pressure illustrates the point. In medical schools students learn that high blood pressure is produced by atheromatous vessels or poor kidney function. Yet strategies to prevent either are given little attention compared to strategies for pushing down the blood pressure, which of course does not treat the underlying condition.

The Director-General of WHO summed up the problem in 1977:

Most of the world's medical schools prepare doctors, not to take care of the health of the people but instead for a medical practice that is blind to anything but disease and the technology for dealing with it; a technology involving astronomical and ever-increasing prices directed towards fewer and fewer people . . . The medical empire and its closely related aggressive industry of diagnostic and therapeutic weapons sometimes appears more of a threat than a contribution to health . . . the very attempt to

Table 1.1 *Summary of Data on Health in the UK*

Cost[a]

Cost of all health services is £20 000m, or £6 per week per person.

Cost has increased from 3.8 per cent of the GNP in 1949 to 6.8 per cent in 1984.

Cost has increased three times in real terms at 1949 prices since the NHS began in 1949.

60 per cent of all health resources are absorbed by the hospital sector.

Drugs bill has risen 57 per cent in real terms in 8 years, now standing at £2000m per annum.

Demands made on Health Services

Annual number of GP prescriptions per person increased 24 per cent 1949–1977.[b]

Attendance as psychiatric outpatients increased 37 per cent 1949 1977.[b]

600 000 people are waiting for operations; 1 million for operation and consultations.[c]

Twice as many people entering and leaving hospital in 1981 as in 1949.[d]

Health and sickness

More than half of all adults and almost all children take some kind of drug every day.[e]

Number of working days lost through sickness for males increased from 186 million in 1954 to 361 million in 1983.[f]

The number of chronically ill has risen from 20.5 per cent of the population in 1972 to 31 per cent in 1986.[g]

3 000 000 handicapped and impaired people in the UK.[a]

Number of consultations with GPs are increasing at a rate of 3.5 per cent per annum.[a]

Iatrogenesis

1 in 10 hospital patients suffer an hospital-acquired infection.[h]

30 per cent of all hospital patients suffer unwanted side-effects from drugs.[h]

---

[a] Office of Health Economics (1986). *Digest of Health Statistics*, London.

[b] Draper, P. *et al.* (1978). *The NHS in its next 30 years*. The Unit for the Study of Health Policy; Guy's Hospital Medical School, London.

[c] The Consumers' Association (1980). Waiting for the NHS. *Which*? (September issue).

[d] Editorial (1984). The NHS sets patient record *General Practitioner*, 2, (September issue).

[e] OPCS (1974). *Morbidity statistics from general practice: Second national study 1970–71*. HMSO, London.

[f] DHSS (1986). Health and social services, annual statistics. HMSO.

[g] World Health Organization, (1987). Geneva *statistical annual*, WHO.

[h] Weitz, M. (1980). *Health shock*. David and Charles, London.

diagnose and treat one ill may produce another, be it through side effects or iatrogenesis.[15]

Conventional medicine's preoccupation with disease has led to an assumption that treatment is the basis of health, and that progress in health care is synonymous with ever greater consumption of illness services. This assumption results in a failure to understand and promote health. To the conventional practitioner the nature of health is often an unknown, unmeasurable, and uninteresting subject. Yet, if more emphasis was placed on health care and the prevention of disease, conventional medicine would be better able to channel its resources into treating the relatively few who had slipped through the net.

The history of medicine

A brief examination of the history of medicine places the development of both conventional and complementary medicine in perspective.[16]

The basic principle of modern medicine, that human ill health and incapacity is the result of specific identifiable sets of symptoms (diseases), each of which is curable by specific treatments, has been a constant refrain in history from antiquity. However, it has always been offset against systems of thought which view disharmony with nature as the condition to be treated and physical symptoms as secondary manifestations. The two positions emerged in the Ancient Greek period (around 500 BC). Aesculapius, the son of Apollo, was the legendary teacher of Greek medicine, and the priests in his temples diagnosed, mixed medicines, and healed diseases by correcting imperfections. However, in the same period, the god Hygieia was worshipped by those who believed that good health resulted from man's understanding of how to live. The ascetic Pythagoras introduced the Hygieian concept of physiological harmony, seeing disease as an imbalance of the constituent elements of man. Hippocrates, to whom lip service is paid as the father of modern medicine, in fact followed Pythagoras and held Hygieian views diametrically opposed to modern medicine. He believed that health was restored by equilibrium—*crasis*—within the fluid essences—*humours*—of man. In his view, the healing process was designed only to aid the body's own self-healing capacities: the *vix medicatrix naturae*. He placed great emphasis on natural living and correct habits, and used drugs more to support healing than to cure disease.[17]

Modern medicine owes more to Galen of Pergamum (AD 130–200), the rationalist and synthesizer, than to the earlier Greeks. Galen retained the concepts of humours and the Hippocratic life force, adding to them body functions such as ingestion. He also developed many drugs to restore body functions when they went awry. However, it was the development, during the Renaissance, of anatomy and pathology, which were practised alongside the traditional purgings, leechings, and Galenical remedies, which heralded the rise of scientifically-based medicine. Medical theory and diagnosis began to move away from the concept of 'harmony' towards the 'specificity' position, although in practice therapy still mostly involved humour-balancing until about 100 years ago.

The development of new drugs, such as aspirin, digitalis, quinine, and opium (derived, incidentally, mostly from traditional herbal lore), dramatically increased the popularity of scientific medicine. The new drugs had spectacular results, making coughs stop, fevers plummet, and pains disappear; with such symptomatic relief the traditionalists were left with principles but not patients. Humours, secretions, vital energy, balance, and *vix medicatrix naturae* were consigned to dusty books and the herbalist's manuals. With the new drugs as tools, physicians could abandon self-healing through harmonization in practice as well as in theory. Each disease that arose could be overcome with a specific cure. The patient had become a battlefield on which the war against disease was waged.[18]

Yet historical perspective shows that medical systems are transient and that modern medicine has only dominated medical practice for the last 100 years. It may represent no more than a swing of the pendulum from Hygieia to Aesculapius; indeed there are already signs that medicine is beginning to move back from the scientific extreme.[19]

Complementary medicine, as we know it today, grew from the same roots as conventional medicine. Six-thousand-year-old herbal prescriptions still survive from Egypt; the Ebers papyrus is one example. Supposed acupuncture needles made of bone have been unearthed in northern China and are believed to date back to the same period. Bonesetting, shamanism, massage, and dietary control leave less evidence for posterity; however they are practised by the few primitive Stone and Iron Age cultures which survive today.

Most of the modern therapies are formalized systems derived from primitive practices. Most were developed in the last century at a time of considerable medical upheaval, when both physicians and traditionalists were exploring new forms of therapy as the inadequacies of blood-lettings and purgations were revealed. For example homeopathy was founded by a Doctor Hahnemann, who was dismayed by the savagery and risk that characterized treatment of disease at the time. His system was a mirror image of medical treatment of the age, using minute doses in contrast to violent medicines and caricaturing symptoms rather than suppressing them.

The development of both branches of medicine, since the Renaissance, has not been at all peaceful, both sides of the medical divide being intolerant and prejudiced. In the middle of the nineteenth century those who held that there were specific drugs for specific diseases were called quacks; a century later the traditionalists were called quacks. In the seventeenth century the early 'Chymists' were harassed by the herbal Galenicists for using poisonous concoctions, yet in this century it is the herbalists who are persecuted by the chemists. A 100 years ago scientific medicine was damned as irrational and irresponsible ('out of the false pride of the laboratory . . . has arisen the worst evil of therapeutic nihilism'[18]); now those practising on traditional lines are branded in precisely the same terms.

During the first half of this century complementary medicine was all but outlawed in this country. The medical profession had a standing regulation that a doctor could be struck off for sending a patient to a practitioner who was not medically qualified. This prevented doctors learning from, or even studying the methods of, complementary practitioners whom they shunned and branded as quacks. Persecution was not as blatant as in America, where osteopaths and chiropractors were harassed in court and out, and where Wilhelm Reich (the founder of bioenergetics) and Ruth Drown (one of the founders of radionics) spent many years in prison for their discoveries; nevertheless it was persistent and effective. Bonesetters were continually accused of harming patients and were starved of resources and respect, hypnotherapists had to run the gauntlet of repeated parliamentary attempts at restriction, and healers were seen as freaks. When acupuncture arrived from the East the medical journals labelled it, too, as witchcraft.

The medical establishment's disapprobation created a very poor public image for the therapies, which has persisted until recently. Even in 1978 a medical public figure felt able to say:

Jabbering, obscurantist, mysticism . . . most of fringe medicine today is simply survival of techniques used in antiquity because there was nothing better. They're pathological stages in human development, grotesque failures to understand. To go back to them now is like striking flints to light the gas fire.[20]

The language of opposition has changed over the years. When conventional medicine was still largely empirical it objected to its predecessor's 'irrelevant and arcane doctrines'. When it developed a scientific rationale, it charged herbalism, homeopathy, and manipulative therapies with being unsystematic. Today, conventional medicine condemns the therapies' lack of experimental verification by means of standard laboratory and clinical methods.

The manner in which the language has changed suggests that the only constant factor in the history of medicine is the defence of professional boundaries, which is then justified by whatever arguments or phraseology comes to hand at the time.

Revival of complementary medicine

The 1960s witnessed the birth of a strong grass roots health movement. It was especially popular with young people, who saw complementary medicine and self-care as the obvious answers to the degenerative diseases of the age. It arose primarily out of frustration with conventional medicine whose new discoveries were, at the time, occasionally turning into life-threatening manipulations. Other important factors were the increasing environmental deterioration, particularly in relation to impure and unnatural foods, and the sterility that characterized much of modern life. Complementary medical knowledge was welcomed as part of a search for new values.[21]

The health movement is no longer a movement; it is more a part of cultural life. Its focus is now changing from criticism of modern medicine to a search for alternatives. Baiting the sacred cow is yesterday's activity, today some people are leaving the arena altogether. A national public opinion poll carried out in 1984 found that 10 per cent of the population 'believed strongly' in alternative medicine. By 1985 this number had increased to 13 per cent, and the same percentage replied that they had used alternative medicine or medicines. When these figures are broken down into social groups, it appears that those using alternative medicine tend to be those setting social trends.[22] The Consumers' Association welcomes complementary medicine because of the extra choices it gives to the consumer. No less than one in five of its members had used complementary medicine in 1985. Furthermore, a national Gallup poll commissioned by the Council for Complementary and Alternative Medicine found that 78 per cent of the UK population wanted complementary practitioners to be state registered. Other European countries are showing the same trend—only more so. For example, in 1979 75 per cent of the Dutch population wanted complementary medicine included in the national health insurance scheme, and 80 per cent said that there should be freedom of choice in medicine with all systems of equal status.[23]

GPs have found themselves caught between their obligation to cater for the health needs of their patients and their adherence to scientific medicine. Some did refer patients, albeit quietly. The Threshold Survey found that in 1981 10 per cent of the patients of lay therapists arrived through a recommendation from their GP despite a British Medical Association (BMA) ruling discouraging connections with complementary practitioners, which was in force at the time. Today, the situation is quite different. The majority of GPs refer patients to complementary medicine, no longer making a secret of the fact that they are relieved to have somewhere to send their difficult cases. A survey of GPs in the county of Avon found that no less than three-quarters referred patients to therapists. Above half of the 145 doctors wanted complementary medicine on the NHS and more than half felt that acupuncture and hypnosis were useful or very useful.[24] Why are GPs *en masse* doing something that would have been unthinkable 15 years ago? What made them change their minds? The answer, according to the Avon study, and as reported in *The Times* of 13 March 1985, is simple: the doctors themselves are receiving treatment from complementary practitioners, and they like it.

More doctors wish to learn about complementary medicine, although all too often their resulting knowledge is superficial. A 1983 survey of doctors training to be GPs showed that 70 out of 86 wanted such training.[25] By 1987 two out of five GPs had attended classes in complementary medicine.[25] The Threshold Survey found that over 2000 doctors (out of a total of 50 000) in the UK practise some form of complementary therapy, including 160 who practise acupuncture, 200 who practise osteopathy, and at least 1000 who practise hypnosis.[26] However, very often the courses available to doctors to train them in complementary medicine are perfunctory, often no more than two or three weekends compared to the several years' training required for lay therapists in the major therapies to gain the appropriate qualification.

Even the attitude to healing, so long the *bête noir* of physicians, has changed from one of classical outrage against sorcery to an agnostic wait-and-see with a dash of curiosity thrown in. Twenty years ago, when healers were allowed into hospitals to visit patients by the hospital management committees, the *British Medical Journal* wanted to know how people who use spirits to cure disease had infiltrated themselves into the system. Now the General Medical Council has stated that it has no objection to a doctor sending his patient to a spiritual or other healer provided the doctor retains overall control of treatment (see p. 70).

In 1983, the Prince of Wales was elected president of the BMA. Much to the chagrin of that august body, Prince Charles, in a careful yet forceful manner, exhorted doctors to re-examine the basic assumptions of technical medicine and to be more open-minded about alternatives: 'Sophistication is only skin deep, and it seems to me that account has to be taken of those sometimes long-neglected complementary methods of medicine which in the right hands can bring considerable relief, if not hope, to an increasing number of people.'[27] Encouraged by Prince Charles the BMA had no choice but to launch an inquiry into complementary medicine. After three years work the team of eminent specialists, which failed to include anyone who knew anything about the subject, scored a much publicized own goal. Their report is a defensive polemic in support of scientific medicine. It lumps the way-out fringe (who gave evidence) with the main therapies (who did not) dismissing them as primitive, untested, ineffective, sometimes harmful, and inconsistent with natural laws.[28] The report served to create a powerful backlash, concentrating the minds of therapists, the public, the press, and Government so as to give complementary medicine a new boost. An Early Day Motion deploring the BMA report and calling for an enquiry was signed by almost 25 per cent of the House of Commons. Ironically, as the report was published in May 1986, the Minister of Health himself opened an international congress on acupuncture in London.

In some ways these changing attitudes are testing complementary medicine, for they necessitate a rapid development of organization and teaching to cope with the demand. They require the removal of extreme and unrealistic attitudes (especially to the applicability of each therapy), which survived unhindered when the therapies were on the fringe. Above all, the concepts used in the therapies may need to be updated. Previously, therapists were reluctant to tamper with the purity of their systems for fear of losing them altogether. Therapists now find themselves burdened by some outmoded concepts which they find hard to adapt to the modern age: the innate intelligence and even the subluxation itself in chiropractic, the physicomedicalism of herbalism, or the tubercular miasmas of psionic medicine and homeopathy.

However, a new generation of young therapists is actively involved in bringing the therapies into the late twentieth century, inspired by the lofty ideals of the holistic medicine movement. Through this movement, for the first time since the birth of modern medicine, the boundaries between specialities can be thoroughly broken down, and like dominos, in turn bring down other boundaries between mind and body, inner and outer, therapist and patient, conventional and alternative. European complementary medicine has generally retained specialization into separate professions, although as discussed later (Chapter 3, p. 48) there is a gradual movement towards bringing different therapies under one roof. A growing number of trained professionals are lending weight and authority to the holistic movement in the US, because of the way in which holistic medicine does not alienate itself from the dominant system but develops it,[29] and because of the sympathetic reception it has had from government itself which delights in its low cost. Some US Government funding has been channelled into the movement, particularly in relation to research into the novel procedures it uses for the care of chronic and degenerative diseases.

It seems inevitable that medicine will eventually accept the ebb and flow of cultural philosophies, welcoming the alternatives as partners. Whether this will happen quickly or slowly will depend on social readiness, on the rate at which complementary medicine can put its house in order, and on one factor which is continually portrayed by conventional medicine as the sticking point: research.

Research on complementary medicine: 'Let the best man win'?

At a time when almost as many Westerners with back trouble are going to chiropractors and osteopaths as to doctors, the basis of vertebral manipulation remains uninvestigated. The total number of published, objective, controlled clinical studies on the effectiveness of chiropractic, osteopathy, healing, naturopathy, homeopathy, Alexander Technique, radionics, and massage *put together*, is no more than the number usually required to put a single new drug on the market. There have been studies and trials on vegetarian and other diets, on biofeedback and relaxation, on hypnotherapy, herbal preparations, and acupuncture. But these are almost never full evaluations. For example acupuncture research has been largely directed towards anaesthesia and analgesia. Research comparing the value of therapeutic acupuncture to that of conventional medicine in the treatment of defined conditions has almost never been carried out in the West.

One reason for this lack of data is the opposition from the medical establishment to research into complementary medicine. Grants are persistently refused, heads of departments squeeze out embryonic ventures from their laboratories, and neither the Deparment of Health nor the pharmaceutical industry will have anything to do with such research.[30] Even the large medical charities, such as the Imperial Cancer Research Fund or the British Heart Foundation are not prepared to fund evaluations of complementary medicine, despite the fact that it is helping thousands of sufferers.

The UK Medical Research Council (MRC) has consistently refused to tread into what it considers to be the dangerous waters of research into complementary medicine, despite being asked to do so in two Parliamentary debates. Only when the Cochrane Committee on back pain requested formal comparative trials of chiropractic and conventional medicine was the MRC moved to enter into a dialogue with chiropractors, which is still continuing. It has, however, supported the appointment, together with the Research Council for Complementary Medicine, of a Fellow in Research Methodology for Complementary Medicine, at Glasgow University, to examine how in fact such research can be done.

Therapists find it irksome that the medical world continues to call for controlled clinical trials while at the same time refusing to carry them out. The BMA Working Party clearly stated that 'it would be for practitioners of alternative therapies to mount any trial'. This is like Goliath challenging David to a contest in which Goliath makes up all the rules while David pays the costs. It is cynical to call out, in these circumstances, as the *Lancet* has done, 'Let the best man win'.[31]

No wonder the Dutch Minister of Health, exasperated with this situation, stated that she could not wait for scientific verification of the therapies, and that she would bypass the medical blockade altogether and consider legalizing complementary medicine purely on the basis of public demand (see Chapter 5, p. 92). It is often forgotten, in the heat of the argument, that much of modern medicine has never been properly verified by science.

Even where there is the will to research into complementary medicine there may be no way. Science is beset by so many obstacles in exploring systems of treatment that do not obey scientific principles, that many in the conventional and complementary camps do not know how to begin. With which experimental tools, for example, can the relationships between acupuncture meridians and health, the actual results of chiropractic manipulation, or the use and effect of homeopathic potencies be investigated?

In particular, since the basic notions of health and disease are different, it is often not possible to come to an agreement on whether a therapy has produced an improvement in health, let alone the nature of this improvement. A patient might arrive at an acupuncturist who diagnoses a severe kidney-yin deficiency and other associated imbalances. He may not have any symptoms that are classifiable in Western terms. The patient is cured and discharged. A Western medical observer might not have noticed any change whatsoever except, perhaps, a slightly better complexion. Or a patient may see a natural therapist about a persistent symptom, say a cough, and the therapist discovers much deeper problems or vulnerabilities which if left untreated would eventually erupt into a life-threatening disease. In this case the presenting symptom is the main one in Western terms but a minor one to the therapist. On which basis does one judge success? Medicine does not even, as Professor Chapman noted, have a vocabulary to describe health.[32] Nor can it easily define functional states, such as vitality, upon which human well-being is based. Yet any real testing of success of natural treatment would have to measure just those categories of well-being and disease resistance, which are beyond the capacity of conventional medical research.

It might be argued that groups of people with a certain disease, for example high blood pressure, could undergo various kinds of treatment depending on the severity of their condition, and the clinical results be compared. This sounds reasonable, but in reality it opens up a Pandora's Box of troubles. The chief problem is that in complementary medicine each patient is treated individually. The patient, the therapist, the therapy, and the patient's total environment form a constantly changing situation within which the treatment operates.[33] Therefore it is difficult to isolate specific therapies and even harder to match patients for comparative purposes. Furthermore, since alteration of the patient's lifestyle is often of the essence in therapy, it is not always clear with what part of the therapy conventional medicine should be compared—a single herb? a series of herbs? a series of herbs plus instructions as to diet? or all that plus ancillary treatments by one or more practitioners of different kinds? If the trial is to be 'double-blind' neither patient nor researcher must know whether they are actually being treated. But the psychological dimension in most complementary therapies is part of the therapy, and to attempt to cancel it out invalidates the treatment. Finally, since complementary treatments are often undertaken over a considerable period of time, a comparative study might have to cut some arbitrary slice out of a lengthy return to health. These problems have led many researchers to abandon the clinical trial as an appropriate research method as the following example illustrates.

In the mid-1970s, a team in Glasgow explored the effect of homeopathy on 54 rheumatoid arthritis patients compared to the effect of conventional aspirin on 41 similar patients. The control group were given a placebo. Homeopathic treatment was given by the homeopathic doctors, conventional treatment by the conventional doctors, and an independent assessor reviewed progress. It turned out that both doctors and patients agreed that progress was at least as good with homeopathy as salicylates (aspirin) and homeopathy produced substantially less side-effects. Both groups did better than the placebo group.[34]

However, this trial engendered a bitter debate, with some justification.[35] How can a single conventional treatment be compared with a whole system of homeopathic treatments in which a total of 200 remedies were used? Yet single homeopathic remedies cannot usefully be tested as they are continually changed according to the individual and his changing symptoms. A comparison between all homeopathic remedies and all possible conventional treatments is unmanageable. There is also the problem that the homeopathic, salicylate, and placebo groups could not be exactly matched.

It was argued that since homeopathic remedies were given by the homeopathic doctor the trial was not controlled as the homeopathic doctor would have a vested interest in the success of his treatment and would communicate this to the patients. But who else could plan homeopathic treatments? There is the question of the wisdom of giving a placebo to arthritis patients in pain. There is the complex problem of whether to allow the homeopathic patients to continue their previous conventional treatment. Finally, there is the question of assessment. In this, trial factors such as joint mobility were used. However, many other signs of health or sickness which are read by the homeopathic practitioner were ignored. The controversy raised by this trial was discouraging for research and researchers.

Practitioners who are quietly getting on with the business of treating people sometimes ask whether research is worth doing at all. Yet investigation is always needed. Without it neither conventional nor complementary medicine would exist beyond the folk remedy level. Society would not know which therapy would do what, and conventional medicine would not understand in what way other therapies could be complementary to it. The problem lies not with the need for research but with the methods.

If we accept that scientifically-based research can only give answers to scientific questions, the use of clinical controlled studies to evaluate the therapies is futile. Even where conventional medicine is concerned some consider that the clinical trial is an over-rated instrument. By attempting to eliminate all but that influence on the patient which is under test, treatment is similarly reduced to little more than the proven remedy. The clinical trial frequently backfires against its users. For the reliance on randomized groups and statistical means hides the effects and side-effects of the treatment on each individual. When the treatment is used in practice on *individual* patients all kind of new problems come to light.

In any event, there are other options available to test complementary medicine. There is always basic research. There are long-term prospective assessments of groups or communities under different forms of treatment. There are new methods under development which are more specifically designed for use in a holistic framework; these include co-operative enquiry in which the investigator and subject form a team to explore the ways in which the treatment affected them both.[36] There is also 'the observation' which is how most significant discoveries in science and medicine are made, even today. These methods have given us a good deal of research data on the therapies already, some of which is presented in the chapters on each therapy.

Sophisticated pure science is extremely powerful and flexible. It is not as hamstrung by its *modus operandi* as applied medical research. Laboratory discoveries that healing energies can affect adhesion of cultured cells and red blood cell haemolysis,[37] or that acupuncture treatment at true (as opposed to false) loci can specifically alter the level of certain chemical messengers between brain and body,[38] are examples of new work at the forefront of biology applied to unconventional healing methods. The benefits of research accrue both ways—to the therapies and to science itself. When complementary therapies have been scientifically investigated new principles have emerged. For example, a new understanding of pain arises from acupuncture research, of brain function from biofeedback studies, and of metabolism and biochemistry from following naturopaths' leads on vitamins. The addition of a scientific approach to complementary medicine could pay dividends in diagnosis. Were science to explore the subtle non-invasive diagnostic methods of the complementary practitioner it would gain a deeper understanding of the entire human physiology. Were therapists to add laboratory tests to their current observations of external signs, [39] they could also add a new dimension to their readings of states of health.

References

1. For general descriptive reviews of complementary medicine see: Hill, A. (ed.) (1979). *A visual encyclopedia of unconventional medicine*. New English Library, London. Inglis, B. (1979a). *Natural medicine*. Collins, London. Stanway, A. (1982). *Alternative medicine. A guide to natural therapies*. Penguin, Harmmondsworth, Middlesex. Hastings, A.C. (ed) (1981). *Health for the whole person*. Westview Press, Boulder, Colorado. Lewith, G.T. (ed.) (1985). *Alternative therapies. A guide to complementary medicine for the health professional*. Heinemann, London.

2. For good summaries of the conceptual basis of complementary and holistic medicine see: Bannerman, R.H., Burton, J., and Wen-Chieh, C. (1983). *Traditional medicine and health care coverage.* World Health Organization, Geneva. Sobel, D. (1976). *Ways of health: Holistic approaches in ancient and contemporary medicine.* Viking, New York. Kaslov, L. (ed.) (1978). *Wholistic dimensions in healing.* Doubleday, New York. Inglis, B. (1979*b*). *A history of medicine.* Fontana/Collins, London.

3. Kriege, T. (1969). *The fundamental basis of iridiagnosis.* Fowler, London. Jensen, B. (1978). Iridology: Its origin, development and meaning. In *Wholistic dimensions in healing (ed. L. Kaslov).* Doubleday, New York. (See chapter 18.)

4. Regush, N.M. (ed.) (1974). *The human aura.* Berkeley Medallion, New York.

5. Bresler, D.E., Oleson, T.D., and Kroenig, R.J. (1978). *Ear acupuncture diagnosis in musculoskeletal plain: Final report of a preliminary investigation.* Institute of Noetic Sciences, San Francisco. Sullivan, S.G. (1985). Evoked electrical conductance on lung acupuncture points in healthy individuals and confirmed lung cancer patients. *American Journal of Acupuncture,* 3, 261–6.

6. Karagulla, S. (1967). *Breakthrough to creativity.* De Vorss Press, California Marina del Ray, Scarecrow Press, New Jersey. Jacobson, N. and Wiklunds, N. (1976). Investigation of claims of diagnosis by means of ESP. In *Research in parapsychology* (eds Morris, J.D., Morris, R.L., and Roll, W.G.).

7. Moss, T. (1979). *The body electric.* Granada, St Albans.

8. Pietroni, P. (1986). 'Spiritual' interventions in a General Practice Setting. *Holistic Medicine,* 1, 253–62. Sobel, D. (1976). *Ways of health: Holistic approaches in ancient and contemporary medicine.* Viking, New York. Kaslov, Leslie (ed.) (1978). Wholistic dimensions in healing. Doubleday, New York. Pelletier, K. (1979). Holistic medicine: From pathology to prevention. *Western Journal of Medicine,* 131, 481–2.

9. Hastings, A.C. (eds) (1981). *Health for the whole person.* Westview Press, Boulder, Colorado.

10. Ardell, D. B. (1977). *High level wellness.* Rodale Press, Emmaus, Pennsylvania. Null, G. (1984). *The complete guide to health and nutrition.* Arlington, London.

11. Dubos, Rene (1968). *Man, medicine and environment.* Praeger, New York. Illich, I. (1976). *Medical nemesis: The expropriation of health.* Penguin, Harmondsworth, Middlesex.

12. Office of Population Census and Surveys. (1974). *Morbidity statistics from general practice: Second national study 1970-71.* HMSO, London. Howe, G.M. (1976). *Man, environment and disease in Britain.* Pelican, Harmondsworth, Middlesex.

13. Inglis, B. (1981). *Diseases of civilisation*. Hodder and Stoughton, London.
14. Eustrom, J.E. and Austin, D.F. (1977). Interpreting cancer survival rates. *Science,* **195**, 847–51.
15. Mahler, H. (1977). Editorial. *WHO Chronicle,* **31**, 60–2.
16. Inglis, B. (1979*a*). *Natural medicine*. Collins, London. Inglis, B. (1979*b*). *A history of medicine*. Fontana/Collins, London.
17. Brock, A.J. (1921). *Greek medicine*. Dent and Sons, New York.
18. Rosenberg, C.E. (1977). The therapeutic revolution: medicine, meaning and social change in the nineteenth century. *Perspectives in Biology and medicine,* **20**, 485–506.
19. Dubos, René (1968). *Man, medicine and environment*, Praeger, New York.
20. Miller, Jonathan (1978). Interview. *Vogue*, November, London.
21. Seminal books that represented the resurgence were: Clark, L.A. (1968). *Get well naturally*. Arco, New York. Forbes, A. (1976). *Try being healthy*. Health Science Press. Holsworthy, Essex.
22. Taylor Nelson Ltd (1985). *The monitor programme*. Epson, Surrey. Annual survey of social trends using a base of 2135 adults throughout the UK.
23. *Opinions about natural therapists* (1980). Report of Opinion Research, Lagendijk, Foundation Central Bureau NWP, The Netherlands. The survey which led to this report was carried out in November 1979 among 1030 Dutch males aged over 18 years.
24. Wharton, R. and Lewith, G. (1986). Complementary medicine and the general practitioner. *British Medical Journal,* **292**, 1498–500.
25. Reilly, D.T. (1983). Young doctors' views on alternative medicine. *British Medical Journal,* **287**, 337–9. Anderson, E. and Anderson, P. (1987). General practitioners and alternative medicine. *Journal of the Royal College of General Practitioners*, **37**, 52–5.
26. Fulder, S.J. and Monro, R. (1985). Complementary medicine in the United Kingdom: patients, practitioners and consultations, *Lancet,* **2**, 542–45.
27. *The Times*. 30 June 1983.
28. Board of Science and Education (1986). *Alternative therapies*. British Medical Association, London.
29. Null, G. (1984). *The complete guide to health and nutrition*. Arlington, London.
30. Tonkin, R. (1987). Research into complementary medicine, *Complementary Medical Research,* **2**, 5–9.
31. Editorial (1981). At the centre and on the fringes. *Lancet,* **2**, 1209.
32. Chapman, J.S. (1974). Health and Medicine. *Archives of Environment Health,* **28**, 356–7.

33. Conway, A.V. (1986). Assessment of complementary medicine—revolution or evolution. *Journal of Complementary Medicine, 3,* 47–51. Heron. J. (1986). Critique of conventional research methodology. *Complementary Medical Research,* 1, 12–22.

34. Gibson, R.G., Gibson, S.L.M., MacNeill, A.D., Dick, W.C., and Buchanan, W.W. (1978). Salicylates and homeopathy in rheumatoid arthritis: Preliminary observations. *British Journal of Clinical Pharmacology,* 6, 391–5.

35. Huston, G. (1979). Salicylates in homeopathy. *British Journal of Clinical Pharmacology,* 7, 529–30. Dick, W.C., Gibson, R., Gray, G.I.L., and Buchanan, W.W. *ibid,* 7, 530 (1979).

36. Reason, P. and Rowan, J. (eds) (1981). *Human inquiry: A sourcebook of new paradigm research.* Wiley, Chichester. Reason, P. (1986). Innovative research techniques. *Complementary Medical Research,* 1, 23–39.

37. Hickman, J.L. (1979). *Experiences with Matthew Manning.* Washington Street Research Centre, San Francisco.

38. Pomeranz, B. and Cheng, R. (1979). Suppression of noxious responses in single neurones of cat spinal cord by electroacupuncture and its reversal by the opiate antagonist naloxone. *Experimental Neurology,* 64, 327–41. Editorial (1981). How does acupuncture work? *British Medical Journal,* 283, 746–7.

39. Lamont, K. (1975). The value of blood tests in diagnosis. *Journal of the Research Society for Natural Therapeutics.* (July issue.)

2

The patient

How many people go to complementary practitioners?

This is a question upon which future health policy decisions will turn. It is therefore unfortunate that such a simple question has not been asked by official medical or sociological research bodies in the UK. One cannot avoid the comment that it would cost a small fraction of the total medical research expenditure to find out what proportion of the population have deserted modern medicine, and why.

Two unofficial polls do give an indication of how many people go to complementary practitioners. The Taylor Nelson survey, mentioned in Chapter 1, and a poll by the Research Surveys of Great Britain both show that 13 per cent of the UK population seek such treatments.[1] There is an even greater usage in Europe. An influential national survey carried out by The Netherlands Institute of Preventive Medicine found that no less than 18.2 per cent of the Dutch population had consulted therapists, 6.9 per cent in 1980.[2] Table 2.1 shows the number consulting each therapy. In The Netherlands, 1 out of every 15 adults have consulted a homeopath, while in the UK about the same number have consulted an osteopath.

Various US surveys of chiropractor usage have appeared in recent years, as a result of the controversy between chiropractors and the medical establishment. A well-executed blanket survey of a town in Iowa found that 13.5 per cent of the adults questioned had paid at least one visit to a chiropractor in 1976.[3] Overall, some 20 million people pay an annual visit to a chiropractor in the US. To this, of course, should be added visits to all the other complementary health professionals.

Another way of gauging how much complementary medicine is used is to assess the total numbers of consultations. This is a less formidable project since it requires answers from practitioners rather than the public. However, it usually suffers from the inevi-

Table 2.1   *Percentage of the adult population, in the UK (1984–85) and The Netherlands (1980), who have consulted complementary practitioners*

Therapy	UK population (%)[a]	Dutch population (%)[b]
Homeopathy	4	6.9
Healing	2	6.5
Naturopathy	–	3.4
Herbalism	12[c]	3.0
Chiropractic and osteopathy	8	2.4
Acupuncture	3	2.1
Hypnotherapy	2	–

[a] From the Research Surveys of Great Britain survey of a random sample of 2000 adults.[1]
[b] From the The Netherlands Institute of Preventive medicine/Technical Industrial Organization survey of a random group of 3782 adults.[2]
[c] This figure includes those purchasing herbs for self-treatment.

table failure to canvass those therapists who keep a low profile. The Threshold Survey found that there were from 11.7 to 15.4 million consultations in the UK in 1981. This represents, for comparison, between 6.5 and 8.6 per cent of the number of GP consultations. The difference arises because in the Oxford, Cambridge, and Exeter areas, there was more extensive use of complementary medicine than in areas such as those in Sheffield and Cardiff.[4] Because the survey showed an average of eight treatments in a course, it indicated that therapists gave courses of treatment to two million people in 1981. These figures exclude radionics practitioners and healers, who often provide therapy without personal face-to-face consultations. If they were included the numbers would be much higher. Acupuncture, chiropractic, and osteopathy are the therapies most commonly consulted with two million annual consultations for each. This is followed by naturopathy with 1.2 million, then hypnotherapy, herbalism, homeopathy, and the others. Healing is frequently used but hard to quantify. A similar independent survey of practitioners in 1983 arrived at similar figures with the additional information that numbers of consultations were increasing by about 15 per cent per year.[5] In other words, the above figures may have to be increased by up to 50 per cent to bring them up to date.

The total number of UK consultations, at about 0.3 per person per year, demonstrates again that a significant second system, apart from conventional medicine, exists. It is still, of course, far less than GP consultations which are now running at about four per person per year. However, it should be remembered that consultations with GPs are free and are used for treatment, enquiry, and vaccination. Therefore, it may be more appropriate to compare complementary medical consultations with those of conventional medical specialists, as in both cases patients are likely to have a history of illness, and are better described as second rather than first resort. This is the point made by the Dutch survey, which only used specialist consultations as a comparison.[2] Consultation rates for specialists are not published in the UK.

Available statistics indicate a much heavier use of medical alternatives than had previously been suspected and should be brought to the attention of health planners. The actual rate of annual increase in the public use is roughly equal to the 11 per cent per annum rate of increase in the number of trained practitioners.[1] The point at which some one in ten of the population consulted practitioners in both The Netherlands and the US coincided with a major revision of restrictive legislation. If that level of public use pulls the social trigger, we can expect a UK medical upheaval in the near future.

Why do people go to complementary practitioners?

Are people who consult complementary practitioners only demonstrating ideological support for the alternative health subculture, or are they cured by it? Are they attracted by some popular image of the complementary practitioner, or have they encountered suffering and failure at the hands of conventional doctors? Are the patients simply medical rejects, incurable chronic cases which the medical world is glad to pass on?

Whenever this question has been asked, two answers are given: people are usually driven to seek alternatives after disappointing experiences with conventional doctors, and are recommended by a successfully treated friend or colleague. Thirty-nine per cent of Dutch complementary patients gave the former as their main reason while somewhat less had been motivated by the success of complementary treatment with someone known to them. The *Three city study* in Australia, carried out by a team from the University of Queensland, found that disappointment with other forms of treatment and personal recommendation of a friend or relative were the two main reasons for consulting therapists.[6] A number of patients first went to a practitioner as a last resort, for example to chiropractors when in pain, but only a relatively small proportion gave belief in complementary medicine as their motive. It is evidently necessity, not ideology, which draws people to the consulting rooms. Studies in both America[3] and UK[7] have also put paid to the notion that alternative practitioners flourish in medically under-served areas. Indeed, both studies point to the opposite conclusion—that where conventional medicine increases its coverage, complementary medicine follows suit.

The inescapable conclusion is that complementary medical patients are mostly refugees from conventional medicine. Not only do the patients themselves say this, but the Dutch[2] and Australian[6] surveys show that most patients receiving complementary treatment have first been to see a medical practitioner for the same ailment. A 1978 US study showed that 83 per cent of patients going to homeopaths did so because of distaste for conventional medicine:

the patients seeking homeopathic care are not ignorant, unsophisticated or under-privileged, nor are they excluded from access to conventional care. Rather they seem to be 'dissatisfied customers' who seek homeopathy in large part because of negative perceptions of and experiences with mainstream medicine.[8]

A patient, frustrated with medical care, is ready to try something new. How does he first hear of a complementary practitioner? Is he attracted by advertising and enticing health magazines? How often does a doctor actually suggest a visit to his erstwhile rival? The Dutch survey found that 71 per cent of the patients had first heard of a complementary practitioner from friends or relatives.[2] Only 14 per cent first thought about it as a result of books or media coverage, while for 12 per cent of the patients it was their medical practitioner who put the idea forward—a surprisingly high proportion. These figures demonstrate that patients arrive largely as a result of a groundswell of opinion and shared experience. The flight to medical alternatives is a grass roots phenomenon, solidly based on personal experience. It is not a temporary media-enhanced fashion.

Who are the patients?

There are a number of myths about the types of people who go to complementary therapists and the kind of relationships that result. For example, some doctors of the author's acquaintance assume that complementary therapy patients are either neurotic or hypochondriacal, or that they go to therapists for sympathy rather than treatment.

The Threshold Survey's data on therapists' patients indicates that they tend to be predominantly young to middle-aged, an impression confirmed by the Dutch and Australian studies.[2,6] There are few infants and few elderly patients. This is in contrast to conventional medicine, where more patients are derived from the two ends of the lifespan than the middle. Possibly the aged are less willing to experiment with complementary medicine and have less money with which to do so, while the very young tend to have acute rather than chronic diseases.

Patients appear to come from all social classes. However, in the UK there are slightly more patients from socio-economic grades A and B (professional, managerial, technical, business, academic, etc.) than the others. However, healing (often free) is weighted towards the less well off, as is herbalism and to some extent hypnotherapy.[4] There are somewhat more women than men among complementary patients compared with doctors' patients.

Complementary medicine is more widely practised in the more prosperous areas of the UK. Oxford, with its students and proximity to a large acupuncture college, and Exeter, with many retired people, both have considerable numbers of acupuncturists. Exeter and Hereford have a high proportion of naturopaths and osteopaths, and few hypnotherapists. In industrial areas there is less complementary medicine, with the exception of the North which is traditionally strong in hypnotherapy and herbalism.

According to the Dutch and Australian reports visitors to complementary therapists tend to be slightly better educated than doctors' patients.[2,9] Sixteen per cent had higher education as opposed to twelve per cent of doctors' patients. There is some difference between the therapies—healing and herbalism draw more poorly educated patients and anthroposophy the most highly-educated.

There are certainly no grounds for believing that the alternative health system battens on the less educated, elderly, or poorer people who are somehow enmeshed in its promises. If anything, the reverse is true, for patients are generally sufficiently knowledgeable to make discriminating choices, old enough to act on them, and rich enough to pay for them.

The health problems treated by complementary practitioners

Since the major proportion of complementary practitioners' patients come for consultation following unsuccessful treatment elsewhere, we might expect that most of the conditions with which they arrive are those which conventional medicine finds hard to cure. There are several such areas:

1. Musculoskeletal, including chronic backache, rheumatic, arthritic and structural problems, slipped discs, etc.
2. Chronic pain, including headaches and migraine, sciatica, and neuralgia.
3. Chronic infections, such as cystitis and bronchitis, which are only manageable by constant use of antibiotics.
4. Allergic conditions.
5. Cardiovascular problems such as hypertension and arteriosclerosis.
6. Neurological diseases such as multiple sclerosis.
7. Sleep disorders, fatigue, and debility.
8. Stress-related and psychosomatic disorders.

These are health problems which conventional medicine can palliate but not cure. Despite continual medical care, it soon becomes clear to the patient that he or she still has the condition. Complementary therapists present an almost irresistible opportunity to a 'root treatment' of the disease. The patient with a persistent ailment will also be more likely to be prepared to make the curative alterations to his lifestyle demanded by complementary medicine, and more attracted to therapies which do not themselves gradually undermine health. One would therefore expect almost all complementary medical clients to have chronic ailments of the type described above, apart from the healthy who go for preventive purposes.

Checking this supposition is far more difficult than it might appear. Practitioners do not necessarily diagnose patients using terminology, classification, or concepts in common with conventional medicine. They diagnose in their own terms (such as 'blood impurities', 'yin-yang', 'vertebral adhesions') and, if pressed for a medical diagnosis, often simply quote what the patient has told them concerning some previous medical contact. In 1976, a survey of the most recent 1000 cases among naturopathic and osteopathic practitioners, carried out by the British Naturopathic and Osteopathic Association, reported the statistics on patients' problems listed in Table 2.2. At about the same time, the University of Queensland research team carried out a poll of no less than 17 258 new patients of practitioners throughout Australia.[9] Their list of major symptoms seen is also given in Table 2.2.

It should be remembered that the majority of patients come to complementary practitioners complaining of a set of symptoms

Table 2.2 *Health problems presented to complementary practitioners*

Naturopaths and osteopaths[a]		Chiropractors and others[b]	
Diagnostic area	Patients (%)	Diagnostic area	Patients (%)
Back	46	Aches and adhesions in back, limbs	35
Neck, shoulders, arms	18	Neuralgia, sciatica	11
Arthritis and spondylitis	14	Postural and joint problems	10
Hips, legs, feet	9	Migraines, headaches	8
Headaches and migraine	6	Respiratory, nutritional and digestive	7
Anxiety and depression	2	Sprains and strains	7
Asthma, bronchitis, hay fever	2	Muscular problems	5
Sinusitis, tinnitus, menieres, facial pain	1	Arthritis, bone disease	5
Skin conditions	1	Nervous and mental disorders	2
Angina, hypertension, chest pain	1	Skin conditions	1
Multiple sclerosis, Parkinson's, nervous diseases	0.5	Others	9
Eyes	0.5		
Obesity	0.5		

[a] From the British Naturopathic and Osteopathic Associations (1976).
[b] From Boven *et al.* (1977), see reference 9.

rather than one single main problem. However, looking at the main diagnostic areas, it is obvious that the majority of patients, 75 per cent in fact, arrive with musculoskeletal problems. In the UK these problems only account for 12–13 per cent of general illness but are the major causes of physical impairment, causing some disability in 1 200 000 people.[10] For example, two million people go to their GP complaining of back pain every year. Even allowing for the preponderance of manipulative therapists in the two surveys, it seems as if complementary practitioners take on a very large number of the chronic and potentially crippling musculoskeletal cases that conventional medicine, by its own admission, is poorly equipped to help. Of the other conditions seen, headache and migraine are common and the rest fall into the groups of chronic medically intractable conditions discussed earlier.

How are the diseases distributed among the different kinds of practitioner? Obviously hypnotherapists and meditation/relaxation instructors see an increasing number of the anxious, stressed, tense, depressed, addicted, or headache patients who are mostly given only tranquillizers and other palliatives by conventional practitioners.[11] Table 2.3, derived from the Australian study, looks at three other key therapies.[6] Table 2.3 indicates a preponderance of chronic musculoskeletal problems, and that these are mostly treated by the chiropractors. Acupuncturists see a much wider spread of condi-

Table 2.3   *Distribution of patients' diseases among complementary Practitioners in Australia 1977 (%)*[6]

Diagnostic classification	Therapy			General practice
	Chiropractic	*Naturopathy*	*Acupuncture*	
Respiratory	3	8	8	26
Musculoskeletal	77	47	31	10
Cardiovascular	1	–	2	11
Genito-urinary	1	–	4	5
Central nervous system	12	16	11	12
Gastro-intestinal	1	5	4	5
Psychological	1	11	19	2
Other	4	13	21	29

Note: There is, in addition, a 10 000 to 1 probability that complementary patients' conditions will be chronic or recurring, and a 5000 to 1 probability that they will report severe pain.

tions, similar to that seen in general practice, but again, more chronic in nature. This evidence shows that chiropractic is more of a supplement to conventional medicine, while acupuncture and naturopathy are more of a substitute. Doctors see far fewer musculoskeletal patients but several times as many patients with respiratory problems than therapists, reflecting the fact that these infections—particularly bronchitis, pneumonia, influenza, and tuberculosis—are still very much a medical preserve. Naturopaths and acupuncturists take several times as many patients with psychologically-based problems as either doctors or chiropractors. This indicates, perhaps, a growing realization of the psychogenic component of illness, and a desire to seek treatment involving both mind and body.

Therapists and doctors are beginning to take on different roles in national health care. Is this a sorting out of roles according to the strengths of each system? If so, it is an important phenomenon which will be likely to develop further as more people are informed of each system's areas of competence.

Patient satisfaction with complementary and conventional medicine

It would be interesting to obtain some indication of patients' opinions of their treatment by various kinds of practitioners. This would take account of the patient as consumer, a point of view gaining in importance as medical care in Western countries comes under increasing pressure. Naturally, patient reports are subjective interpretations, full of any number of biases. They do not constitute objective data on the quality of health care. Yet the experience of the patient is crucial in medicine, and evaluation by the patient should be given no less prominence than evaluation by detached professionals.

According to the Consumers' Association[12] nine out of ten of their members who have used complementary medicine would use the same method again. While 75 per cent of almost 2000 of its members who had been to a complementary therapist claimed that they had been cured or improved by the treatment. The result of this is obvious—the same proportion said they would recommend the treatment to others.[13]

The Dutch study found that more than 80 per cent of the people who had used complementary medicine would recommend it to others. These findings point to a high degree of satisfaction with complementary medicine. They are joined in this conclusion by the more sophisticated Australian studies, which asked complementary therapy patients whether they were satisfied with their current treatment.[6] Ninety-three per cent stated that they were. Complementary therapy patients were then asked about their previous treatments. Of those who had previously been to medical practitioners, only 8 per cent were very satisfied with the treatment they had received, while of those who had previously been to a different complementary. practitioner, 51 per cent were very satisfied.

It is somewhat misleading to compare the degree of satisfaction that patients experience with conventional and complementary therapists by asking only those patients who had been 'converted' to complementary medicine. Naturally, they give overwhelming support to their current therapy. In fact, when the University of Queensland team compared the satisfaction of patients seeing complementary therapists with that of patients seeing medical practitioners, they were both equally satisfied with their current practitioner, even though many more of the doctors' patients had reservations about the treatment. Those people who were not happy with their complementary practitioner were found to be uncured, but unharmed, while those dissatisfied with their doctor were not necessarily unharmed. It is at least possible to conclude that although all patients have a strong loyalty to their practitioner, complementary therapy patients are generally more satisfied with their overall treatment than doctors' patients.

In Australia, the stereotype of the doctor that exists in the public imagination is now less flattering than that of the chiropractor. This was the conclusion of the University of Queensland team in another report on public experiences and attitudes.[14] It surprised the researchers concerned who found that members of the public felt it more difficult to see chiropractors, who were also more expensive than GPs.

The Australian government-sponsored study found that 50 per cent of patients were 'greatly improved' and another 40 per cent 'improved' or 'slightly improved' after complementary medical treatment, a figure that the authors found surprisingly high given the chronic nature of most of the patients' conditions. When the question became more specific, relating to particular symptoms such as pain, limitations to work, or social activity and depression, the reported improvements were consistently in the range of 85 to 90 per cent.[6]

Does this improvement stand the test of time? The New South Wales team evaluated the response of patients both straight after their treatment and 10 weeks later. Eighty-eight per cent still experienced improvement after 10 weeks, which not only indicates a high degree of improvement, but that the therapists' treatments are also long term, although it should be pointed out that the less chronic cases might have returned to health during this period whether or not they saw a practitioner. This result does indicate that patients are pleased with complementary therapists because of their actual results, not simply because they enjoyed the treatment.

How does this compare with patients of medical practitioners? The Dutch study[2] compared the general effectiveness of complementary therapists and medical specialists in the eyes of their patients. It then continued with an analysis of the range of symptoms. In general, people arriving at a complementary practitioner regarded their health as slightly poorer and the improvement slightly greater, than those using medical specialists. Patients were then asked which complaints they had experienced and the success of their treatment. The results are given in Table 2.4. Like other studies before this the major symptoms reported particularly by the complementary therapy patients, were musculoskeletal, tiredness, nonspecific sickness, pain, tension/depression, and insomnia. There were only minor differences between the complementary practitioners and the specialist. For example, the complementary practitioner was better than the specialist in relieving insomnia, dizziness/fainting, and shortness of breath, while the specialist did better in relieving poor vision and hearing. One could conclude that complementary patients feel at least as successfully treated as patients of medical specialists, if not more so.

Are patients so satisfied with their complementary treatment that they abandon their conventional doctor? According to the American study of homeopathic patients[8] one in six had abandoned conventional medicine completely while three out of four said they would rely on conventional physicians for acute illnesses or emergencies only. In Australia the government-sponsored survey[14] found that 33 per cent of all complementary patients would not use conventional medicine. In answer to their questions, these patients stated that they would go to a complementary therapist first for any kind of symp-

Table 2.4   *Comparison of the success rate in the treatment of symptoms by complementary practitioners and medical specialists in the Netherlands, 1980*[2]

	Patients of complementary practitioner		Patients of medical specialist	
Symptom	% reporting symptom	% improved	% reporting symptom	% improved
Palpitations	19	12	17	10
Stiffness	39	26	24	13
Feeling very ill	36	27	27	21
Itching or burning sensation	14	10	10	5
Tiredness and lethargy	57	40	47	28
Fever	7	6	9	9
Pain	64	45	55	32
Tension and depression	48	33	43	28
Coughing and chestiness	17	13	14	7
Blood loss	3	3	10	10
Tingling, numbness	27	16	20	8
Shortness of breath	26	20	19	10
Nausea and vomiting	14	10	12	8
Diarrhoea and constipation	12	8	10	5
Poor vision and hearing	13	4	19	9
Paralysis	5	4	3	2
Insomnia	40	23	31	14
Dizziness and fainting	20	16	17	9
Anxiety	26	17	28	18
Rash	12	7	8	4
Emotional instability	16	9	16	10
Sexual problems	7	4	7	4
Other	12	9	9	5

tom, including cancer, chest pain, internal bleeding, or influenza. This group tended to be young, female, and health conscious and saw complementary medicine as a true alternative primary health care system. However, the majority still appear not to be so converted, but to be attempting to get the best of both systems. Time will tell whether this represents an end point, or a transitional moment, catching in mid-stream a major shift in health care systems.

If complementary therapies are indeed being used as complements rather than substitutes it augurs well for both systems. The individuals concerned are ceasing to be mindless consumers of drugs and services, becoming more discriminating and aware in their choices. They are also bringing their new options back home to their family physicians, and contributing to an awareness among doctors of the existence and potential of natural therapies. It is the patients, rather than organized lobbies, who will bring about the co-existence and mutual respect between the various medical systems which is as obvious as it is inevitable.

References

1. Editorial, Research Surveys of Great Britain Ltd. (1984). Survey reported in *Journal of Alternative Medicine*. (July issue). Taylor Nelson Ltd, (1985). *The monitor programme*. Epson, Surrey.
2. Oojendijk, W.T.M., Mackenbach, J.P., and Limberger, H.H.B. (1980). *What is better? An investigation into the use of, and satisfaction with, complementary and official medicine in The Netherlands.* The Netherlands Institute of Preventive Medicine and the Technical Industrial Organization. This has been translated into English and is published by the Threshold Foundation, 19a Cavendish Square, London W1M 9AD. The survey took place at the beginning of 1980 among 3782 Dutchmen aged 18 and over; 300 people were followed up later.
3. Yesalis, C.E., Wallace, R.B., Fisher, W.P., and Tokheim, R. (1980). Does chiropratic utilisation substitute for less available medical services? *American Journal of Public Health,* **70**, 415–7.
4. Fulder, S.J. and Monro, R. (1985). Complementary medicine in the United Kingdom: Patients, practitioners and consultations. *Lancet,* **2**, 542–5.
5. Davies, P. (1984). *Report on trends in complementary medicine.* Institute of Complementary Medicine, London.
6. This is the third study of a series of four carried out by Professor Western, Professor of Sociology at the University of Queensland, and his colleagues. A total of 484 patients derived from complementary practitioners in Perth, Brisbane, and Melbourne were interviewed at length. The study forms Appendix 8 of the Report of the Committee of Inquiry into Chiropractic, Osteopathy, Homeopathy and Naturopathy, Parliamentary Paper No. 102 (1977). Its title is

Current patients of alternative health care—A three city study by Boven, R., Lupton, G., Najman, J., Payne, S., Sheehan, M., and Western, J.

7. Hewitt, O. and Wood, P.H.N. (1975). Heterodox practitioners and the availability of specialist advice. *Rheumatology and Rehabilitation,* **14**, 191–9.

8. Avina, R.L. and Schneiderman, L.J. (1978). Why patients choose homeopathy. *Western Journal of Medicine,* **128**, 366–9.

9. Boven, R., Genn, C., Lupton, G., Payne, S., Sheehan, M., and Western J. *New patients to alternative care.* Western Report No. 1 published as Appendix 6 to the Report of the Committee of Inquiry on Chiropractic, Osteopathy, Homeopathy and Naturopathy, Parliamentary Paper No. 102 (1977). This study concentrates on questionnaires sent out to new patients.

10. Office of Health Economics (1979). *Compendium of health statistics,* London.

11. Richman, J. (1987). *Medicine and Health.* Longman, Harlow, Essex.

12. The Consumers' Association, *Which?* August (1981).

13. The Consumers' Association, *Which?* October (1986).

14. Parker, G. and Tupling, H. (1977). *Consumer evaluation of natural therapies.* Parker Report No. 2, Appendix 11 of the Report of the Committee of Inquiry into Chiropractic, Osteopathy, Homeopathy and Naturopathy. Australian Government Publishers. The survey was based on 144 completed questionnaires from complementary therapy patients.

3

The therapist

Who are the therapists?

The public image of a complementary practitioner has been at a nadir for over a century. However, there has been a considerable change in recent years. The public is now more ready to see therapists as true professionals. The therapists themselves, especially if young and recently qualified, are more confident, more forthcoming, and more politically and socially active in the furtherance of their profession. Their older colleagues are less concerned with their public status and keep a low profile, tending to devote themselves completely to their practice. Complementary practitioners are usually male, and in early middle age. A survey of UK osteopaths put their average age at 37 years and had been in practice for an average of 13 years.[1]

Characteristics of therapists would seem to be similar to those of any other set of health care professionals although they come from diverse backgrounds, certainly more diverse than the average professional, who tends to come from a middle-class home. No less than 80 per cent of Australian therapists have had previous occupations of one kind or another.[2] One can understand why, for the profession of complementary practitioner is marginal, holding an uncertain status. Entrants are usually motivated more by the calling itself than by any of the ancillary social benefits that may result. Entrance to medical school, by contrast, usually occurs immediately after completion of secondary education, at an age when social and parental pressures are still determining factors on careers, and status is an important goal.

Numbers of therapists practising in the UK

In 1981 the Threshold Survey made a serious attempt to estimate the total number of therapists in the UK. Questionnaires and follow-up forms were sent to all the organizations representing or training complementary practitioners. Every organization was contacted or eliminated as defunct or irrelevant. Steps were taken to eliminate therapists appearing on more than one register and distinguish practising UK members from retired, honorary, foreign, or associate membership. The figures are given in columns 1 and 2 of Table 3.1 and refer only to practising UK therapists. However, this is only half

Table 3.1   *Complementary practitioners in the UK (1981)*

Therapy	Medically qualified[a]	In professional association	Not in professional association	Total
Acupuncture	160	548	250	958
Alexander Technique	5	170	50	225
Chiropractic	1	156	200	357
Hakims, Chinese doctors	0	40	40	80
Healing	20	6300	13000	19320
Herbalism	10	228	200	438
Homeopathy	425	41	230	696
Hypnotherapy	1000	507	170	1677
Massage/manipulation[b]	350	1000	1500	2850
Misc. physical therapies[c]	0	300	800	1100
Music, art, drama therapy[d]	0	815	90	905
Naturopathy	5	204	200	409
Osteopathy	212	777	150	1139
Radionics	21	98	100	219
Totals	2209	11 184	16 980	30 373

[a] Implies doctors. However, as organizations mostly failed to distinguish between doctors and other health professionals, it is possible that in some cases paramedical and auxiliary medical professionals will also have been included in column 1. Otherwise they would be included in column 2 or 3.

[b] Excludes beauty therapists.

[c] Includes reflexology, rolfing, metamorphic therapy, polarity therapy, and applied kinesiology. As there are no proper professional bodies with registers in these therapies, and they are taught to the public, the number given in column 2 is an estimate of the number of instructors plus full-time practitioners. The number in column 3 is an estimate of the part-time and occasional practitioners. All estimates are derived from the organizations themselves.

[d] These therapies are included as they are arguably alternatives to conventional rehabilitation and are based more on anthroposophical than medical principles.

Certain other therapies such as colour, aroma, and sound therapies are not specifically included, but practitioners have been incorporated into the estimates in column 3 of naturopathy, homeopathy, and herbalism. Data derived from the Threshold Survey (see ref. 4).

the story, because many therapists choose not to join professional bodies. Furthermore they may be full-time therapists or part-time untrained therapists who treat an occasional person in their spare time. Their numbers were obtained by combining rough estimates from the various organizations, and are given in column 3. They are basically informed guesses.

In 1981, there were over 11 000 therapists belonging to professional bodies practising in the UK, including all possible therapies. This was no less than 41 per cent of the number of general practitioners in the UK. If healers are eliminated as an inappropriate comparison with medical practitioners, and the creative therapies (art, music, and drama) as outside the definition of complementary medicine, there were 4069 full-time professional therapists, which was 15 per cent of the number of GPs. This was a minimum: if one takes into account the estimated numbers of therapists who do not belong to professional bodies, it increased to 33 per cent of the number of GPs. There are no data on the number of practitioners in practice in 1987. However, allowing for an increase of 10 per cent a year (see below) it is possible that there are approximately 6000 therapists in professional bodies, corresponding to 20 per cent of the number of GPs.

The 1981 Threshold Survey found that over 2000 doctors, or 8 per cent of the number of GPs belonged to complementary medical professional bodies. This figure seems to be underestimated, however, as a recent study reported in the *British Medical Journal* indicated that no less than 45 per cent of GPs in one area of the UK practised some kind of complementary medicine.[3] These GPs, however many there are, play an highly important part in the spread of complementary medical services.

There is a very large number of healers in the UK; organizations in the field agree upon a figure of around 20 000. However, this figure includes healing circles in churches and healing by prayer groups. Healing has a much stronger tradition in the UK than in other Western countries. The largest complementary profession is osteopathy, which has always been regarded as the most senior, respected, and powerful of the therapies. However, acupuncture is rapidly catching up and is now in second place, despite its relatively recent appearance in the UK.

Numbers of therapists have been increasing rapidly. The annual trends in numbers of practising UK therapists were calculated from

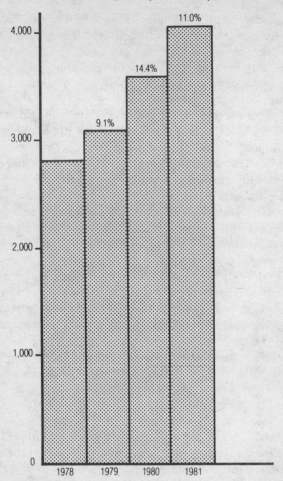

Fig. 3.1: Trends in numbers of professionally organized lay therapists.

membership organizations for 1978–81 and show that acupuncture is indeed the fastest growing therapy, doubling its number of professional practitioners between 1978 and 1981.[4] Homeopathy has also increased considerably, as a result of the establishment of a body of lay homeopaths. No therapy has declined. Figure 3.1 indicates that the increase in numbers of therapists belonging to professional bodies rose by 11.5 per cent a year from 1978 to 1981. This is nearly *six times* the annual increase in the total number of UK general medical practitioners. There are indications that this growth is continuing unabated.[5]

The cost of complementary medicine

In 1981, the Threshold Survey found that most first consultations fell within the range of £6–£15 and almost all subsequent consultations within £6–£10. These fees are less than those of a medical specialist and roughly twice the total cost per consultation of providing general practitioner services, excluding drugs. They are likely to be 30 per cent greater in 1987.[5]

If we assume that the average fee is £10 for each visit to a complementary practitioner, and 15.4 million consultations are given annually[6] then £154 million are spent annually on consulting complementary practitioners. The additional cost of vitamins, supplements, herbs, X-rays, and mechanical aids could reasonably bring the figure to £250 million per year. This is equivalent to only 1.2 per cent of the total health services bill, despite serving some 2 million people annually.

Europeans as a whole spent over £1200 million on complementary medicine in 1986, 60 per cent of which was for consultations and physical therapies and the rest for remedies and supplements.[7] The amount is forecast to rise by about 10 per cent a year in the next few years.

How many patients do therapists see?

The demand for therapists is an indication of the popularity of the practices, the popularity of the practitioners, and the room for future expansion. The Threshold Survey's statistics are given in Table 3.2 together with those from the University of Queensland alternative practitioner study,[2] as a comparison.

In the UK, a surprising number of practitioners, 16 per cent, saw hardly any patients. This reflects the proportion of part-time and occasional therapists who obtain their livelihood by other means. The Australian figures tend to ignore part-time practitioners, since the research team restricted their study of practitioners to professional organizations. In the UK, more than half the total consultations are accounted for by less than a quarter of the practitioners.

Table 3.2   Numbers of patients seen by complementary practitioners per week in the UK[a] and Australia[b]

No of patients seen	UK practitioners (%)	No of patients seen	Australian practitioners (%)
<5	16	<20	22
6–20	24	21–60	38
21–50	31	61–100	16
51–100	19	101–200	14
101–200	10	<201	1
>201	0		

[a] From the Threshold Survey.[6]
[b] From the Queensland survey of complementary practitioners.[2]

Chiropractors and osteopaths see the greatest number of patients. This is both because treatment takes less time than other therapies and because the therapists themselves tend to be more organized. Acupuncture and naturopathy follow, then hypnotherapy, and finally, healing. Many healers see very few clients. The average number of weekly consultations overall was 43 in 1981[6] and according to a more recent report is now about 50.[5] This is between one third and one half of that of general medical practitioners, who see 21 patients per day.

The consultation

At a first consultation with a complementary practitioner, the patient will usually be required to give a full personal history. The individualistic nature of complementary medicine, in which the practitioner takes time to decode the origin of the disease from the cipher of character and constitution, makes this necessary. First consultations in traditional acupuncture and homeopathy can take up to two hours. The Threshold Survey found that most first consultations take between 30 and 60 minutes and average time for all consultations is 36 minutes. This is *six times* that of a general practitioner. We need look no further for one of the reasons for the popularity of complementary medicine. Modern medicine, outside the hospital, does not require lengthy personal contact with the physician. Although GPs rightly claim that they are too overworked to give sufficient time to patients, if they were given 36 minutes per patient per visit it is doubtful if many of them would know what to do with it.

Because a complementary practitioner sees one-third to one-half of the number of patients as a GP, but for six times as long, he would have, on average, two to three times as much total patient contact as a GP. Even allowing for the house calls of the latter, we can conclude that complementary practitioners are as busy as GPs and that demand is considerably outstripping supply.

Courses of treatment

The once-only visit to a complementary practitioner is a rarity. The practitioner is involved in a programme to steer the patient to his state of maximal health. Often the patient will be suffering from chronic or deeply rooted conditions which require lengthy management. The practitioner in virtually all the therapies is concerned with the fundamental causes of a patient's condition and thus his patients should expect continuing, rather than *extempore*, all-at-once, treatment.

The statistics reflect this. The Threshold Survey found that the numbers of visits in a linked series (during less than a year) were highly variable, especially in the case of acupuncture. Acute cases generally needed 3–4 visits, chronic cases 10–12. Some healers, hypnotherapists, and radionicists gave up to and over 30 treatments in a course: the average was 9.7.[6] The Dutch study found that an average patient made 7.5 visits to his complementary practitioner per year.[8]

Clinics, health centres, and hospitals

Many professional therapists practise from private houses, with simple treatment rooms that would remind one of a family doctor with a small practice, minus receptionist. In fact, it would be quite difficult to tell therapists apart, were it not for their equipment. Osteopaths have a padded raised table and medical-looking diagnostic instruments; chiropractors usually have a much more complex hinged, spring-loaded table, and sometimes an X-ray room; herbalists their tinctures and bottles; naturopaths their charts; radionicists their instruments; homeopaths their bottles of little pills; and acupuncturists, packets of sterilized needles and perhaps electro-acupuncture apparatus.

There is a growing trend for therapists as well as GPs to share their treatment facilities rather than work in isolation. Two or more therapists of the same or different discipline may work together in a shared clinic at which they are likely to be able to employ a secretary and provide a more efficient service to the public. Half of all therapists now work in a group practice of this kind.[6] It is worth remembering that complementary therapists do not have any general administrative infrastructure to channel patients to them and their code of ethics does not permit advertising. So they are, like GPs, dependent on patients' recommendation through the local grapevine to provide new clients. When therapists pool resources their influence increases. For example, an acupuncture clinic at Farmoor near Oxford was established for a number of years, building up sufficient clientele to be able to support no less than nine acupuncturists. The existence of this centre was instrumental in the growth of an awareness of acupuncture itself throughout Oxfordshire. There are now 15 full-time acupuncturists serving the city of Oxford and its immediate surroundings.

A growing number of therapists feel that practice in clinics is only a prelude to a much more powerful establishment: the natural or holistic health care centre. Such a centre (which under a new ruling cannot be called a 'health centre' to avoid confusion with NHS health centres) employs the services of several therapists practising different disciplines. There are often classes in yoga, relaxation, diet, or other self-care methods. It is an attractive arrangement to both therapist and patient as it can deal with a wider range of problems more effectively. For example, acupuncturists and osteopaths both treat a large number of back pain cases. However, while the osteopath can provide relief and the opportunity for repair of the physical frame, the acupuncturist can deal with underlying metabolic or energetic disturbances. A mixed treatment of this kind is better than the sum of its parts. For the patient, this kind of centre is a boon. It drastically reduces the laborious search for the right therapist, which understandably discourages so many potential patients. The patient can instead put himself in the hands of a group of natural therapists whose skills complement each other, enabling them to guide the patient to the most appropriate therapy for his condition. The Nature Cure Clinic in London is perhaps one of the best known examples of this kind of polyclinic, but there are now hundreds throughout the country.

A centre that is solely a group practice of professionals is still to some extent a sickness centre. A health centre that is true to its name should play a preventive, health-promoting role in the community, and there are a growing number that do this. Like the US Holistic Health Centres, these places become a focus where lectures, workshops and classes are held, self-help groups meet, and techniques for developing human health and well-being, such as yoga or T'ai-chi, might be taught. Examples include the Wellbeing Centre in Cornwall and the Bristol Natural Health Centre. Some centres, in fact, are dominated by instructional and educational activities, to which may be added the more consciously social goal of the spread of natural health measures and complementary medicine among the public.

While the number of these centres is fast increasing, there is little to offer in the way of natural therapy hospitals or residential clinics. This is a sad state of affairs, for many people with chronic conditions, such as high blood pressure, could be substantially cured by intensive residential natural treatment combined with a drastic alteration in their lifestyle. There are very few naturopathic hospitals, and none of them are bigger than 100 beds.

The best known and most successful is the Tyringham Clinic near Newport Pagnell in Buckinghamshire. Set up as a charity in the mid-1960s, this manor house is booked up virtually all the year round by both in- and out-patients. On admission a patient is seen by a multi-disciplined consultant and therapies are assigned according to individual need. A large number of therapies is available and careful attention is given to a patient's diet. The Kingston Clinic in Edinburgh is noted for its purificatory procedures and emphasis on nature-cure. Other clinics include Shrubland Hall in Ipswich, Enton Hall in Godalming, and Grayshott Hall in Hindhead. There are, of course, health resorts too, the best known being Champneys at Tring. However, these are less naturopathic hospitals than health farms or health resorts at which relatively healthy people can clean out the residues of their indulgences in an amenable but expensive environment.

The training of complementary practitioners

There are basically two ways to learn the healing arts. At one extreme is the apprenticeship. A student learns his skills through a gradual process of osmosis from long periods of working with accomplished therapists. This experiential training is more suitable for the intuitional healing arts which involve special sensitivities, for example healing, radionics, Alexander Technique, or reflexology. At the other extreme is the highly formal and standardized training.

At one time complementary therapies were virtually always taught by apprenticeship. The knowledge was passed down as a semi-secret art from therapists to disciples, whose only entrance requirements were enthusiasm and endurance. Under these circumstances, there was every opportunity to be very good or very bad. Small colleges were set up, but they too were of greatly differing qualities, depending on the competence and ability of their founders. The colleges taught different interpretations of each therapy, fragmenting the knowledge and preserving the fragments with professional rivalries. Attempts to set up standards were fruitless. Therapists therefore arrived into the mid-twentieth century as a mixture of the highly competent and incompetent, highly trained and untrained.

Modern medicine started its colleges in a somewhat similar vein. However, its education is now at the other extreme: precisely delineated teaching sequences, producing similarly trained practitioners, all of reasonable competence. The lack of standardized training in the complementary therapies has given, and still gives, the medical profession ammunition with which to criticize the therapies. The therapists reply: 'Why should the medical school be an appropriate model for other healing arts?'

Today, complementary therapists are rapidly becoming more professional. Their new attitude is producing an intense preoccupation with education and training; the therapists are attempting to found new, and upgrade existing, teaching establishments and the Government and organized medicine is using education as a test of complementary medicine's acceptability. This is a mixed blessing. While the need for acceptance by professional peers is undoubtedly improving education, it also produces a subtle shift in the way a therapist is judged by society at large. Instead of being judged by results, as in the pre-professional era, a therapist will be judged on qualifications. This does not matter too much in conventional medicine, where doctors share a single canon. It might, however, matter in complementary medicine, which does not have a single, crystallized body of knowledge.

If, as is the case with complementary medicine, there is no single standard body of knowledge, there can be no single standard training. The fluid world of the complementary therapies requires great flexibility in matters of training and assessment. Otherwise the very strengths of these systems—their adaptive and unconventional healing strategies—will be crushed. Admittedly, there is no substitute for therapists who are selected as to ability, who are carefully and intensively trained, and who have built up a resource of experience, sensitivity, and understanding. Even spiritual healing can be, and is, taught so that healers learn to amplify their energy and channel it into the required therapeutic form. There are entry standards into the profession just as with other therapies. However, training should always expand ability, not distort or reduce it.

The current state of therapists' education

The author's first contact with a complementary therapy college was as a young patient seeking osteopathic treatment. The college used a large and rather gloomy Victorian house. The secretary who made the appointments also seemed to run the entire establishment, from a partitioned office on the ground floor. Nearby were classrooms with ancient books in glass-fronted bookcases, old wooden desks, and a skeleton or two dangling in the corners. Apart from the secretary, the place had a rather quiet, sleepy air, with an occasional student in a crisp white jacket calling patients for treatment. The course there was a full-time, four-year course, which students might enter straight after school, with certain minimum O- and A-level entrance requirements. The students were mostly in their late-teens or early-twenties. They gave a pleasing impression of devotion and dedication to their therapy.

It turned out that this first impression was rather typical of the full-time colleges, although they are more modern now. Anthroposophy, chiropractic, herbalism, naturopathy, and osteopathy are all available as full-time courses of at least three years' duration. Acupuncture and homeopathy are taught in part-time courses of equivalent duration. All the therapies, with the exception of anthroposophy, can also be studied in a briefer, part-time, and often more superficial manner. This includes correspondence courses.

Standards are set by the practitioners' associations in each therapy. Usually, students must pass an examination and undergo a certain prescribed amount of clinical training before being awarded a Diploma or Licentiate, such as DO (Doctor of Osteopathy) or Lic. Ac. (Licentiate of Acupuncture). The diploma entitles the student to practise; however, sometimes the student is required to practise under the supervision of a senior therapist for a set period before being included on a register.

Just as there is no legal hindrance in the UK to an individual setting himself up in practice, so there is none to prevent him teaching others to do so, and setting the standards to boot. There has been a continuous splintering process in all the therapies as therapists succumb to the temptation of founding their own colleges. Naturally this has resulted in a proliferation of courses and colleges whose standards vary from the excellent to the abysmal. In no case would the teaching come up to the academic level of universities, but in no case is this an ambition of the colleges. Rather, the best of teaching standards, for example at the Anglo-European College of Chiropractic, the British School of Osteopathy, the European College of Osteopathy, or the revised National Institute of Medical Herbalists full-time course, are equivalent to polytechnic or technical college standards.

In Part 3 all the courses are listed, together with their length, the amount of attendance required, and the type of qualification awarded, giving a summary of the teaching available in the UK. It should be pointed out that some subjects do not require extensive courses—a four-year, full-time course in reflexology, for example, would be a ridiculous idea. On the other hand, where full-time courses of several years' duration exist in a subject it is an indication that that subject needs it, and colleges offering only minimal training in the same subject should be looked at with suspicion.

Two other kinds of teaching are also available. The first is the short course, which is given to laymen to acquaint themselves with the rudiments of a therapy for first-aid or self-care purposes, or given to other therapists to broaden their knowledge of different therapies in the mosaic of overlapping complementary systems. These courses are a unique and important facet of complementary medicine. The second kind is postgraduate teaching, which in some cases is very extensive indeed. Acupuncturists, in particular, seem never to stop learning more of the deep mysteries of Chinese medicine. Other therapists also continue to develop their skills, part of the tradition of apprenticeships in complementary medicine.

There is a great deal of argument dividing therapists from each other concerning the minimum length and depth of training courses. The colleges which provide full-time, four-year courses are somewhat righteous about this. Others counter that as much can be taught part-time. There is also a perpetual debate about the wisdom of the scientific/medical model within teaching. For example, some naturopaths are keen to adopt the American-style multidisciplinary 'Doctor of Naturopathy' (ND), training, which generates practitioners which are almost indistinguishable from holistic doctors. The more traditional naturopaths see the way the NDs hand out vitamin pills as a mirror of the symptomatic treatment offered by conventional medicine. They want to preserve the emphasis on diet and hygienic methods which allow proper self-healing, and to teach a purer course.

One consequence of being on the medical fringe is a lack of government support for complementary medical education. This means that practitioners must establish the colleges themselves and teach in them. There is rarely a possibility of attracting full-time professional lecturers. Therefore, teaching is usually part-time and carried out by practising therapists. On the one hand this compromises standards. On the other hand it has had the result of keeping teaching closely connected to practice, preventing the development of excessive esotericism at the expense of the patient. Some local authorities will give discretionary grants to students at the major chiropractic, naturopathic, and osteopathic colleges. However, they are the lucky few, and most students must pay their way, in contrast to conventional medical education, which is free. This is certainly unfair, although in the long term it may not make much difference and may even help the budding professions by selecting the more motivated as entrants.

Unhindered by the need for accreditation, each college has set about designing education for its own therapy in an original and individualistic way. At one extreme this has produced some novel and exciting courses tailor-made to the unique situation of an 'alternative' therapy inside a modern, scientific-based, cultural milieu. For example, one might pick out the two main traditional acupuncture colleges and the new College of Herbal Medicine. At the other extreme it has generated some chaotic establishments where the students are subjected to burdensome amateur teaching by egotistic practitioners whose schools are set up mostly for financial gain.

Let us examine the teaching of acupuncture. This rich and sophisticated therapy requires a world view of elements and energies, yin and yang, radically different from that in which the students have grown up. It needs elegant and sensitive teaching, and special methods to develop subtle skills like pulse diagnosis. It is, however, also possible simply to insert needles in prescribed places in order to relieve certain symptoms. This 'formula acupuncture' is the one doctors learn if they are taught by the British Medical Acupuncture Association and the Western College of Acupuncture in its weekend courses.

The British College of Acupuncture takes the subject more seriously. It also requires all acupuncturists to have some prior qualification in another healing area, either conventional or complementary. A prior knowledge of basic medical sciences is assumed. The course lasts a minimum of two years at the end of which students receive the licence to practise. In the first year, the students learn the rudiments of the philosophy and the Chinese view of the body, the acupuncture points and basic principles of diagnosis and treatment. In the second year treatment is explored more deeply and combined with clinical work in the associated London clinic. Attendance is on occasional weekends and there is an examination at the end of each year. There are some 200 students in the entire college, including those taking further study for the bachelor or doctor degree. The course can be criticized for its brevity, which limits the practitioner in his use of acupuncture. Practitioners tend towards a modern adaptation of traditional acupuncture, including the use of electrical equipment.

At the College of Traditional Acupuncture, in Leamington Spa, the student is taken through a full three-year course, assuming no prior knowledge of acupuncture or any other therapy. In this college, acupuncture is taught as a complete therapy with a full traditional grounding in Chinese concepts and therapeutic practices. During the first two years the students attend at the college for 20 weekend sessions in all, together with extensive home study. They receive teaching in the theory and laws of traditional medicine, the five element system, the meridians, and the basis of diagnosis and treatment. They also take parallel courses in conventional surface anatomy and physiology, which aim to be of a standard equivalent to nurses and physiotherapists. The third year has weekly attendances for clinical training for six months, after which the student sets up in supervised practice for a further six months. Basic conventional medical pathology and diagnosis is also taught at this time, as well as the rudiments of conventional drug treatment so that students understand something about the effects of modern drugs and their interactions with acupuncture treatment.

The students find the course profound, exciting, and even dramatic. It is felt that the part-time nature of the course is not a disadvantage, since the student has time to absorb what he has learnt, relating the initially outlandish concepts to his own experience.

The founder and head of the college is a charismatic and authoritarian figure, J.R. Worsley, who has personally built up the college and the associated register of practitioners to reflect his own interpretation of traditional Chinese acupuncture (the 'five elements' system). This is the norm rather than the exception in complementary medicine. The students often dislike the therapy being stamped with a personal mould, especially when it creates rivalries which prevent intercourse with other schools of thought. However, as soon as students leave college they begin to expand their knowledge into other areas, especially since teaching at Leamington appears to inspire the students to continue exploring the subject.

The other main college of traditional acupuncture, the International College of Oriental Medicine, was also set up by a founding father of acupuncture in Britain, J.O. van Buren. The college embodies his own alternative variant, known as the 'eight principles' system. Teaching is more intensive, involving at least two days' class attendance per week, as well as a great deal of home study—over three years. Traditional Chinese acupuncture is explored more fully and in a more traditional manner than in any other college. There is also a thorough grounding in Western medical pathology in which, interestingly, diseases are examined simultaneously from conventional and Oriental medical positions. Clinical practice is carried out during the second and third years and requires a minimum of 100 hours in each of these years, by far the most of any UK acupuncture college. There are not many students, perhaps 60 undergraduates as well as some post-graduates, and the stated intention of the college is to produce an élite, well grounded in the rich and complex basis of Oriental medicine.

Although this is one of the most comprehensive acupuncture courses to be found anywhere in the Western Hemisphere, perhaps students receive too much new knowledge in a manner which can cause confusion and disorientation. However, by the same token this college provides excellent postgraduate tuition to acupuncturists initially taught elsewhere.

This summary of the teaching of acupuncture must in fairness state that there are one or two establishments that are not recommended by competent and properly qualified acupuncturists. For example there is one case, reported in the *News of the World* on 21 February 1982, where a 'failed salesman' has claimed; 'Give me £2250 and I can turn you into a qualified acupuncturist in four weekends'. He trained entrants through weekend courses in a hotel, supplies equipment, and then franchised an area in which an individual can use the name of his 'college'.

With the current expansion of complementary medicine, and the focus on education, one can expect some rapid developments, in particular the eventual spread of complementary medicine from its bedrock of private colleges into the state-controlled educational sector. As the therapies are consciously non-academic, it is the polytechnics that are the natural home of such teaching. For example, in 1984 the Polytechnic of Central London opened an osteopathy degree course in co-operation with the British School of Osteopathy. Sheffield Polytechnic teaches a course in complementary medicine as part of its health sciences degree. Exeter University has opened a unique centre for Complementary Health Studies, an interdisciplinary research, teaching and resource unit, in July 1987.

The biomedical content of therapists' education

How much medical science should be taught? This is a thorny question. All but the most extreme natural medicine zealots now accept that there are some diseases or body repairs that are best left to doctors and surgeons, although naturally there is a continuing contention about how much. Some degree of daily accommodation with the medical world is essential. If a diabetic comes to a naturopath for treatment the therapist cannot ignore the patient's dependence on insulin. A traditional acupuncturist needs to know the effect of medical drugs on the pulses and Oriental diagnostic signs. Therapists who are unable to diagnose certain serious conditions, such as venereal disease, tuberculosis, or multiple sclerosis, imperil the patient and themselves. If complementary professionals are to care for the public they must have sufficient medical knowledge at least to diagnose those conditions which require referral elsewhere.

There are wide variations in the extent to which colleges fulfil this responsibility. The larger ones are sometimes able to provide extensive teaching and even laboratory study of preclinical medically-oriented subjects. The smaller ones sometimes do little more than pay lip service to this aim, hoping that the practitioners will pick up the necessary experience as they go along. In addition, the pressure for recognition and status has led to some padding of the curriculum; for example, the study of anatomy and physiology might be included in the prospectus, but in reality the students are flung a couple of weighty tomes and told to get on with it.

One of the most medical of courses is the four-year three-month course at the Anglo-European College of Chiropractic. Preclinical basic medical science teaching averages 17 hours of theory and practical per week for the first two years. The preclinical section is run by a full-time director of studies who is an experienced university teacher and academic. There is no dissection, but histology, biochemistry, and physiology are well covered by laboratory studies. Moving on to the clinical studies, the student will still find the course intensive and highly scientific; it includes endocrinology, toxicology, neurology, paediatrics, dermatology, and orthopaedics.

Dutch and Australian Government committees (see pp. 93–100) have recommended that teaching of complementary medicine be carried out in each country's normal higher educational establishments. They point to the teaching of physiotherapists as a convenient yardstick. The Dutch stated that such a course would act as a point of reference for the teaching of the therapies in private establishments throughout the country. The Australians, on the other hand, imagined such a course as the sole legitimate training, which would lead to the closing down of all other existing teaching establishments. They were, however, only referring to chiropractic and osteopathy, the other therapies not being worthy of recognition in their eyes. Therapists have misgivings about the use of degree courses as a necessary standard, for the result would be a tendency to assimilate the therapy into the dominant scientific-medical academic framework.

A full tertiary scientific-medical preclinical course is only necessary if the therapist intends to use those principles in his practice. Therapists must have the knowledge to interface with doctors, but not to be like doctors. It is only the fact that modern medicine happens to be the dominant system today that requires therapists to learn the principles of medicine but does not require doctors to learn the principles of natural therapies. The call for therapists to be taught more than they need for interfacing is for political rather than educational reasons. Having said that, there is, of course, no reason not to use the education resources of tertiary institutions to share teaching of the more medical complementary therapies, providing it is fully tailored to the needs of the public and the therapists rather than the medical profession. The International College of Chiropractic in Australia has been sending its students for some time to the preclinical courses of the local Preston Institute of Technology, and the system works well.

The trained, the untrained, and the quack

There is no statutory register of complementary practitioners who have reached an agreed standard of competence, as there is with physicians, nor are there laws in the UK which restrict members of the public from practising any therapy they choose. This creates an environment in which quackery, the practice of medicine for profit by the untrained and incompetent, can flourish. In actual fact real quackery is relatively rare. The Threshold Survey found only 4 untrained practitioners out of 137, and these claimed to have been in practice for some time and to have been taught by apprenticeship. The Australian studies have come up with a similar analysis. They found that 80 per cent of the 600 active therapists who returned their questionnaires had a formal diploma or doctorate. Most of the others were older therapists who had miscellaneous kinds of training and qualifications. The average number of years in practice of the therapists who were not formally trained chiropractors was 15. Out-and-out quacks are unlikely to last that long.

Although quackery is not a great problem, the superficially trained therapists who belong to impressive-sounding organizations cause more serious disturbance, both to the therapy they practise and often to patients. For example, there is one hypnotherapy organization in the UK which trains practitioners in a brief correspondence course, after which it gives them recorded tapes and a franchise on an area of the UK. The practitioners advertise hypnotism as a cure for smoking or over-eating, and the public pay dearly for what can only be described as utterly inadequate treatment. In a slightly different case, a student can also receive a diploma in a number of complementary therapies, including, for example, psychotherapy, solely through correspondence courses. The school makes it clear that their courses are introductory, yet they do nothing to stop someone hanging their elegant Latin diploma on the wall and starting a practice.

There is little that can be done about this except to make sure that the public is well informed. Patients can certainly sue incompetent therapists, but they never do. In the absence of legal registration of therapists, it is, in the last analysis, a case of *caveat emptor*.

Another kind of poorly trained therapist who sometimes plays at professionalism, is a member of the public who has taken a bit of self-help instruction and has been tempted to take on patients. The author has witnessed one typical episode of therapeutic theatre in which a middle-aged lady chased someone around the house with bottles of Bach Flower Remedies, to which she had been recently converted. Since complementary medicine gives so much more responsibility to the patient than conventional medicine, there is the inevitable risk that the patient grabs more responsibility than he or she ought to. This probably does little harm, and may even be helpful in raising more interest in self-care, providing it is kept to a domestic scale.

The organization of complementary medicine

Professional associations of therapists have usually borrowed a structure from medical associations. They have an elected council, a management committee, a code of ethics, a register to which only suitably qualified practitioners will be admitted, and sometimes a research section. Some are charities, others companies limited by guarantee. For example, the strongest acupuncture organization started off as the Association and Directory of Acupuncture Ltd, and became the British Association of Acupuncture by permission of the Board of Trade in 1977. Its Executive Council sets standards and appoints examiners. Acupuncturists can only be admitted to the Association and included on its published register if they have passed the examination of the British College of Acupuncture, which the association has set up to train its practitioners. If acupuncturists have been trained elsewhere, they have to satisfy the examiners as to their qualifications.

All the organizations are described in Part 3. There are some 60 professional bodies in the UK, with members ranging from half a dozen to several thousand. Virtually all the professional associations have codes of practice which are mostly voluntary, although some organizations state that they would be prepared to use the only sanction available, dismissal from the register, when a member was in breach of the code. The larger and more established bodies are stricter in relation to membership and will normally only draw their membership from specific approved colleges. Very few associations hold examinations for membership, but it is quite common for budding practitioners to be required to practise for a certain period, say a year, before being admitted to the association and inscribed on its register. It is, of course, the stringency of entry requirements that select the major from the minor organizations.

Complementary medicine is beset by divisiveness. Many parallel organizations, often having little to choose between them as far as standards are concerned, have been at loggerheads for years, although the situation is changing rapidly. For example, the osteopaths are the most established therapists in the UK, yet have eight professional bodies. The largest organization, the General Council and Register of Osteopaths (GCRO), has recently joined forces with an earlier rival, the Society of Osteopaths on the basis of their equivalent standards.

They are now in the midst of a seemingly endless dialogue with the British Naturopathic and Osteopathic Association (BNOA), previously shunned because of its more naturopathic and less medical orientation. This may result in a merger, but at present (1987) there is much uncertainty. The British Osteopathic Association and the Osteopathic Medical Association, which both represent the medically qualified osteopaths, are not only set off against each other, but also against the remainder of the osteopathic organizations because they are not sufficiently medical. Meanwhile the College of Osteopathy, the British and European Osteopathic Association, and the Natural Therapeutic and Osteopathic Society and Register are not accepted by the former organizations because of a disagreement on standards. Therefore these organizations have formed the Association of Osteopathic Practitioners as an umbrella body. It bickers continually in public with the GCRO, and leaves the BNOA somewhat uncomfortably suspended in between them. Members of each register appear on other registers in a confusing way. One or two outsiders have been omitted as they are completely unacceptable to any of the above organizations.

The rivalry between those therapeutic organizations whose members are medically qualified and lay therapist organizations is perhaps more understandable, although nonetheless unfortunate. The societies of medical osteopaths, acupuncturists, and hypnotists still strongly hold the position that they alone should dominate the therapy and that lay practitioners be banned. However, the secretary of the Faculty of Homeopathy recently made a courageous recommendation to its medically qualified members to co-operate with lay practitioners for the benefit of the therapy as a whole.

Disagreements have, of course, been highly damaging to the political development of the therapies (see p. 72). For example, when Joyce Butler MP put forward a motion in Parliament in 1976 for the statutory registration of osteopaths, it was undermined by the failure of certain osteopathic groups to support it. However, it should have been clear by that time that lay therapists did not need to continue to behave so defensively as attitudes were changing. The Threshold Survey noted that 42 per cent of therapists polled utilized more than one therapy. This included all the naturopaths and masseurs, and about 33 per cent of the acupuncturists, although few chiropractors or osteopaths. Organizations are still disputing over therapeutic boundaries which are rapidly disappearing.

References

1. Burton, A.K. (1977). *A work study of the osteopathic association of Great Britain: Part I: The structure of practices; Part II: The characteristics of patients*. Osteopathic Association of Great Britain.
2. Boven, R., Lupton, G., Najman, J., Payne, S., Sheehan, M., and Western, J. *A study of alternative health care practitioners*. Appendix 7 of the Committee of Inquiry, Parliamentary Paper No. 102 (1977). This is the second report by the University of Queensland team, based on interviews with 594 practitioners throughout Australia.
3. Wharton, R. and Lewith, G. (1986). Complementary medicine and the general practitioner. *British Medical Journal*, **292**, 1498–1500.
4. Fulder, S.J. and Monro, R. (1982). *The status of complementary medicine in the United Kingdom*. Threshold Foundation, London.
5. Davies, P. (1984). *Report on trends in complementary medicine*. Institute of Complementary Medicine, London.
6. Fulder, S.J. and Monro, R. (1985). Complementary Medicine in the

United Kingdom; patients, practitioners and consultations. Lancet, **2**, 542–5.

7. Frost and Sullivan Ltd. (1987). *Alternative Medical Practices in Europe*, Report No. E874. Sullivan House, Grosvener Gardens, London SW1W 0DN.

8. Oijendijk, W.T.M., Mackenbach, J.P., and Limberger, H.H.B. (1980). *What is better? An investigation into the use of, and satisfaction with, complementary and official medicine in The Netherlands*. Netherlands Institute of Preventive Medicine and Technical Industrial Organisation.

4

Complementary medicine, government, and the law

The practice of medicine and the law

A complex ordinance introduced by Hammurabi, a king of ancient Mesopotamia, decreed that physicians mismanaging their patients could be punished by mutilation. In dynastic Egypt, a malpractising or incompetent physician whose patient died was arraigned for trial and might be executed. No doubt certain critics of the medical profession, such as George Bernard Shaw, would have delighted in these measures, but times have changed. Modern legislation controlling medical professionals has been instigated and influenced in part by the professions themselves. The result is that it protects the doctor as much as the patient. The doctor is given power over the patient, power over other 'auxiliary' or 'paramedical' professions such as nurses or pharmacists, part protection from the consequences of possible incompetence, and a monopoly over health care. The patient is given protection from quacks and charlatans, and protection from avaricious or unethical activities.

Until just over a century ago, the profession of medicine in the UK was largely self-regulating. Licences were issued by various established bodies, such as the Royal College of Physicians, to those who had completed the required course of instruction. Heavy pressure was brought to bear on doctors who practised unorthodox or unscientific methods, in particular homeopathy or hypnotism, but this was a struggle within the profession. It ran in parallel with a centuries-long jostling for power between physicians, apothecaries, and surgeons. Unlicensed 'folk' practitioners of traditional medicine—bonesetters, herbalists, and healers—were not deemed a threat to the physicians. They treated the poor, who were anyway unable to afford the attentions of physicians. Indeed, many a country doctor would send cases to the local bonesetter.

Parliament has always been reluctant to map out the boundaries of professional activities, partly because such legislation cannot guarantee competence and public respect and partly because it is hard to enforce. However, Parliament was, and still is, drawn in to shore up the status of different professional groups or settle their squabbles, for example those between the drug prescribers (physicians) and drug dispensers (apothecaries). When legislation establishing a medical profession was eventually passed in 1858 it was intended to rationalize a chaotic system of multiple licensing, hierarchies and rivalries, the end result of centuries of self-regulation.

The 1858 First Medical Act laid down that all qualified doctors should be entered on a single register, and that only registered practitioners could practise conventional medicine or surgery. A General Medical Council (GMC) was established with powers to set standards, control entry to the register, and outline and enforce appropriate ethical requirements. In its first reading, the bill made it possible to strike off any doctor practising unconventional forms of therapy. This clause was rejected in the House of Lords and the rejection upheld in the House of Commons, to the chagrin of the medical profession. The bill then allowed any doctor to practise whatever form of therapy he wished. However, the GMC took steps to ensure that all mention of alternative forms of therapy was excluded from the education of doctors, a situation which persists in the UK.

Registration has now been extended. There are separate acts registering the profession of dentist (1956) and optician (1958) with their separate registration authorities. Nurses and midwives have their own legal mandate and licensing procedures, and eight other paramedical professions (radiographer, dietician, occupational therapist, orthoptist, physiotherapist, remedial gymnast, chiropodist, and medical laboratory scientific officer) are grouped under the Professions Supplementary to Medicine Act (1960). This sets up a separate registration board to oversee standards in each profession, all of which report back to one council.

The effect of registration varies. It confers on doctors the sole right to describe themselves as doctors, physicians, registered medical practitioners, and so on. Although a doctor who is struck off the register may still practise outside the NHS, he would find it almost impossible to gain patients. In other cases, such as those of dentists or midwives, an unregistered person may not practise at all.

With nursing, or the professions supplementary to medicine, an unregistered person may practise and may use the title for which he is trained, e.g. nurse, dietician. However, he cannot be employed or remunerated by the Department of Health and Social Security and the National Health Service.[1] In all these cases, since it is illegal to pretend to be registered, the lack of registration profoundly inhibits both employment prospects and public respect.

The lay complementary practitioner and the law

On his own ground, the lay practitioner has almost complete freedom: a customary right to practise any form of therapy apart from a few exceptions defined below. This right is part of common law; that is, a traditional freedom to carry out those kinds of activities which are not expressly restricted by Act of Parliament. The freedom under UK common law is an enviable freedom not shared by therapists in other European countries that largely follow the Napoleonic code, in which activities are generally restricted unless regulations expressly permit them. The restrictions that do exist are designed to protect the public from charlatanism and confusion and are of no great hindrance to the complementary practitioner. Certain functions are limited to those on the relevant registers, namely the practice of dentistry, midwifery, veterinary surgery, and the treatment of venereal disease. Mental health legislation prevents any but registered medical practitioners and psychiatrists from carrying out certain procedures related to mental health such as electroconvulsive therapy. However, all kinds of verbal, hypnotic, or psychological techniques are not restricted.

It is illegal under the Cancer Act (1933) to advertise treatments or remedies for cancer, although it is not illegal to treat it. A clinic in the UK offering natural therapy and advice to cancer patients, calls itself a Cancer Help Centre and is therefore within the law. The law also prohibits the advertisement of aids for certain specific diseases including Bright's disease, cataracts, diabetes, epilepsy, glaucoma, locomotor ataxy, paralysis, or tuberculosis.

Legislation under the Companies Act (1982) now prevents any new centre, except those employing doctors and nurses, from describing itself as a 'health centre' to avoid confusion with the 1000 National Health Service health centres.

Naturally, complementary medical practitioners are subject to the laws, both criminal and civil, which apply to all professions, for example, the laws concerning misrepresentation and trade description, health and safety at work, or professional negligence. Misrepresentation could arise if a practitioner attracted members of the public by announcing that he could cure a disease or achieve a result. If he is unsuccessful, he is laying himself open to civil action by those induced to take his services. This is normally avoided by practitioners observing voluntary codes of behaviour which prohibit advertising. Yet the author has seen many hypnotherapists advertising liberation from smoking or obesity, a claim which would seem to be most unwise. The Health and Safety at Work Act (1974) requires employers, professionals, and others to ensure that injury to employees or members of the public on their premises does not occur. On the other hand, the small inspectorate which enforces this law is unable to cover all possible premises to which the law applies.

Professional negligence, or malpractice, may arise if someone is injured as a result of inadequate care by a professional. When a client or patient visits a therapist he automatically enters into an agreement in which the practitioner, for his part, must observe a minimum reasonable standard of competence. This standard is difficult to define but is usually taken to be the quality of treatment 'professed' by the profession, and that expected from the qualifications of the therapist. Doctors and therapists are usually protected by professional indemnity insurance against actions for damages brought by their clients. Contrary to the US, in the UK actions for professional negligence against therapists are rare, and this is reflected in the level of insurance premiums which complementary therapists pay. For example, an osteopath earning from £10 000–£15 000 per year would pay only £50 per year for insurance of up to £250 000. Complementary therapists argue that this is low, not because of the rarity of civil action, but because such therapies are extremely safe and unlikely to injure a patient.

The use of civil laws concerning malpractice has been a means whereby the medical establishment can harass lay practitioners in spite of their common law rights. There was a famous case before the World War I, where the medical profession persuaded a patient to sue the highly successful society osteopath Herbert Barker. Barker lost the case but the GMC was roundly attacked by the media as a result. As Brian Inglis put it: 'A valuable form of treatment has been left out of the medical curriculum, yet here was the profession seeking to crush a man for providing it'.[2] Complementary practitioners in the UK have been fortunate in being spared this form of harassment in more recent years. It has happened much more frequently to their colleagues in Australia and the US.

Relations with the Department of Health and Social Security (DHSS)

The DHSS obtains its advice from the medical profession, and has traditionally shown itself to be hostile to most forms of complementary medicine. A notable exception to this is the mutual respect between the DHSS and herbalists, won during the course of an arduous, singleminded, and energetic campaign by them to ensure their inclusion in medicines legislation (see p. 80). Also, the assigning of two DHSS officers at the end of 1983 to supervise relationships between the Department and complementary medicine indicates some softening of attitude.

The National Health Service (NHS) cannot employ unregistered practitioners of any kind. However, there are exceptions. For example, lay osteopaths are employed as part of special NHS back and neck units at two hospitals. In one case, at Guy's Hospital, London, the osteopath quipped that he was regarded as a kind of respected charlatan. There is, however, nothing to stop medically qualified health professionals from incorporating complementary medicine into their NHS practice. Acupuncture is available at several pain clinics in NHS hospitals, for example, in Poole, Birmingham, and Liverpool. Hypnosis is also occurring more frequently for pain relief or to prepare patients for surgery. Physiotherapists sometimes include techniques such as massage, osteopathic-type manipulation, and even acupuncture in their repertoire.

The most interesting development of complementary medicine within the NHS is in general practice. Four out of ten GPs polled in one area of the UK said that they had trained in one or other of the complementary methods and used them on occasion. However, they generally admitted that their training (often weekend courses) was inadequate.[3] A large NHS holistic health centre in North London, the Lisson Grove Health Centre, has carried out a spectacularly successful experiment in holistic general practice. Together with conventional medicine, patients are given regular instruction in relaxation, stress education, diet, and meditation. The results, which have been monitored, are improved health awareness and reduced medication for the patients, and a more workable system for the staff. The centre has now moved to bigger premises and received a large grant for research. Complementary practitioners are included on the team.

Sickness and death certificates

Sickness certificates are notes to the DHSS that a named individual is sick, and therefore potentially eligible for sickness benefit. These certificates are traditionally signed by the individual's doctor. Can a lay complementary practitioner sign them too?

Until recently, most complementary practitioners have assumed that they could not. Local DHSS offices and their medical advisers were happy to reinforce this assumption. Where certificates were supplied from, for example, a patient's chiropractor, they were often refused. The law, however, states otherwise. Sickness certificates can be supplied by any competent person who is in a position to state that an individual is sick. Complementary practitioners can supply sickness certificates. Under the Social Security and Housing Benefits Act of 1982 it is the responsibility of the employer not the DHSS to decide whether or not to accept a certificate. In case the employer is in any doubt, the DHSS has issued specific instructions in its leaflet N1227 that non-registered medical practitioners, including acupuncturists, osteopaths, and herbalists, are quite entitled to issue certificates.

Death certification differs, however. Although any person may furnish such a certificate, the coroner will not normally accept it unless it is provided by a medically qualified practitioner. Nevertheless, on at least two occasions death certificates have been accepted from complementary practitioners.

The fees of chiropractors, osteopaths, and occasionally even naturopaths are being reimbursed with ever greater frequency by the Criminal Injuries Compensation Board, the Industrial Injuries Board, and ex-servicemen's bodies. Certificates and reports from these practitioners are also being accepted as evidence in court cases. After some wide publicity concerning industrial injuries treated by chiropractic, some firms and trade unions, such as those whose members are employed by British Leyland, now consistently reimburse the charges of chiropractors and osteopaths.

Relations with official medical bodies

The medical profession hoped that the 1858 Act would cement their monopoly position. When the law failed to do so, the newly set up General Medical Council (GMC), dominated by members of the medical profession, instituted the harsh ruling that medical practitioners consorting with, or aiding, unregistered practitioners could be struck off. This spelled the beginning of a difficult period for complementary practitioners. Patients had to go to therapists more or less in secret for fear of jeopardising their relationship with their medical practitioner. Therapists hardly dared advertise their existence for fear of 'exposure' by the media or the threat of a malpractice case, as happened to Herbert Barker.

Osteopathy gained strength briefly before the Second World War. At one point, the osteopaths even felt able to take their case to the House of Lords and presented a bill for their registration. This was a disaster. Cross-questioning destroyed the osteopaths' claim to treat all diseases, their claim of education to a high standard at the British School of Osteopathy and the reputation of osteopathy as a whole. The osteopaths retreated in disarray.

The first half of this century also saw a rapid decline in the fortunes of homeopathy, even though homeopaths worked from within the medical profession. If a doctor wished to study homeopathy, he was (and is) required to finance this further study himself, and his eventual prospects became poorer as the corps of homeopathic professionals and hospitals dwindled. Similarly, the acceptance of homeopathy by and for doctors in the US in 1939 was soon followed by its suffocation.

The founding of the National Health Service in 1949, under Aneurin Bevan, only augmented the physicians' monopoly. It did so by offering patients free treatment in orthodox medicine only, thus restricting freedom of choice. The patient could not request treatment by any parallel or alternative method. The herbalists were the only group who requested entry to the NHS. They were refused, and were informed that even if a future application was successful, they would always be auxiliaries to doctors.

However, as we saw in Chapter 1, the attitudes of doctor, patient, and therapist to each other are changing. The formal barrier was removed during 1974-7 when the GMC dropped its notorious clause preventing doctors from making contact with complementary therapists. The Council's new position is that a doctor may send a patient to someone who is not medically qualified, if it would benefit the patient, provided the doctor retains overall responsibility.

The British Medical Association (BMA), which promotes the interests of the profession more directly than the GMC, cannot quite bring itself to accept the GMC's more relaxed position. The Handbook of Medical Ethics simply repeats the GMC's statments. But the BMA also believes that since a doctor does not know what a complementary practitioner does, he cannot retain overall control of the patient. This is made clear in a statement in a letter in 1979 from the BMA to Sydney Rose-Neil, then director of the British Acupuncture Association:

. . . instruction in the technique of acupuncture has not formed part of the medical syllabus of doctors in training and we cannot see how a doctor could exercise such responsibility when he is ignorant of the techniques applied by the acupuncturist. Therefore . . . we must continue to recommend doctors to medically qualified acupuncturists unless they are sufficiently familiar with the technique to be able to exercise responsibility for the management of the case.

The inaugural speech of its president, Prince Charles, in 1983 has forced the BMA to take another look at its position in relation to complementary medicine. Immediately after the publication of an editorial in *The Times* headed 'Physician, heal thyself'[4] the BMA announced it was setting up a working party under Professor James Payne to consider ways in which the contribution of complementary medicine could be assessed. In a call for information on the therapies Professor Payne stated: 'Our minds are open. Much success is being claimed for alternative therapy so we believe the time is right to gather information'.[5] The secretary of the BMA indicated that 'doctors were now much more open to the idea that other methods of treatment could be successful, including acupuncture and homeopathy'.[6] The report of the working party, as seen in Chapter 1 (see p. 17), did not reflect this open attitude to the slightest degree. It was, as the Research Council for Complementary Medicine indicated, produced by a: 'committee struggling to understand new concepts, failing to do so and falling back defensively upon what they were brought up with'. There are signs that the report irked doctors in general practice as well as complementary practitioners, and even the DHSS remarked, unofficially, that the report was premature, biased, and generally unhelpful.[7] It appears that the BMA has drawn its traditional opponents into the open in order to do battle. The result may be precisely what official medicine is seeking to avoid—the Government taking complementary medicine seriously.

Approaches to registration of complementary practitioners

'I am free to practise as I wish, I have more patients than I can cope with, why should I bother to change my status?' 'If the National Health Service can manage without us, we can manage without them.' These are frequent refrains from individual therapists and there is a clear division in attitude among therapies. On the one hand, the more established therapies, such as osteopathy and chiropractic, are eager to regularize their status by some form of statutory recognition. On the other hand, therapies, such as naturopathy, which are further away from the medical model see neither prospects nor benefit in registration. Therapies, such as acupuncture, which are split between medical and traditional camps tend to be correspondingly split on the registration question. To make matters more complex, each school within each therapy has different views, or rather aspirations, on whether they would like to be inside or outside the NHS, which kind of registration they envisage for themselves and whether they see themselves as complementary to, auxiliary to, or rendering superfluous the medical profession. In fact registration is as yet only a pipedream. The message from the Government comes over loud and clear: we are not yet ready.

The advantages of registration are obvious. It gives status in the form of a 'Parliamentary-approved' persona to practitioners and therefore attracts the confidence of the public. It protects the profession from quackery (although not incompetence) and ensures standards. It secures for the profession a recognized niche or therapeutic territory, and it opens the door into the NHS.

The disadvantages are not so obvious. Registration implies official control over training standards and practices, some supervision by the medical profession, a possible gradual medicalization of the therapy's basic tenets and incorporation into what many feel is a sickness service rather than a health service. Practitioners are often loath to give up their current independence, an attitude which has some justification if one considers the ways the medical profession first recognized, then swallowed up, osteopathy in the US.

The osteopaths have always felt themselves closest to the medical establishment, to the point of emulation. They have also been the most persistent in approaches to the Government, their abortive attempt in 1935 being only the first of several. This attempt proved most instructive as they were told that in order to attain registration, they must first put their house in order. This meant primarily upgrading the standard and rigour of their training establishment, the British School of Osteopathy. Secondly, it meant introducing an acceptable corporate structure and professional body, with a register and voluntary self-regulation of standards and ethics. The osteopaths established the General Council and Register of Osteopaths in 1936, successfully defeating challenges to the title by other groups. The lesson was not lost on the rest of complementary medicine. Therapists coalesced into professional bodies, however diminutive, with their own registers, codes of ethics, regulations, and infrastructure.

In 1957, the osteopaths asked those involved in drafting the Professions Supplementary to Medicine Regulations whether they intended to include osteopathy. They were told that osteopathy was not envisaged as a Profession Supplementary to Medicine. Having come to terms with the notion of a somewhat humiliating professional destiny as auxiliary to physicians, and then being refused, osteopathy went back to exploring independent registration. In 1963 they were told informally by the Minister of Health that there were neither plans nor intentions of registering osteopaths, and that registration could only happen by 'natural processes', i.e. when a consensus existed between the profession, the public, and the DHSS; no amount of lobbying beforehand would hasten the process.

Some osteopathic organizations tried again in 1976, the centenary of the birth of American osteopathy. A Private Members' Bill to set up an osteopathic register was introduced by Joyce Butler MP.[8] She stressed the competence of osteopaths both to diagnose and treat conditions without reference to conventional medicine, thereby putting osteopathy outside the Professions Supplementary to Medicine. The Secretary of State for Health and Social Security again felt that registration was premature; this remains the state of play today. In a House of Lords debate on registration in 1985[9] the

Government recorded its position that there was no reason to afford complementary medicine further powers nor to impose on it further regulations. The attitude of the Government was one of 'benign neutrality'.

The extent to which complementary medicine should be obliged to prove itself efficacious is a difficult question usually raised in such debates. In 1976, in relation to osteopathy, the Secretary of State for Health and Social Security stated that before legislation could be considered:

. . . the practitioners themselves would have to demonstrate, by objective scientific evidence, firstly that their system of therapy was valuable, and secondly that registration was necessary for the protection of the public against persons not qualified to practise it.[10]

This sounds like trial by ordeal because the GMC ruling in force at the time, by prohibiting doctors from working with unlicensed therapists, denied osteopaths both the opportunity and the resources to carry out such research. Even if they could carry it out, it would be an uncommonly difficult task. If these therapies could be entirely amenable to scientific verification they would not have been alternatives in the first place. In other words, the request bears the stamp of medical protectionism. Fortunately, Parliament itself has usually seen through illogical arguments advanced to protect groups of professionals. Its position on the 'prove your worth' issue was well put by Lord Glenarthur, Parliamentary Undersecretary at the DHSS.[9] He stated in the debate in the House of Lords in 1985 that the therapies should be able to prove that they were based on a systematic body of knowledge, which while not wholly scientific, must be compatible with the general body of knowledge that forms the basis of contemporary medical practice.[11]

Herbalists, too, have sought independent registration several times by means of Private Members' Bills, presented in the nineteenth and early twentieth centuries.[12] Since they were all unsuccessful, the herbalists have left that tack and put their energy into defending their products rather than registering their practice (p. 80).

In theory, at least, registration as a Profession Supplementary to Medicine is open to complementary practitioners. The DHSS has often recommended it to one or other of the organizations representing therapists, in both correspondence and meetings. It would appear to be an easier path to follow than full registration, as the Professions Supplementary to Medicine are subsidiary to doctors, receive their patients after diagnosis, and are certainly no threat to the medical profession. Complementary therapies, however, would stand to lose their independence to diagnose and treat their own patients.

This is, nevertheless, the course the British Acupuncture Association has pursued. However, in its contacts with the Professions Supplementary to Medicine Council it has found that the general criteria for entry (including a membership of at least 500, a minimum of three years' full-time training at established colleges, an acceptance of and familiarity with scientific medicine, the maturity and status of the professional body, the involvement of doctors in the running of the profession, and—the big stumbling block—approval of the profession by the medical establishment) were unrealistic. Also, the more traditional acupuncture bodies, who refuse to consider the sophisticated and ancient science of therapeutic acupuncture to be an auxiliary to medicine, would not be prepared to be registered under the Professions Supplementary to Medicine.

The herbalists were similarly discouraged despite a DHSS invitation to join the Professions Supplementary to Medicine. However, the most unfortunate case of all is that of the chiropractors. Chiropractors were prepared to be supplementary to medicine and the British Chiropractors' Association made a formal request for entry. They had fulfilled the general requirements in relation to training standards, the maturity of their professional body and so on. They were refused. No reason was given. 'There was an absolute refusal to this apparently reasonable request. This induced an appeal to the Privy Council, which said it could not compel the Professions Supplementary to Medicine Council to disclose its reasons', stated Lord Ferrier later in the House of Lords. He continued: 'My personal view is that the Professions Supplementary to Medicine Council's refusal to state their reasons can only spring from a guilty feeling that is founded on bigotry'. Lord Harris put it even more strongly: 'The Council', he exclaimed, 'acted in the spirit of a monopolist, the mean, narrow exclusive spirit of a medical trade union, slamming the door on specialists who might tackle some infirmities better than general practitioners or even surgeons themselves.[13] The Government will not intervene on one side or the other, unless, as Baroness Trumpington, Parliamentary Under-Secretary of State for the DHSS, stated in the stormy aftermath of the BMA report (see p. 17), 'disagreements between conventional and complementary medicine forced it to, to protect the public'.

Time for registration is not yet ripe. Yet there is general agreement on how registration ought to proceed once it is agreed upon. Registration would set up a supervisory council and all qualified therapists would be invited to join a register. The unqualified could also join under a 'grandfather clause', provided they had been established in practice for a number of years. Registration would apply to all the therapists in the discipline, whatever their organizational affiliations. It would proceed in much the same way as the registration of dentists in 1956 and opticians in 1958. This is exactly the way in which chiropractors and osteopaths are now registered in Australia and New Zealand (see p. 103).

The path sounds reasonable, except for one fundamental problem. The structure that governs medicine may not be applicable to non-medical therapies. How, for example, would it deal with therapists who use some or all of the therapies eclectically, depending on the individual patient? How would it set standards for therapies, such as radionics and healing, that rely more on intuition and 'grace' than on knowledge? Could the medical profession as a whole ever come to terms sufficiently with, say, naturopathy or traditional acupuncture, which use an utterly different language, to assist in their regulation? It would be preferable to see a more open system, such as that found in India, in which parallel councils govern the main segments of national medicine. The councils would be answerable to the Health Ministry but would otherwise have wide powers to license practitioners, however diverse, as well as promote research, education, and public awareness. Brian Inglis has put forward a similar idea in the form of a Council for Professions Complementary to Medicine, to be run on similar lines to the Council of the Professions Supplementary to Medicine.

Advertising standards

Almost all complementary therapists have imposed voluntary constraints upon themselves, preventing advertising of the benefits of their treatments. Like doctors, therapists usually limit their advertising to a name plate with a note of their speciality. The Advertising Standards Authority, in the British Code of Advertising Practice, used to state that advertisements were acceptable from registered osteopaths and members of the British Naturopathic and Osteopathic Association but not from any other therapist. The Code today makes no mention of therapists. It only states that in respect of herbal, homeopathic, and other non-allopathic medicinal products, claims must be assessed in the light of expert opinion within the fields concerned.

Insurance

Private medical insurance in the UK is generally within the medical mould. The statutes of BUPA, Private Patients Plan, and Western Provident limit reimbursement to medically qualified personnel. Yet there are signs of a revision of the rules. All three insurance companies admit to reimbursing naturopathic, osteopathic, or chiropractic fees on occasion provided the therapist concerned is well established and respected. The Private Patients Plan has announced that it will reimburse patients who go to a complementary practitioner of approved status, provided that the patient has a recognized and admissable medical condition.

In relation to accidents, or insurance of life and limb, insurance companies expect a doctor's assessment of injury or incapacity. Therapists normally send patients to a medical practitioner for this purpose in order to avoid prejudicing the patient's claim. However, both chiropractors and naturopaths have on occasion supplied reports to insurance companies which have provided the basis for claims.

Homeopathy—medicine's unwelcome bedfellow

In 1949, the Minister of Health gave 'an absolute guarantee' that homeopathy would be allowed to continue within the National Health Service as long as patients demanded it. Despite this assurance, homeopathy continues to be squeezed by assaults on its facilities by allopathic doctors and administrators. In 1977 a homeopathic clinic was planned at the newly built Royal Liverpool Hospital, to replace an earlier facility which was closed down. Dr. G. Martin was to head it. At a meeting of the area health authority medical consultants it was insisted 'unanimously' (after Dr Martin had been requested to leave) that:

. . . undergraduates should not be exposed to any unorthodox medicine before qualification, that the very existence of such a clinic in the hospital's prospectus would cause alarm and . . . under no circumstances would the Departments of Medicine of Clinical Pharmacology . . . accept a Homeopathist as a teaching hospital professional colleague.[11]

There was an immediate response in the House of Commons where Tom Ellis MP stated that: 'for sheer blind prejudice and bigotry, crass ignorance and highly questionable ethical behaviour, it would be hard to find a better example, even from the minutes of the Wapping Bargees' Mutual Benefit Society, let alone a body of professional men.'[15] Strong words. The Liverpool clinic was opened, and has a achieved an international renown. Yet even in 1986 the local District Health Authority requested it to close down two days a week.

Another restriction suffered by homeopathy is that the Council for Postgraduate Medical Education does not provide funding for courses in homeopathy as it does for other subjects. At the same time, since the Royal College of Physicians refuses to accept homeopathy as a speciality, there are no consultant-grade appointments and no career structure.

The Royal London Homeopathic Hospital itself has also been at risk. Only some frantic lobbying and marshalling of public support has managed to forestall drastic action by its Area Health Authority. The first occasion was in 1979, when the Area Health Authority decided to close down most of the hospital as part of a long-term plan. An Early Day Motion was signed by 230 MPs requesting that the hospital be saved, and later, a petition containing no less than 116 781 signatures was laid before Parliament. The result was successful. The hospital was kept open. Yet the Area Health Authority, followed by the District, Authority Health persisted. Its later attempts to close down half the hospital's wards, and in 1981 its operating theatre, have all been forestalled by direct parliamentary or ministerial intervention.

There are few homeopathic doctors, and facilities are minimal and stretched to the limit by an accelerating demand for homeopathy from the public. 'The distribution of funds within the health service', laments Dr Michael Jenkins, of the Royal London Homeopathic Hospital, 'is not related to patient need specifically. It is related much more to the decibel count put up in committees by powerful groups'. At present, even the modest goal of a clinic in every town seems unobtainable.

Unsuccessful steps to control hypnotherapy

It has been difficult to control the practice of professionals who treat the human body. It has been impossible to control the practice of those who treat the human mind. Apart from the Mental Health Acts (1959 and 1975), which have placed boundaries on the more forceful kinds of management of the mentally disturbed, Parliament has been unable to agree on the means by which psychotherapy can be controlled or even the desirability of doing so. There are fundamental issues at stake relating to personal freedoms of exploration and expression, and there are powerful ambiguities which, fortunately, make it absurd to draw lines between therapy and guidance, between psychology and religion, and between hypnosis and conviction.

Since the time of Mesmer, Charcot, Coué, and others, the medical profession has found hypnosis an uncomfortable subject. Hypnosis has a history of spectacular demonstrations, passionate converts, and emphatic denials from the medical world. Like homeopathy, it has largely been introduced by heterodox doctors, making it a subject for attempts at suppression from within the profession rather than for legislation from without. However, doctors no longer doubt that hypnosis works. Indeed the British Medical Association's Psychological Medicine Committee now regards it as a treatment 'of choice' for psychosomatic conditions, psychoneuroses, and the 'removal of morbid patterns of behaviour'.[16] It recommends that hypnosis be taught to medical undergraduates although this has not yet happened.

In 1952, the Hypnotism Act, concerning stage hypnotism, gave responsibility to local authorities. In future, local authorities would need to supply licences for public performances of hypnotism. There was no attempt to restrict private or therapeutic hypnotism. However, if Parliament could not decide whether hypnotism was harmful it is hardly likely that the local authority would be able to do so; some local authorities grant licences freely, others, particularly in the

London area, never grant licences.

In 1979 Lord Kinnoul introduced a bill which went further. It was intended to tighten up the control of stage hypnosis by including clubs, to control hypnotists' advertisements, and to ban the sale of hypnotic tapes or records. During the debate, Lord Wells-Pestell and others suggested that the bill did not go far enough; hypnotism should be banned altogether except when performed by medical experts. However, the Government stated that it could not see what all the fuss was about, and it had no evidence of harm, even from stage hypnotism.[17] The bill went to committee where the Lords were reminded that hypnotherapy was a useful therapeutic tool. The result was an amendment that removed the ban on advertising and tapes by lay hypnotherapists. Hypnotherapy emerged untouched and, without ammunition, there are no signs of inclination for further attacks.

Acupuncture—the case of the dirty needles

No therapy has taken the authorities by surprise in the way acupuncture has. One can almost speak of the acupuncture 'phenomenon', an illustration of the fluidity of the medical *status quo* today. Twenty years ago acupuncture was assumed to be mere trickery. Fifteen years ago it was somewhat more acceptable provided it was practised on the other side of the planet. Today, it is one of the dominant complementary therapies. The medical profession accepts its effectiveness but restricts its validity to the relief of certain symptoms, in particular pain. Lay acupuncturists use it as an entire therapeutic system in its own right and maintain that medical symptomatic acupuncture does more harm than good.

In 1977, events in Birmingham forced acupuncturists into the limelight and the authorities to take them more seriously. An outbreak of hepatitis was traced back to a lay acupuncturist who had previously been denied entry to acupuncture associations. He had been using dirty needles. Questions were asked in the House of Commons about registering and controlling the practices of acupuncturists.[18] The Under-Secretary of State for Health answered that registration would not necessarily prevent dirty needles, and anyway might have the side-effect of giving statutory support to the acupuncture profession before it has established itself. He put forward the Health and Safety at Work Act (1974) as existing legislation which could prevent acupuncturists 'endangering the public' but it was realized that the overworked and small Health and Safety Inspectorate would be unable to enforce the Act by inspecting all the acupuncturists' premises. It so happened that the West Midlands County Council had already put a bill before Parliament requesting powers to control standards of hygiene by licensing acupuncturists, tattooists, massage parlours, and similar activities. Parliament was glad to leave it to the local authorities to worry about.

The West Midlands bill met stiff resistance from acupuncturists, who forced the DHSS in committee to admit that they had no evidence that there was any health risk from a trained acupuncturist. The acupuncturists won the battle but lost the war when the House of Commons overturned the recommendation of an exemption for acupuncturists put forward by its own committee, and the bill became law.[19] Fortunately, acupuncturists had another chance in the similar Greater London Council's General Powers Bill which they, together with other therapists, fought successfully. A promise has been made that complementary therapists who are members of a professional body which has control over its members will be exempted from the bill when it next does rounds in Parliament. This was all very well except that in 1986 one of London's local councils reneged on the promise and requested complementary therapists to be licensed and inspected by them. Therapist organizations fought, and won again—the exemption remains.

These events demonstrated the DHSS's ignorance of the nature and purpose of acupuncture by lay practitioners. However, this has proved a benefit as the threat to their practice has taught acupuncturists to feel the political pulse with a little of the sensitivity that they normally reserve for wrist pulses.

Herbs and medicines

Government has trodden gingerly in the boggy territory of the licensing of the healing professions. But it has stepped more confidently to regulate the substances they use. An inscription on the Acropolis, dating from the fourth century BC, announces that one Evenor the physician had been appointed inspector of drugs. A similar function has existed in the West ever since. One of the main problems has always been the development of methods to detect adulteration and substitution, and a standard helps in this. A pharmacopoeia, in which standards are defined for the preparation and purity of specific drugs and herbs, has existed in the UK from the early seventeenth century.

Medicines legislation is extremely complex, and will not be reviewed here other than where it relates to the complementary practitioner. A number of Acts, including the Pharmacy and Poisons Act 1933, the Therapeutic Substances Act 1956, and the Dangerous Drugs Act 1965, resulted in a system in which certain defined remedies were to be available from a pharmacist on prescription only, and some poisons were placed under special restrictions. The Acts also described the measures to be taken to ensure purity. However, the control of safety and of advertising claims was a purely voluntary arrangement. After the thalidomide tragedy in 1972 the Government realized that voluntary controls were no longer sufficient. In 1968 it sponsored the Medicines Bill which became law in 1971. This required manufacturers to prove to the Licensing Authority of the Medicines Division of the DHSS that a remedy was both safe *and* effective before a licence could be issued to supply it to the public. The claims made in the advertisement had to conform to those granted in the licence. These controls took effect immediately with new drugs. However, drugs that were already on sale before 1971 were given automatic Licences of Right, allowing sales using the previous claims. At the same time a Committee on the Review of Medicines was established to review the safety and efficacy of all pre-1971 remedies. It will take years to re-examine them all.

Prior to the Medicines Act, herbal medicines could be sold openly, with the exception of a few that were more or less accidentally found to be toxic. When the White Paper preceding the Medicines Bill was published, the herbalists mounted an unprecedented national campaign to ensure that herbalism was not drowned in a sea of medicines legislation. The British Herbal Medicine Association, made up of firms engaged in the manufacture and supply of herbs, together with professional bodies, was set up to co-ordinate the fight, and a number of MPs and Peers were enlisted to support the herbalists' case.

When the Medicines Bill was debated in Parliament, clauses were substantially altered to give exemptions for herbal products. Undertakings were made to consult with herbalists before the various subsequent orders embodied in the bill were laid. These measures were supported by speeches from MPs of all three major parties, led by Joyce Butler. A Herbal Remedies Subcommittee of the Prescriptions Only Committee examined the current use and dosages of herbs supplied by herbalists, and listed them in the Herbal Remedies Report. They were then incorporated into law in the Herbal Remedies Order of 1977. The current law is as follows:

There are three categories of herbal remedies which have some restriction placed on them. Those in Part I of the schedule of the Herbal Remedies Order are full Prescriptions Only Medicines, and may only be prescribed by a doctor, for example ergot, scopalia, or digitalis. Those in Part II may not be retailed to the public; they include all the herbs for which any restriction exists. Those in Part III may be supplied by herbal practitioners (who are not defined, and would also include naturopaths) to their patients, within the dose levels indicated in the list. They include *Atropa belladonna, Ephedra sinica* or *Datura stramonum*. They must be prescribed from the herbalist's private premises after personal consultation with the patient, and they must be labelled with names and addresses of the herbalist and patient, together with dosage details and directions. The herbalist must also keep records and notify his practice to the 'enforcement authority'. At first this authority was defined by the DHSS as the Pharmaceutical Society. However the herbalists complained that a society of retail druggists could hardly be an impartial enforcement authority, and the Secretary of State for Health and Social Security became the enforcement authority.

Any herbs that are not entered on the above three lists can be freely supplied by herbal practitioners and sold in all retail outlets, provided that they are properly labelled. There is also a General Sale List, containing both herbal and non-herbal remedies (e.g. aspirin, vitamins), sometimes with maximum dosages appended. These can be freely sold in retail outlets, and are exempt from licensing restrictions, although they must conform to any relevant regulations concerning safety, purity, and efficacy.

Substances are defined as medicines if they are supplied with a *therapeutic intent*, even if they contain nothing but salt. Many substances with a quasi-medicinal value are sold in health food shops. Provided that the substances do not appear on the Herbal, Homeopathic, General Sale, or Prescriptions Only lists, they are classed as vitamins and food supplements and are allowed an unrestricted sale. They are outside the Medicines Act altogether. However, as soon as a herbalist opens one of the packs and supplies its contents to members of the public, a therapeutic intent exists and the substances are brought into the sphere of the Medicines Act. This does not mean very much, for vitamins and similar food supplements would either be on the General Sale List or not mentioned on any list and therefore exempt. However, the herbalist must obtain a licence, normally granted automatically after his qualification. The licence is termed an Assembly Licence.[20]

The position of homeopathic remedies under the Medicines Act 1971 is fairly simple. The Medicines Commission considered that any medicine which is diluted to one part per million or greater is harmless. Therefore they advised that, even where a medicine is on the Prescriptions Only List, at a 6x dilution or greater, it is exempt from restriction and can be supplied by lay practitioners and sold in shops. The Medicines Commission also published a list of materials which, despite being restricted at full strength, can be supplied freely at a dilution of one part per thousand (3x) or greater.

Herbal remedies also come in for some special consideration in the part of the medicines regulations which relates to purity, safety, and efficacy. All manufacturers, wholesalers, and importers of drugs need to obtain licences, the most difficult being the product licence that the manufacturer or original supplier must obtain for each and every medicinal preparation, even those on the General Sale List. A very great deal of evidence on safety, purity, and especially effectiveness (including clinical trials) is needed for a new drug. The research involved costs many millions of pounds. Obviously it is inappropriate to demand that herbal and food supplement products should be given the same tests. The Committee on Safety of Medicines have listened to herbalists and have decided that a simple unprocessed herb (that is not on one of the restricted lists) sold without claims does not require a product licence at all.

Licences are required for manufactured herbal products sold to the public as medicines. Most of the products of that kind now on sale were given a licence before 1971 and they will be required to be reassessed by the Committee on Review of Medicines within the next few years. New products require a Product Licence from the Committee on Safety of Medicines and an application must be made from scratch. These committees have so far been quite confused as to how much laboratory and clinical research to call for before granting a Product Licence. They have adopted delaying tactics and almost no new licences for herbal medicinal products have been issued since the Medicines Act became law. In 1981 the committees decided on a policy, outlined in their proposal MLX133. It stated that the safety and quality of herbal and traditional products should be examined with the same rigour as conventional drugs. However, they recognized that they could not call for the same evidence of effectiveness for a herb as for a chemical drug. It would be ridiculous to ask for a expensive hospital trials of chamomile tea before allowing it to be sold, and it would, of course, put the entire herbal and natural medicine industry out of business. Therefore, effectiveness will be assessed on the basis of whatever information is available, including traditional experience. The amount of evidence will also be in proportion to the claim the manufacturer wished to make. For minor or 'self-limiting' conditions traditional evidence may suffice. For claims that relate to more serious conditions, much more scientific evidence will be required. In other words clinical trials would be required for a herbal blood pressure pill, but not for a herbal stomach upset pill.

On the one hand this is a significant step forward. For the first time the DHSS has recognized that herbs are more subtle, long-term, and preventive; the current pharmacological methodology may be inappropriate to assess them, and the herbal industry unable to do so. Their new attitude has been proved. When a manufacturer of garlic capsules requested a new licence in 1986 the DHSS not only allowed the previous claims (for colds, catarrh) but even suggested a new one (rhinitis) without requesting any scientific evidence of effectiveness at all. They said that traditional usage was sufficient evidence. On the other hand none of the members of the various commissions are experts on herbs or herbal practitioners. Furthermore, the lenient attitude stops short of permitting all herbal preparations to pass easily through the net; only those for minor conditions. This means that herbs which are more strongly curative may be effectively knocked off the shelves when they come up for review—possibly half of all the herbal products now on sale, according to herbal manufacturers.

The herbal manufacturers have been up in arms about this, and formed a pressure group to lobby Parliament. An Early Day Motion requesting the Health Minister to include experts in the practice of natural, homeopathic, and herbal medicines on the relevant DHSS committees was signed by more than 200 MPs. Nothing came of it and the DHSS could not see what all the fuss was about. The Parliamentary Under-Secretary for State said at a meeting early in 1986 that; 'We wholeheartedly support the freedom of the individual to seek the benefits of alternative medicines and therapies. It is not our intention to use the Medicines Acts to restrict the general availability of alternative medicines'. The problem seems to be that the intention to permit natural medicines may be there, but when this is translated into practice, many traditional remedies and small firms could be removed by the small print. According to the herbal manufacturers, the end result can only be a proliferation of cheap 'cowboy' herbal products which through various loopholes (such as being sold as a food) escape the licensing regulations altogether. Indeed, this is already happening; the shelves of the health shops are full of herbal products of indeterminate species, origin, and purity, sometimes of quite inadequate amounts of active ingredients and of ineffective dosage.[21]

Herbal manufacturers would like the DHSS to adopt a West German system, in which there are commissions of experts on herbal, homeopathic, and anthroposophical medicine to advise the health ministry. The DHSS feels that it has already gone a long way towards recognition of herbs, for example, by continual dialogues with representatives of herbal users, by recognition of the British Herbal Pharmacopoeia as a guide, and by employment of herbal advisers in the drafting of the current laws. The recognition, voiced in MLX133, that herbal products reduce trivial consultations with doctors, and prevent people from using more toxic conventional remedies unnecessarily, is not openly afforded to any other complementary therapy by the DHSS. It has only come after years of strenuous efforts by F. Fletcher-Hyde, the head of the National Institute of Medical Herbalists. Other therapies would do well to learn from the herbalists, that the key to official acceptance is a continual dialogue on a professional level. Familiarity breeds respect.

It would, however, be wise to end on a cautionary note. In 1976 a committee advising the Medicines Commission proposed that all injectable substances be put on the Prescriptions Only List. This would for the first time prevent lay practitioners from giving injections.

Complementary practitioners were caught unawares and hastily defended themselves in the ensuing parliamentary debate,[22] and obtained a postponement. After a great deal of dialogue between the

DHSS and the practitioners, further postponements and meetings,[23] the DHSS finally decided that those practitioners who had been giving injections before February 1978 would be exempted.

However, the victory may be a Pyrrhic one, because new practitioners will not be allowed to give injections until the therapists' organizations present an accepted scheme for 'the validation of their members' training and competence by some nationally recognised training body in the medical or paramedical field'. As this implies both medical and official recognition of the therapies, it is unlikely to happen in the foreseeable future. Indeed, when it does happen the therapies would presumably be registerable and the whole question of exemptions would then be irrelevant.

The injection saga shows that the Government could nibble away at practitioners' common law rights if it needs to. It is clear that unless practitioners are vigilant and politically active, their sphere of activity may be eroded bit by bit even though their common law right remains the same. Some practitioners take this as a sign of a gloomy future in which they are within the law but are so hedged around with restrictions that it would be better to be outside it. Others see themselves becoming increasingly aggressive in the protection of their interests. The reality probably lies somewhere in between.

References

1. *Times Health Supplement.* 21 November 1981.
2. Inglis, B. (1979*a*). *Natural Medicine.* Collins, London.
3. Wharton, R. and Lewith, G. (1986). 'Complementary medicine and the general practitioner.' *British Medical Journal,* **292**, 1498–1500.
4. *The Times.* 10 August 1983.
5. British Medical Association (BMA). 16 August 1983.
6. *The Times.* 30 June 1983.
7. Editorial (1986). Pressure grows in parliament. *Journal of Alternative Medicine,* **4** (7), 1.
8. *Hansard.* 7 April 1976, Column 142.
9. Editorial (1985). Lords debate alternatives: no action until BMA report. *Journal of Alternative Medicine,* **3**(4), 2.
10. The DHSS position has recently been summarized in: Trumpington, The Baroness, (1987). Alternative medicines and therapies and the DHSS. *Journal of the Royal Society of Medicine,* **80**, 336–8.
11. *Hansard.* 7 April 1976, Column 441. Baer, H.A., (1984). The drive for

professionalism in British osteopathy. *Social Science and Medicine,* **19**, 717–25.
12. Fletcher-Hyde, F. (1978). The origin and practice of herbal medicine. *MIMS Magazine,* **2**, 127–36.
13. *Hansard.* Chiropractic and the NHS. 21 November 1979, Column 248.
14. Meeting of the Medicine Division of the Liverpool Area Health Authority Central District, March 1977.
15. House of Commons Adjournment Debate. 7 April 1977.
16. Asher, R. (1956). Respectable Hypnosis. *British Medical Journal,* **1**, 309–13.
17. *Hansard.* Hypnotism Bill. 20 November 1979, Column 54.
18. *Hansard.* 16 December 1977, Column 1174.
19. *Hansard.* 19 February 1980.
20. The Medicines (Prescription Only) Order 1977, No. 2127; The Medicines Act 1968 Order 1977, No. 2128; The Medicines (Supply of Herbal Remedies) Order 1977, No. 2130; The Medicines (General Sale List) Order 1977, No. 2129.
21. Fulder, S.J. (1986). Ineffective herbal remedies in the UK market. *Journal of Alternative Medicine*, 4–5. (February 1986).
22. *Hansard.* 31 January 1977.
23. *Hansard.* 20 February 1978, Column 1175.

5

International complementary medicine

In this chapter the social and legal positions of the therapies in several countries are reviewed. No attempt is made to give a classified and comparative survey. Instead countries have been picked out either because they are Western countries in which the status of complementary medicine is undergoing critical changes (Europe and Australia) or because their treatment of complementary medicine carries particular weight throughout the West, or because they have an ambivalent attitude to complementary medicine which it is instructive to consider (the USSR), or because they have been notably successful in welding traditional and modern medicine together and so exemplify solutions to the perennial problem of incompatibility between the systems (China and India).

The legal, social, and political situation of complementary medicine in the US has had to be omitted for lack of space. It is exceedingly complex, with each state deciding its own independent policy. In most cases these describe complementary medical techniques as the practice of medicine, which is proscribed to non-physicians under various Medical Practice Acts. However, in each therapy there are some states that have introduced some kind of regulatory or licensing arrangements. For example, in acupuncture, 34 states only allow practice by physicians. In some cases (e.g. Illinois) physicians are required to demonstrate some acupuncture training, in other cases (e.g. Tennessee) they have to possess a licence. Other states (e.g. Massachusetts) only permit lay practitioners to practise under medical supervision and of these a few states (e.g. Washington) require them to have a licence as well. As of 1982, only eight states allow the independent practice of acupuncture by lay therapists, but in every case only after a recognized course of training and an examination. California is the prime example. The restrictions on the lay practice of therapies such as herbalism, naturopathy, and homeopathy are similar, and only chiropractic has won full recognition, after a hard and bitter fight.

Western Europe

Anyone looking for consistency in the relationship between European governments and their complementary practitioners will find only a frustrating chaos. Each country has moved into the final years of the twentieth century carrying its own special brand of historic friction between medical and non-medical healing traditions. Membership of the EEC has not led to a common policy.

The legal position of individual therapies in each country is summarized in Table 5.1. Countries which adhere to the Napoleonic Code (where an action is generally forbidden unless specifically permitted) have allowed complementary practitioners to remain illegal. However, circumstance, culture and political history have resulted in exceptions such as nature-cure in Germany or chiropractic and anthroposophy in Switzerland.

West Germany

Apart from The Netherlands, the most liberal country in Western Europe is West Germany. Naturopaths have been licensed as a special class of health care professionals (Heilpraktiker) since the Second World War. New Heilpraktikers were forbidden to practise by the Nazi government but the edict was repealed in 1956. Now the Heilpraktikers, who are basically nature-cure/hydrotherapy practitioners, are trained in accredited colleges and granted a state licence after examination. Acupuncture, homeopathy, herbalism (phytotherapy), chiropractic, etc., although actually illegal, now thrive under the banner of Heilpraktik. Any practitioner may use these therapies without restriction provided he first trains as a Heilpraktiker.

Doctors who wish to be Heilpraktikers must also obtain the qualification. However, this has not stopped many doctors from practising and exploring complementary therapies in addition to conventional medicine. Such doctors are in great demand in West Germany. There are at least 700 homeopathic doctors today, along with one large homeopathic hospital and several homeopathic sanatoria. Four universities teach homeopathic courses for medical undergraduates. Medical homeopathy in the land of homeopathy's

Table 5.1 *The legal position of therapies in some West European countries and Scandinavia (1986)*

Therapy	Denmark, Scandinavia	Belgium, Isle of Jersey, Italy, Spain	The Netherlands	West Germany, Luxembourg	France	Switzerland
Chiropractic	Legal but restrictions	Illegal	Illegal but tolerated, law to be changed	Illegal unless also a Heilpraktiker	'Recognized' but formally illegal except in Alsace-Lorraine	Legal
Naturopathy	Legal but restrictions	Illegal	Illegal but tolerated, law to be changed	Legal as Heilpraktiker	Illegal	Illegal except in the Canton of Appenzell
Acupuncture	Legal but restrictions	Illegal	Illegal but tolerated, law to be changed	Illegal unless also a Heilpraktiker	Illegal but substantially taken up by doctors	Illegal except in the Canton of Appenzell
Homeopathy	Legal but restrictions	Illegal	Illegal but tolerated, law to be changed	Illegal unless also a Heilpraktiker	Illegal but substantially taken up by doctors	Illegal except in the Canton of Appenzell
Herbalism (phytotherapy)	Legal but restrictions	Illegal	Illegal but tolerated, law to be changed	Illegal unless also a Heilpraktiker; substantially taken up by doctors	Illegal but substantially taken up by doctors	Illegal except in the Canton of Appenzell

foundation flourishes and is certainly much stronger than in the UK.

A powerful nature-cure organization, the Kneipp system, organized by medically qualified practitioners, flourishes in West Germany. These doctors have set up a national health and therapy movement, based on the teaching of Father Sebastian Kneipp over a century ago. This movement is basically a spa-orientated mixture of water, exercise, and diet cures. It is large indeed. Its main spa is a virtual hydrotherapy town. Bad Worishösen has about 50 Kneipp doctors, 80 masseurs, and 120 trained bath attendants. The movement, which actually might be better named a brotherhood, boasts two scientific journals devoted to supportive studies on nature cures and physical medicine.

Herbalism, or phytotherapy, is also much stronger in West Germany than in the UK. Most pharmacists have displays of natural product remedies which rival those of conventional drugs. Germany is the centre of the international herb trade, and the main traditional source of herbal teas and tisanes. There are, needless to say, very many more doctors practising herbalism than in the UK. The same applies to anthroposophy, which originated in Germany. The Ministry of Health has relaxed its strict pharmaceutical registration laws. Committees on anthroposphical, herbal, and homeopathic remedies, including practitioners as members, have been set up in 1986 to advise the Ministry of Health on safety and efficacy.

France

France does not have authorized exceptions to the rules against non-medical practitioners, although chiropractic is in a very strange position of Gallic indeterminacy. A 1978 survey revealed that 13 per cent of the French population go to chiropractors, and they are reimbursed by many social security and insurance schemes. Despite this *de facto* recognition, chiropractic remains illegal and the law has deterred laymen from careers in complementary medicine, thus leaving it open for French doctors to add a good deal of complementary medicine to their exclusive domain. However, in France, unlike the US, the doctors have retained the purity and independence of the therapies and taken their principles seriously.

Acupuncture was brought to the West by the French, 1000 doctors are trained in it, and it has been practised widely in France in hospitals and clinics for almost 50 years. The international acupuncture body (SIA) was started in France by Dr J. Schatz, who is a major figure in the development of acupuncture in the West on rational yet traditional lines.

Doctors also practise extensively in phytotherapy and homeopathy. 10 000 doctors prescribe homeopathic remedies, 30 times more than in the UK. Four schools train 1000 doctors a year in established 3 year courses. There is a section on homeopathic remedies in the French pharmacopoeia. Almost every pharmacy is stocked with homeopathic remedies which are manufactured on a large scale by three pharmaceutical companies. Homeopathic prescriptions qualify alongside conventional ones for a state subsidy of 70 per cent of their price, and they are used by one in six of the population. Only the esoteric therapies, healing, and radionics, are rare, compared to the UK.

The French spend extravagantly on health. Their health services cost some 8 per cent of the Gross National Product, which is 2 per cent more than in the UK. However, the health shops, the ubiquitous herbal teas, the sudden rise of complementary medicine, and the serious attention to fitness programmes are evidence of a change.

The Netherlands

In 1977 the State Secretary for Health, J.P.M. Hendriks, set up a Commission for Alternative Systems of Medicine. Its task was to investigate the significance of alternative medicine in The Netherlands and make recommendations to the Government on the basis of its findings. The Commission was the end result of a runaway public campaign for freedom of choice in medicine, a campaign helped, unwittingly, by the Government itself through its health centres. The public made clear to the Government the anomaly of the promotion of natural health in a society that bans natural medicine. The Ministry of Health took their views seriously, and a 1970 State Commission on Medical Practice took the unprecedented step of recommending that only where public health was at risk should the unqualified be prevented from practising. This led to the drafting of a new Individual Health Care Occupations Bill, in 1977, which embodies this so-called 'Scandinavian' option. Wisely, the Secretary of State for Health wished to understand fully the social, legal, practical, and political dimensions of complementary medicine before actually putting the bill before Parliament. The Commission for Alternative Medicine was set up for this purpose.

Dutch law, as in all the European countries, stated that only qualified doctors were permitted to practise medicine, giving them effective monopoly. Professor Muntendam, the head of the Commission, pointed out in his introduction to the report that: 'The consensus of public opinion is no longer behind the monopoly, and the law is broken a thousand times a day as sick and disabled people seek the help of people who are not legally authorized to provide it'.[1] Naturally, the medical profession was opposed to the Commission. It attempted to keep the legal monopoly by the argument that the therapies were not scientifically proved. The Health Minister boldly stated that the argument was not good enough; that the public demand for freedom of choice in medicine is more important in generating new laws than scientific verification. The public could not wait for, and were uninterested in, the question of scientific verification. The Commission itself stated that it:

. . . believes that the division between alternative and orthodox medicine is not—or is not principally—of a scientific nature . . . The demand that alternative practitioners must demonstrate the effectiveness of their treatments before they can be granted any form of recognition thus seems to the Commission to be indefensible.

The Commission sent full questionnaires to all the organizations involved, and then held hearings. It sponsored a world survey of the scientific and subculture literature on complementary medicine. It carried out a survey of the legal position of complementary medicine in other countries, and sponsored a detailed sociological survey of distribution, statistics, population use, and practices of complementary medicine.

The Commission's report was comprehensive and powerful. No Government has ever made such a comprehensive attempt to understand the practice of complementary medicine. Its basic conclusion was that: 'alternative medicine is such an important factor in health care in The Netherlands, that government policy cannot disregard it'. Accordingly, the Commission advised the Health Ministry specifically to include trained practitioners of complementary medicine as one of the qualified classes of health professionals defined in the 1977 bill. Those who could not be considered qualified, for example, because they belonged to a therapy that did not provide adequate training, would not be prevented from practising but could not use certain appellations. The report suggested a novel idea of arranging sponsored courses in basic medicine for these practitioners to reduce any potential public risks. It saw expansion of training as the key to the successful integration of complementary medicine. The organizations representing therapists were strongly exhorted to maintain solidarity. The recommendations of the commission are quoted in Table 5.2. They constitute a first blueprint for the full incorporation of complementary medicine into the national life of any Western country.

It is taking a long time to implement the recommendations of the Commission, and there are many problems still to be solved. The details of the replacement of the old Medical Act are still under discussion. However, the Government has instituted courses for complementary practitioners in tertiary educational institutions, and it continues to encourage the various therapies to improve their organization and standards. The Health Minister himself opened the 1986 first Joint Conference on Natural and Alternative Health Therapies with that message.

The rest of Europe and Scandinavia

Of the other European countries, Belgium, Italy, and Spain tend to follow the French pattern, with Belgium the most conservative. In 1973 the complementary therapy world was shocked by dawn police

Table 5.2 *Recommendations of the Dutch Commission on Alternative Systems of Medicine (1977)*

The commission recommends that the Government:

1. Set up a consultative and advisory committee under the auspices of the Minister of Health and Environmental Protection to consult and advise the Government, *inter alia*, on the elaboration and implementation of its recommendations and on problems pertaining to alternative medicine.

2. Institute a national information and documentation centre, which will subsequently be referred to as the IDC.

3. Include alternative medicine as an additional item in the budget of the Ministry of Health and Environmental Protection for 1982 and subsequent years.

4. Promote research into alternative forms of treatment.

5. Promote the provision of information on alternative forms of treatment in existing university and university-type courses, with special

Table 5.2 *(Continued)*

emphasis on the responsibility borne by the medical profession for supplying such information to the public.

6. Undertake an immediate study to determine whether, to what extent, and on what conditions alternative practitioners who are unqualified under the present legislation can be given the opportunity of acquiring legal status.

7. Take steps to ensure that the practitioners of alternative therapies, whether qualified or unqualified under the Individual Health Care Occupations Bill, have undergone an adequate or basic course of training.

   (a) As regards those who are qualified to practise under both the present and the new legislation, it is recommended that the government ensure that only those who have received the appropriate training will be permitted to practise an alternative system of medicine.

   (b) As regards those who are not competent to practise at present and will also be unqualified under the new Act, it is recommended that the Government ensure, by giving financial support to training establishments with a suitable curriculum, that these alternative medical practitioners are also given the opportunity to acquire a basic medical knowledge.

   (c) As regards persons who wish to train in an alternative medicine with the object of being admitted to a professional group as qualified practitioners under the new Act, it is recommended that the Government take steps to ensure that the establishments referred to in (b) receive the financial aid needed to enable them to provide training for this group also.

8. Vigorously oppose charlatanry as defined in Chapter 2 of its final report.

9. Address an immediate request to the Health Insurance Funds Council to study the recommendations in the Commission's report and to put forward proposals concerning the inclusion in health insurance schemes of alternative systems of medicine specified in the request, and concerning the categories of practitioners of those systems of medicine.

10. Introduce the Individual Health Care Occupations Bill without delay.

11. Pending the Government's decisions on the proposals contained in the report, no proceedings should be instituted against alternative practitioners except in instances where such practitioners have seriously impaired the health of patients or in obvious cases of fraud.

raids on the premises of 28 Brussels chiropractors (it is said that the policemen who posted the closure notices arrived later for their usual treatment). In 1986, 75 per cent of Belgian practitioners in complementary medicine were medically qualified and only with these practitioners will the patient's expenses be returned under the state social security system. Scandinavia is extremely liberal and has licensed practitioners, although there are certain forbidden areas, for example surgery, obstetrics, and anaesthesia. Since 1975 Finland has, uniquely included acupuncture as a standard part of its medical curriculum following the Soviet model.

The EEC and complementary medicine

Britain's entry into the Common Market caused widespread alarm in the complementary medicine movement. The International Federation of Practitioners of Natural Therapeutics, now disbanded, warned therapists of the supposed imminent dangers of joining the EEC, and tried to fight for practitioners' rights in Brussels. The main fear, of course, was that the UK common law right would disappear under EEC harmonization plans. Even when it became clear that there would be no wholesale imposition of Napoleonic law onto the UK, a more specific concern took its place. Practitioners from countries where complementary medicine was illegal would have the right to practise their profession in the UK, but not *vice versa*. At the same time, herbalists and those practitioners using medicines were worried that medicines legislation in the UK would be harmonized with that abroad and all the special consideration won by herbalists and homeopaths would be lost again.

In fact all these concerns have proved unfounded. There is nothing in the Treaty of Rome which would require a rewriting of medical or medicines legislation. Certain changes have been made in procedures for the licensing of drugs, but these have not affected the general position of traditional products. From 1967 to 1970 the International Federation had a series of meetings with the section of the EEC concerned with the professions. They attempted to obtain paramedical status for complementary practitioners within the EEC. The EEC officials gave the usual answer that a disunited complementary medicine cannot expect a united status. They also said that the only complementary medicine training standards formally accepted by an EEC country were those of the Heilpraktikers in Germany. In the absence of any others, this standard would be taken as the universal EEC standard if recognition occurred. The matter was dropped, but surfaced briefly in 1979 in the European Parliament. A question was put forward by French chiropractors who said that since their profession was still illegal in France, but not in certain other member states, they were discriminated against within the EEC.[2] The EEC's answer, predictably, was that as no harmonization of laws had occurred, member states were free to pursue their own policies which were outside the jurisdiction of the EEC. In those countries where chiropractic is legal, there should be no discrimination against chiropractors from any other member states. In those states where it was illegal, the law would apply to all nationals anyway.

In 1984 the Council of Europe issued a Directive on alternative medicine.[3] Its basic position is favourable to non-conventional medicine (which it found impossible to define). 'In view of the frequency with which sick people nowadays seek help from non-conventional practitioners, this phenomenon can no longer be regarded as a medical side-issue', reported the EEC committee, 'it must reflect a genuine public need'. The Directive requests member states to reimburse complementary medicine within each country's social security system: 'the emancipation of patients is resulting in the patient's right to choose the therapy and the therapist he considers best, and also the right to receive this health care on the same financial conditions as any other medical care'. This appears to have an advantage over The Netherlands Commission on Alternative Medicine, with its concentration on freedom of choice in medicine. It is, however, unlikely that the more conservative member states will start to subsidize visits to herbalists, whatever the Council of Europe says, and there is enough ambiguity in the report to support actions for or against complementary medicine. For example, the Directive states that only those in 'general medical practice' should be allowed to provide medical services under each state's social security system—but this term is not defined. This alarmed the complementary medical community in the UK so much that they successfully requested a debate on it in the House of Commons. After all, if this term meant 'registered medical practitioner' it would mean a permanent ban on patients of lay practitioners ever receiving treatment under the NHS. Other potential restrictions exist in relation to permissible titles, and 'preventing the issue of inferior diplomas'. Therapists may justifiably be rather nervous about moves that permit more patients to consult them, but limit their freedom to treat these patients when they arrive.

The USSR and Eastern Europe

The USSR encompasses a diverse conglomerate of peoples: the Mongolians, the Siberian tribes, the Europeanized Slavs, and the Turko-Tartar Moslems of the south. Its medicine reflects this: it is a bizarre jumble of the unfulfilled intentions of central government and the unfulfilled desires of its constituent peoples.

The present medical system was established about 50 years ago, with the urgent priority of bringing epidemics such as cholera and typhus under control. A very large number of physicians were trained and, like China, a system of rural paramedical health workers (Feldshers) dealt with primary care and preventive medicine. However, despite sophisticated centres of excellence in the major cities, conventional medicine in the hinterland is still patchy. Drug supplies, reasonable hospital services, and good quality personnel are often in very short supply. Even the Soviet Health Minister complained in 1981 that 75 per cent of all available X-ray film was useless.[4] Health in the USSR is getting worse. Infant mortality has been rising steadily, and is now double that of the US. The life expectancy of males has dropped to 63 years, some 8 years behind Europe.[5]

All this leaves considerable scope for alternatives, and traditional medicine is present in rural areas of the USSR to an extent unparalleled in any Western country. Cupping, plasters, herbalism, and so on are regularly available, supplied by part-time, rural practitioners. Visits to spas are a national pastime. While the average British worker is enjoing an indulgent holiday in Blackpool or Palma Majorca, the Russian worker takes his break at a health spa on the Black Sea. One can still find strongly regional practices. The Mongols, who introduced yoghurt to the West, are still practising their version of Indo-Tibetan medicine and supplying 'Kumiss' (mare's-milk) cures to the chronically sick. Siberian semi-shamanistic folk medicine and the Arabic-Hippocratic Moslem medicine of Turkestan are thriving. Healers practise widely, charging quite high fees. Even the late Party Chairman, Leonid Brezhnev, had a personal healer–hypnotist. Acupuncture is taught in Soviet postgraduate medical colleges by several professors of acupuncture. There is a central acupuncture research institute in Moscow. Soviet doctors use it regularly for a widening sphere of applications including: an accompaniment to surgery and anaesthesia, nervous diseases, allergies, stomach and intestinal conditions, and chronic pain.

However, the official Soviet policy is to restrict traditional complementary medicine as a system, incorporating only what can be scientifically proved into modern state medicine. It has therefore waged an erratic war against complementary medicine, while, paradoxically, studying parts of it in heavyweight institutional research programmes.[6] It is illegal to receive money for the practice of complementary medicine without being a doctor or otherwise licensed, although the law is widely flouted. Occasional suppressive announcements from the Health Ministry state that doctors supplying herbs and medicines which were not approved, could be struck off. Yet announcements concerning new medicinal discoveries from the 'rich herbal wisdom' of the USSR were released to the world press. The 10th Soviet pharmacopoeia still contains several kinds of herbs and crude extracts, perhaps 8 per cent of all the drugs therein. They are mostly herbs such as *eleutherococcus*, traditionally used in Oriental medicine, which have a preventive and tonic action and which are unmatched by any Western drug.[7] The previous pharmacopoeia contained 20 per cent of natural products, most of which were dropped without any reason other than modernization.

Homeopathy can only be practised in a few special clinics. Healers are sometimes called charlatans and those teaching healing risk losing their jobs and suffer low level KGB interference. Yet psychic phenomena are taken very seriously, labelled with scientific catch phrases such as the 'bioplasma field', and studied in modern, well-equipped laboratories. Brezhnev's healer was approved by the state, since she takes part in university-sponsored tests and attends scientific congresses.

Although the state's attitude to medicine is confusing, there is at least no professional dominant caste which attempts to secure a therapeutic monopoly. This has meant that traditional medicine has survived in the USSR to an extent greater than in any European country. The current constraints on complementary medicine are initiated by a bureaucracy intent on rationalization rather than a medical establishment intent on dominance. Hence segments of complementary medicine can survive, stripped down to that part which is provable by scientific methods. In some respects this has led to the inclusion of novel techniques and ideas into science and medicine far ahead of Western countries. For example the USSR is practically the only country to introduce the teaching of acupuncture and reflexology into medical schools. However, it is an acupuncture shorn of the many traditional subtle aspects which are essentially unprovable using current scientific criteria.[8]

In Eastern Europe there is also a rich herbal and natural medicine tradition. Bulgaria is the foremost exporter of herbs, and family medical chests are invariably herbal. UNESCO has its phytochemistry centre in Sofia. As in the USSR, healing and parapsychology are demystified and secularised. The Sofia Institute of Parapsychology and Suggestion Research is part of the university and teaches degree courses. There and at other places research is continuing on altered states of consciousness, healing, hypnosis, and yoga. Hypnosis has been shown to heal wounds more quickly, and as a result it is practised in sanatoria and neurological clinics all over the country.

Other East European countries have a state medicine which lies some way between the hard official line of the USSR and the open traditionalist attitude of Bulgaria.[9] The future may see complementary medicine gaining strength in all Soviet bloc countries, both because of its cautious entry into the laboratories and because of the state's inability to stamp it out. In the last analysis it does take the pressure off their overburdened medical systems.

Australia, New Zealand, and South Africa

'Back to it' ran the heading of a medical journal editorial on chiropractic and the medical profession.[10] The 'it' was the 'chiropractic problems' that the New Zealand Medical Association was having, arising from a favourable report of a Government commission of inquiry into chiropractic. The report spurred the Government into thinking about registration of chiropractors, inducing disquiet in the medical profession. The Government report on complementary medicine in Australia had the same result. Australia, New Zealand, and South Africa are countries where legislative changes could serve as prime precedents for the UK and for this reason are described fully here.[11]

Complementary therapies in Australia are enjoying a boom as great as in the UK and there are more consultations in relation to population than in the UK. According to a recent parliamentary submission by the Australian Natural Therapists' Association, 10 million consultations and treatments were given in 1985. Colleges are highly active and train so many natural therapists that certain areas, such as Sydney which has 900 naturopaths, are already saturated. Medical insurance organizations are paying rebates for manipulative, naturopathic, and acupuncture therapies from selected colleges, but Medicare does not as yet.

Chiropractic is popular, and osteopaths are less well defined and include both the highly trained, from the British School of Osteopathy, and the partly trained manipulators who tend to call themselves osteopaths. Naturopathy is widespread and includes all the varieties of therapy seen in the UK, a major difference being the strength of iridology which is an almost universal diagnostic tool among Australian, but not UK, naturopaths. Homeopathy is not extensive, and most people practising it would be described as naturopaths. Acupuncture is growing rapidly and has been taken more seriously in Australia since the National Health and Medical Research Council Report on Acupuncture (1974) recommended clinical studies.

Until various state Medical Acts were passed complementary practitioners were free to practise in Australia under a common law right similar to that of the UK. The main problem that faced complementary practitioners in Australia was the opposition by the medical profession. This often went as far as the courts. Patients have been induced to bring malpractice actions against complementary practitioners and on at least one occasion a naturopath has been prosecuted for treating cancer, despite his plea that he was treating a condition unrelated to the tumour.

In 1974 the Australian Committee was established by the Ministry of Health in response to the wide public usage of chiropractic.[12] It took 2½ years (2½ times as long as forecast) to review the evidence which consisted of written submissions from individuals and organizations, followed by oral interviews, visits to educational establishments in Australia and abroad, extensive personal meetings with and observations of therapists, and several research projects specially commissioned by the Committee.

The Committee was adamant that chiropractic was a paramedical or auxiliary skill, filling a hole in modern health care, but not a system of therapy in its own right. It therefore recommended that chiropractic and osteopathy should be registered in each state by means of a Manipulative Therapists (Chiropractors and Osteopaths) Act, but not as alternative health systems. A registration board should be set up to supervise standards, ethics, and education. Existing practitioners should be registered providing they had sufficient past experience, and took a test of competence and an up-dating course. As far as education was concerned the Committee recommended that there should be a system of accreditation of colleges, and that a new four-year bachelor course in a tertiary institution in Australia would provide a standard qualification against which other attainments could be measured. Despite vehement medical opposition, chiropractors are now registered in many states. From 1980 the chiropractors were included in the federal health insurance fund.

The other complementary therapies received very different treatment. The Committee described naturopathy as 'a minor cult system' and rejected herbalism in extraordinarily uncompromising terms, pronouncing that the pharmaceutical industry already knew all the plant chemicals of interest. The Committee also rejected acupuncture as a separate therapeutic system, accepting the National Health and Medical Research Council's report of its limited usefulness.

Only the manipulative therapies are now registered in all states. The other therapists, grouped by the Government into Oriental medicine (acupuncture, Oriental herbalism), and naturopathy (the category for all the other therapies including homeopathy and herbalism) remain outside the law, apart from regulations relating to sterilization of needles and certain medical conditions such as cancer which may not be treated. The one exception is Northern Territory which passed a law in 1985 registering naturopaths and other allied health professionals. The existing professional bodies were empowered to oversee the various professions.

However, the situation is very fluid. A major new enquiry has been conducted by the Social Development Committee of the Victorian Parliament. The Committee refused registration of the complementary therapies, but will consider accredition of courses and will introduce a special licensing system for natural remedies and health products.[13]

Complementary medicine in New Zealand has developed in a similar fashion to complementary medicine in Australia. New Zealand's legislation also embodies the precepts of common law.

With the exception of chiropractors, who were licensed to practise in 1960, complementary practitioners operate under common law but outside the statute book. Chiropractors require an annual certificate of practice which falls far short of registration or any form of parliamentary blessing and is more a licensing of premises than an acceptance of the practitioners. The medical opposition to chiropractic in New Zealand was vehement and unbending. In 1978, while the official Health Ministry Commission of Inquiry on Chiropractic was at work collecting evidence,[14] the New Zealand Medical Association quickly inserted its first specific written statement on the subject into its Annual Handbook: 'It is *unethical* for a doctor to refer a patient to a chiropractor for treatment' [author's italics], thus making clear its opposition to any changes favourable to chiropractors which the Commission might suggest. Having decided that referral to chiropractors was unethical, the New Zealand Medical Association was then able to reject the Commission's report on the grounds that it was asking doctors to do something unethical. 'The rules of medical ethics cannot be abolished by statute', stated the chairman of the Association. No doubt it was this that led to the cartoon in the *Otago Daily Times* showing a doctor with his nose in the air and the Commission of Inquiry in the background commenting: 'You ought to see a chiropractor about that stiff neck of yours, doctor!'

However in the last few years there has been a softening of attitudes. A new medical bill registering chiropractors as medical auxiliaries in the manner of physiotherapists became law in April 1983. Some complementary medicine is even taught in medical schools.

South Africa has also regularized complementary medicine in a set of laws that therapists regard as a mixed blessing. Act 63 of 1982 incorporates all complementary practitioners into a register supervised by the South Africa Associated Health Service Professions Board. This register has the same status as, and is independent of, the General Medical Council supervising the conventional medical profession. Practitioners not on this register are not allowed to practice. The register requires practitioners to be trained in a six-year university level course in alternative medicine, which runs parallel to the medical school course except that it replaces drug and surgical treatment in the later stages of the course, with naturopathy/manipulative methods or herbs/homeopathy.

Some complementary practitioners were pleased with the new legalization. To others it was a disaster, and the profession was reduced from 3000 practitioners to 600 more or less overnight. One of the issues which even therapists accepted onto the register find problematic is that they are not allowed to perform acts outside their defined profession. This encourages an unhealthy specialization which runs contrary to the natural eclecticism of complementary medicine, for example, it prevents a naturopath also prescribing homeopathic remedies where appropriate. The acid test will be whether in the coming years complementary medicine in South Africa will maintain its authenticity and independence.

Traditional medicine—its worldwide fate

Third World Countries

Many developing countries have only recently become aware of the fact that it is quite beyond their means to establish a sophisticated modern medical health structure, especially in rural areas. For example, the cost of maintaining 1 physician per 1000 population works out at roughly 1 per cent of the Gross National Product in the US. In less developed countries such as Tanzania or Uganda, the cost would take up to 8 per cent of the Gross National Product and there is therefore very little chance of sufficient medical personnel being available to provide modern medicine for all. In 1987 80 per cent of the world's population used traditional healing methods and it is against this background that an attempt to preserve centuries-old indigenous medicine is being made.

Traditional medicine is a designation that partly overlaps complementary medicine; it is usually applied to indigenous, non-conventional healing practices, including folk and village medicine. A World Health Organization (WHO) study group defined traditional medicine as:

the sum total of all the knowledge and practices, whether explicable or not, used in diagnosis, prevention and elimination of physical, mental or social imbalance, and relying exclusively on practical experience and observation handed down from generation to generation, whether verbally or in writing'. It continued: 'The essential differences among various systems of medicine arise not from the difference in goal or effects, but rather from the cultures of the peoples who practise the different systems.[15]

It follows from this that traditional medicine is no more or less irrelevant and declining than traditional cultures themselves.

It is, of course, true that among this collection of remedies and practices some are ineffective and even harmful, as in all medical systems. In addition, traditional medicine is often overwhelmed by epidemics of infectious and contagious diseases, especially during a breakdown of the stable social milieu. Nevertheless, the effectiveness of much traditional medicine is not in doubt.[16] When modern pharmacologists attempt to obtain drugs from traditional herbs, the inclusion of traditional practitioners in research teams increases the success rate from 1 per cent to 40–50 per cent of all plants tested.[17] (The traditional medicine section of the Bibliography (p. 105) lists further articles exploring the role of traditional medicine.) The value of traditional practitioners is that they are already a part of a people's own health system, with the social standing necessary to reach everybody. They can readily deal with culturally based health problems arising, for example, from diet.

As health experts became aware of the vast resources inherent in traditional medicine, especially in poorer rural communities, they began to see it as an aid to health goals rather than a hindrance to the spread of modern medicine. At the same time local leaders began to see traditional medicine as part of an attempt to rehabilitate their cultural heritage. This new attitude led to the recruitment of traditional birth attendants to help in family planning. Gradually the WHO adopted a historic change of course, taking it towards confrontation, primarily with the drug companies, but also with the professional medical establishments of the West.

The WHO moved its emphasis from disease eradication by high technology medicine to the support of primary health care. A series of conferences led to a resolution at the 29th World Health Assembly to take into account 'the manpower reserve constituted by those practising traditional medicine'. A Working Group on Traditional Medicine was established at Geneva in 1976, and has been highly active in support of programmes to research and develop traditional medical resources.

The International Conference on Primary Health Care at Alma-Ata in 1977 laid down the guidelines for the WHO policy of primary health care. It envisaged a worldwide movement of barefoot doctor or feldsher type community health workers bringing low cost public health and first-line treatment to the villages, a reverse of the expensive, sophisticated and inadequate medicine dispensed by specialists to the privileged few.[18]

A WHO meeting in 1977 published an important document on the manner in which this was to be achieved.[15] The programme would:

1. Give recognition to traditional practitioners and incorporate them into community development programmes.
2. Retrain traditional practitioners for appropriate use in primary health care.
3. Acquaint professional health personnel and students of modern systems with the principles of traditional medicine in order to promote dialogue, communication, mutual understanding, and eventual integration.
4. Educate the community to believe that the provision of traditional remedies was not second-rate medicine.
5. Catalogue all medicinal plants in a country or region and disseminate this information.
6. Retain the traditional forms for prescriptions used in primary health care and carry out relevant research into the traditional systems of medicine.

There are, of course, immense problems with such a programme, mostly political.[19] In many developing countries traditional medicine is excluded or illegal. Only 3 out of 19 African countries possess legislation for traditional medicine, while 15 do not even recognise traditional birth attendants, who are, perhaps, the spearhead of acceptable traditional medical personnel. This lack of interest in traditional medicine is usually the result of physicians' fears of loss of status, or governments' fears of turning the clock back on modernization programmes.[20]

Traditionalists also have doubts about the WHO programme. Practitioners argue that the WHO plan would turn them into paramedical health workers and destroy traditional medicine in the process. There is evidence (see p. 113) that contact with modern medicine often leads traditional practitioners hastily to abandon ancient practices in favour of fast-acting Western drugs. These bring speedy relief of symptoms and easily ensnare folk practitioners and their patients into dependence. Sulphonamides and aspirin are now used by most Third World healers.

The philosophical and cultural bases of traditional and modern medicine are so far apart that integration seems impossible. When the two meet, a cultural shock wave can result which leads in a few short years to alienation and destruction of a sophisticated and ancient teaching. When this happens, as it has with Bedouin, Persian, and Eskimo medicine, reconstruction is virtually impossible.

For these reasons, the countries which have had most success in drawing on traditional medical resources have been those in which traditional practitioners have been given a secure status but left free from the hazards of integration. This is the position of the shamanistic bomohs of Malaysia, who number 20 000 compared to 2300 Malaysian physicians. Many African countries have left their traditional healers alone, neither legislating for nor against them. China and India are discussed in detail as two cases in which traditional and modern medicine seem to have evolved successfully in parallel.

China

China can claim to have the most ancient and sophisticated medical system in the world. It stretches back at least as far as Egyptian medicine, and has been developing in an unbroken line since then. In contrast, Western medicine is the result of cycles of growth, destruction and renaissance. The unique Chinese techniques of acupuncture, herbalism, and moxibustion have folk and shamanistic origins overlaid with Taoist and imperial theory to produce a unique, elaborate and sensitive system of physiology, pathology, and medical skills.[7] Chinese medicine is discussed in Chapter 6.

Western medicine entered China with the missionaries at the end of the seventeenth century. Jesuit doctors confounded and entranced the imperial court with the novelties of Western anatomy and drug treatment, a mirror image of the captivation of French doctors by the mysteries of acupuncture some 200 years later. One early Chinese emperor used to pit the wits of European, Chinese, and Tibetan doctors against each other. Another locked up Western anatomy charts as the potential dynamite that indeed they were, for by the end of the nineteenth century hospitals and Western doctors were so pervasive in the main cities of China that traditional medicine, or Chung-i, was on the brink of disappearing altogether. Lack of resources and communication saved it, for it persisted in the rural hinterland as the sole medical resource.

The Communist Party was originally committed to the final eradication of traditional medicine. It was seen as a superstitious feudalism, standing in the way of progress into the modern world. During the Civil War both sides relied heavily on traditional medicine, the Nationalists willingly, the Communists grudgingly. Subsequently, the Communists had to admit that traditional medicine had proved itself in the ultimate test: the epidemics, injuries, and chaos of the war. As early as 1944, Mao stated, 'to surrender to the old style is wrong; to abolish or discard is wrong. Our responsibility is to unite those of the old style that can be used, and to help, stimulate and reform them.'[21] This was the embryonic stage of a movement to 'unite the old and the new' that Mao pursued throughout the development of the People's Republic. The cardinal principles of the Chinese health care system were defined at the First National Health Conference in Peking in 1950 as follows:

1. Medicine should serve the masses.
2. Prevention should come first.
3. Health work should utilize mass campaigns.
4. Chinese traditional and Western medicine should be integrated.

Traditional doctors were brought back into society, and the barriers of secrecy lifted. Dual clinics were set up in the countryside. Traditional doctors were included in Western hospitals and clinics, and new hospitals, colleges, and research facilities were established exclusively for traditional practitioners; finally, in the midst of the Great Leap Forward, traditional doctors were included in the Chinese Medical Association. Medical doctors were encouraged to study traditional medicine, although this was later discouraged when it was realized that this would undermine the strength of the traditional practitioner.

In fact integration was much more difficult to achieve than any of the party ideologues imagined. Western-trained doctors shirked their duties to research and upgrade traditional practices, and dumped their impossible cases on traditional practitioners. The conceptual basis of Chinese medicine proved to be completely untranslatable in scientific terms. Twenty years after the call to integration, Chinese experts still could not agree on whether the traditional term for 'kidney' (one of the five main viscera) corresponded to the Western anatomical kidney, the testes, or some physiological function that included both. No real progress has been made on the basic question of whether acupuncture meridians correspond to any structure or function of the body known to medical science.

The Cultural Revolution did, however, succeed in integrating traditional medicine where it mattered most—in the clinics and commune hospitals of the countryside. At the same time as attacking the Ministry of Health as a 'Ministry of Urban Health', and throwing doctors into the fields along with other urban élites, the Cultural Revolution established the barefoot doctor programme, the most successful community health system in the world. Barefoot doctors (who are neither barefoot nor doctors) are trained paramedical health visitors who carry on medical work for one third of their time and agriculture for the rest. They offer primary treatment, first aid, public health, preventive medicine, and family planning, and they refer more serious cases to clinics and hospitals. They carry a medicine chest of basic drugs as well as traditional herbs and acupuncture needles. In many cases they are traditional practitioners who have been retrained. They have been given most of the credit for the remarkable increase in health and life expectancy during the last 25 years in China, which now rivals any Western country. Barefoot doctors are the main inspiration for the World Health Organization's vision of community health workers bringing primary health care to the world's poor.

While traditional medicine remains popular today, especially in the countryside, it has taken second place to the echelons of new health workers even there. Within the medical establishment it seems that integration is still beyond reach. The Chinese Medical Association no longer accepts traditional practitioners, who have formed their own All China Association of Traditional Chinese Medicine. The reason given for the split is that the two medicines have two languages and cannot intercommunicate. Thirty per cent of medical education includes traditional medicine but in practice there are only some 10 000 doctors who have trained in traditional as well as modern medicine and there are not many highly experienced doctors of traditional medicine left in the country at present.

All hospitals have a traditional medicine outpatient clinic, but few have proper inpatient facilities for traditional practitioners. In the 'Western' hospitals medical doctors mostly assign serious cases to medical departments, often despite patient preference for traditional medicine. In traditional hospitals, traditional medicine is often found alongside departments which carry out surgery, radiology, ENT, obstetrics, and other modern specialities. The traditional doctors in charge of traditional in- or outpatient facilities are Western-trained doctors with a subsequent traditional training. They use traditional techniques for the less serious conditions and cases such as liver diseases, the treatment of bones, of acute abdominal syndromes, or of cardiovascular diseases, where Chinese research or experience has shown that traditional medicine is highly effective.[22]

More surprising is the fact that modern scientific terminology and the classification of diseases has taken over in traditional treatment centres. Because it has been largely left to doctors and paramedical health workers to bring traditional medicine into the twentieth century the doctors have of necessity imposed their language. For example, the original Chinese pathological designations, such as hot, cold, moist, full, empty, have been universally mapped onto Western nosology, so that doctors now diagnose a condition as a hot or cold, yin or yang, version of, say, high blood pressure.

Traditional methods of increasing the health and lifespan of the individual, through delicate adjustments to organ systems by means of diet and herbs, is an ancient art that is unique to Chinese medicine. Yet it has no place in the modern Chinese doctor's use of traditional techniques. In fact, traditional acupuncturists in the West are often of the opinion that true Chinese traditional medicine is now more authentically practised in places like Hong Kong and Taiwan than in mainland China. The political upheavals and pressing immediate public health problems may have forced traditional medicine into a subsidiary mode. As Marilynn Rosenthal asks: 'Is this integration or is it Western medicine assimilating selected treatment modalities and traditional medicine grasping for a future by enmeshing itself in the structure of Western medical explanation?'[22]

China can be justifiably proud of its medical achievements. It has achieved its health goals, and set a precedent of co-operation rather than destruction of the old by the new. China wishes to export its medical knowledge. It is supported by the World Health Organization in its belief that acupuncture is a powerful health weapon for the Third World. Traditional medicine is still very strong in China. The attempt to bridge the gap between systems is continuing, and given time, more of the old knowledge will be found useful and applicable. Chinese investigations into their medical heritage are 'redolent with the balmy air of spring, budding with life and energy', according to the head of the Shanghai Chinese Traditional Medical Institute, who

also reminds us that there are double the number of Chinese traditional doctors in Shanghai today than at the time of liberation. The
evidence shows, however, that when the ancient cultural base is destroyed and traditional medicine is squeezed into a modern health
care role, it may be weakened in the process.[23]

India

Traditional medicine in the Indian subcontinent consists largely of
Ayurveda, an ancient healing system derived from the Vedas. Like
Chinese medicine, it represents a complete guide for health, well-
being and spiritual energy which dates back several thousand years.
Siddha medicine is an offshoot of Ayurveda and practised almost
exclusively in Tamil Nadu and Sri Lanka. Unani-tibbi is a mixture of
Ayurvedic medicine and Arabic or Persian medicine, largely in use in
north-west India and Pakistan.

Statistics relating to the practice of traditional medicine in India
are amazing. In a country of 640 million population there are no less
than 400 000 Ayurvedic practitioners, 242 Ayurvedic hospitals,
some 11 000 dispensaries, and more than 100 officially accredited
colleges, many of which are attached to universities, to train practitioners. Unani medicine in India is also strong, with 19 hospitals and
903 dispensaries, while Siddha medicine, although local, boasts 65
hospitals and 392 dispensaries.[24]

Until 10 years ago, Ayurvedic medicine was the centre of considerable and often violent controversy. Traditionalist factions saw
Ayurveda as part of the rootstock of Indian culture and had been
lobbying strongly to preserve and expand it. The rural poor and
Indian intellectuals had supported this approach, as had local politi-
cians whose promises of universal health care could only be realis-
tically fulfilled by expanding the traditional Ayurvedic corps. Ranged
against them were the Health Ministry and the medical profession,
who were adamant that modern medicine would eventually provide
exclusive health coverage in India. However, it was transparently
clear that modern medicine was, if anything, getting worse rather
than better. By 1973, the Primary Health Centres, government rural
clinics, provided for two doctors per 100 000 population, 90 per cent
of whom did not find reason to use the centres. While 80 per cent of
the population live in the countryside, 80 per cent of the doctors
work in the towns.[25] Ayurveda was itself in a rather poor state,
for without controls on standards or education, incompetent

practitioners had free reign. Students who were rejected by medical school became partly qualified Ayurvedic practitioners as a soft option. The traditional apprenticeship system gave plenty of opportunity for quackery.

Necessity forced the Indian Parliament to pass legislation recognizing and controlling Ayurveda for it continued to be the only medicine serving a large proportion of India's population. The 1970 Indian Medicine Central Council Act set up a Central Council for Ayurveda which was charged to establish a register of current established and qualified practitioners, and to ensure proper training. Under this Act, new colleges were established and old ones accredited. The qualification was called Bachelor of Ayurvedic Medicine and Surgery; it was a three-and-a-half-year course, and included a basic study of Western medicine. A further three years postgraduate study was required for full qualification. Separate bodies were set up to govern research and development of Ayurveda, and new legislation was introduced to control the manufacture of Ayurvedic and Unani medicines. Each state had a Directorate of Indian Systems of Medicine, in parallel with the Directorate of Medicine and Health Services, which operated the accredition.

The Act has not yet solved the problem of incompetent practitioners, as there are no real measures in the law to prevent the unregistered from practising. Furthermore, 'quickie' colleges offering basic instruction in Indian and Western medicine have sprung up, providing a back door into the medical schools. A survey of practitioners has found that only 12 per cent of practitioners had obtained the degree diploma of a recognized teaching institution, 54 per cent had obtained diplomas at unrecognized institutions, and the remaining 33 per cent had no formal qualifications.[26] Seventy-five per cent of practitioners are now registered. However, although there is much room for improvement, considerable progress has been made in upgrading standards in the 12 years since the setting up of the register.

Following the example of the Chinese, the Government introduced an alternative rural health scheme which attempted to use traditional practitioners to distribute medical services. However, only about one-sixth of these practitioners were willing to join the scheme, as it involved some additional training in modern medicine, family planning, and public health. Those that wished to join the scheme were mostly the unregistered practitioners. Although the rural health scheme was not a great success, it turned out,[27] that a large number of traditional practitioners were using modern medicines anyway, largely at the insistence of their patients. Ninety per cent of practitioners prescribed modern scientific medicines, and over half used these medicines most of the time. However, less than one-third of these practitioners had received training in their use. This data has shown that rural communities like modern medicine but not the doctors that administer them. Traditional practitioners have 'shown a considerable degree of adaptability to fill this vacuum though at no cost to the Government but considerable cost to the consumer'.[26] Those Ayurvedic practitioners who were using modern medicine said that if they did not so they would face extinction.

India has the largest homeopathic establishment in the world. A separate Central Council for Homeopathy was established alongside that for Ayurveda. It has now registered some 200 000 homeopathic practitioners. There are 104 colleges running undergraduate courses for school leavers, with four years to a diploma and five and a half years to a degree. Postgraduate degrees are awarded by a new National Institute of Homeopathy in Calcutta, which is developing and evaluating homeopathic teaching. It carries out an extensive research programme in which clinical research as well as drug 'provings' in the Hahnemannian fashion are carried out. There are 130–150 homeopathic hospitals and some 1500 homeopathic dispensaries, all supported by the Government. Each state has its homeopathic board. There is also a Central Council for Research in Homeopathy which undertakes standardization, prepares a homeopathic pharmacopoeia, and co-ordinates drug 'provings' (that is, homeopathic checking of remedies) and clinical trials.

Homeopathy in India is respected and taken seriously, although it must be said that it is also considered a soft option for those that cannot be medical students. It is interesting that even doctors must start more or less from scratch and study for several years if they wish to become homeopaths. The practitioners practise pure Hahnemannian homeopathy with some admixture of naturopathic instruction. The extent of homeopathy in India ensures that it is taken more seriously world-wide, although Indian homeopaths are chagrined that they are not recognized by the Faculty of Homeopathy in the UK.

Like China, India is a country with a powerful pre-existing medical tradition which has been largely preserved, admittedly more by default than by intention. At the same time there is a natural evolution towards incorporation of some of modern medicine into traditional practice, influenced by popular demand. Although the situation is somewhat chaotic and incompetence is still rife, Indian medicine represents accommodation between traditional and modern medicine, compared to their official marriage in China. Perhaps the ideal solution would be a combination of Indian and Chinese strategies. Indigenous practitioners could be encouraged to train in the lengthy and rigorous traditional manner, supported if necessary by Government funding comparable to that offered to medical students. At the same time, community health workers in each village could provide public health, family planning, and simple health care, activities that would waste the talents of highly skilled traditional and modern practitioners. The community health workers would be drawn from the villages and could provide mixed, integrated primary care using traditional and modern techniques pragmatically, in the style of the barefoot doctor. Conventional doctors would have their role to play. However, if the sophisticated but fragile traditional medical wisdom is to be preserved it is essential that medical schools teach the limitations of conventional medicine as well as its potentials, and ensure the respect for time-tested therapeutic systems that is their due.

References

1. *Alternative medicine in The Netherlands* (1981). Report of the Commission for Alternative Systems of Medicine, Ministerie Van Volks Gezondheid en Milieuhygiene. Available from Staatsuirgeverij, C. Plantijnstraat 2, Is Gravenhage, The Netherlands.
2. Commission of European Communities (1979). Written question No. 100/79.
3. Council of Europe (1984). *Legislation and administrative regulations on the use by licensed health service personnel of non-conventional methods of diagnosis and treatment*. Strasbourg.
4. Holden, C. (1981). 'Health care in the Soviet Union'. *Science,* **213**, 1090.
5. Feshbach, M. and Davis, C. (1980). *Rising infant mortality in the USSR in the 1970s.* US Bureau of Census, Washington.
6. Fulder, S. (1980). 'The hammer and the pestle'. *New Scientist,* **87**, 120-3.
7. Fulder, S. (1987). *The Tao of medicine: Ginseng, oriental remedies and*

the pharmacology of harmony. Destiny Books, Rochester, Vermont.

8. Goidenko, V. (1979). Soviet Health Ministry champions acupuncture. *Acupuncture and Electrotherapeutic Research,* **4**, 61–2.

9. Brelet, C. (1979). *Traditional medicine in Eastern Europe*. Report submitted to Traditional Medicine Section, World Health Organization, Geneva.

10. Editorial (1980). *New Zealand Medical Journal,* **91**, 345.

11. Hocken, A.G. (1980). Chiropractic in from the Cold? *British Medical Journal,* **280**, 97–98.

12. Committee of Inquiry (1977). *Chiropractic, osteopathy, homeopathy and naturopathy*. Parliamentary Paper No. 102, Government Printer, Canberra.

13. Parliament of Victoria, Social Development Committee (1986). *Inquiry into alternative medicine and the health food industry*. The Government Printer, Melbourne.

14. Commission of Inquiry (1970). *Chiropractic in New Zealand*. Government Printer, Wellington.

15. World Health Organization (1978). *The promotion of traditional medicine*. Technical Report Series No. 622, Geneva.

16. Scarpa, A. (1981). Pre-scientific medicines: Their extent and value. *Social Science and Medicine,* **15A**, 317–26. Harrison, Ira E. and Cosminsky, Sheila (1976). *Traditional medicine: Implications for ethno-medicine, ethnopharmacology, maternal and child health, mental health, and public health; An annotated bibliography of Africa, Latin America, and the Caribbean*. Garland, New York.

17. Furst, B.G. *Traditional medicine and indigenous practitioners*. American Public Health Association, International Health Programs, Washington DC. Ampofa, O. (1977). Plants that heal. *World Health*, 26–30, November issue.

18. World Health Organization (1978). *Primary health care*. A Joint Report by WHO and UNICEF, International Conference on Primary Health Care, Alma Ata, USSR.

19. World Health Organization Document, SEA/OMC/Traditional Medicine Meeting. *Inter-regional consultation on traditional medicine programme*, New Delhi (October 1976). World Health Organization Document EB/57/21. *Training and utilisation of traditional healers and their collaboration with health care delivery systems* (November 1975).

20. Velimirovic, B. and Velimirovic H. (1977). The Utilisation of Traditional Medicine and its Practitioners in Health Services: a Global Overview. *Modern Medicine and Medical Anthropology*. Pan-American Health Organization, Washington.

21. Crozier, R. (1968). *Traditional medicine in modern China*. Harvard University Press, Cambridge, Mass. Hillier, S. and Jewell, T. (1987).

Traditional medicine in China, pragmatism and holism. *Holistic Medicine, 2*, 15–26. Fulder, S. (1987). *The Tao of Medicine: Ginseng, oriental remedies and the pharmacology of harmony.* Destiny Books, Rochester, Vermont.

22. Rosenthal, M.M. (1981). Political process and the integration of traditional and western medicine in the People's Republic of China. *Social Science and Medicine,* **15A**, 599–613.

23. Bibeau, G. (1985). From China to Africa: The same impossible synthesis between traditional and western medicine. *Social Science and Medicine,* **21**, 937–43.

24. Bannerman, R.H., Burton, J., and Wen-Chieh, C. (1983). *Traditional medicine and health care coverage.* World Health Organization, Geneva.

25. Ministry of Health and Family Planning (1973). Government of India, DGHS, CBHI. *Pocket book of health statistics.*

26. Bhatia J.C., Vir, D., Timmappaya, A., and Chuttani, C.S. (1975). Traditional healers and modern medicine. *Social Science and Medicine,* **9**, 15–21.

27. Doyal, L. (1987). Health, underdevelopment and traditional medicine. *Holistic medicine, 2*, 27–40.

PART 2

The therapies

6

Acupuncture and oriental medicine

Background

Traditional Chinese medicine is a system of medicine which uses not only acupuncure but herbs, diet, and exercise for the prevention and treatment of disease. The theory of acupuncture is drawn from an ancient Chinese text—*The Yellow Emperor's classic of internal medicine (The Nei Ching)*—probably compiled during the warring states period (770–476 BC), although the mythical Yellow Emperor referred to in the text belongs to a much earlier period (2000 BC). The theories of medicine expounded in the *Nei Ching* remain to this day the most authoritative guide to traditional Chinese medicine.[1]

There is also archaeological evidence which shows that acupuncture dates back to the Stone Age: instruments called *bian* found in China were thought to have been used as very primitive needles. By the Bronze Age acupuncture was already comparatively developed, and needles were made of bronze. Today the needles are made of high quality stainless steel.

Throughout its history acupuncture has experienced periods of popularity and neglect. However, in China today hospitals offer treatment by Western and traditional methods, according to the doctor's judgement of which is more suitable for the individual patient (see Chapter 5, p. 109). Sometimes the systems complement each other, for example the use of acupuncture for anaesthesia or for the relief of pain. However, traditional Chinese medicine stands on its own as a complete system of healing, and its complex theories of diagnosis and treatment are currently beyond explanation by modern scientific analysis.

Fundamental concepts

The Chinese medical system embraces a philosophy very different from that of the West.[2] This philosophy springs from a sensitive awareness of the laws of nature and more particularly of the order of the universe. Life is activated by what the Chinese call *chi*, or vital life force, roughly translated as energy. *Chi* pervades all things: in man this energy is derived partly from heredity and partly from the air we breathe and the food we eat. As long as *chi* flows freely through the body, health is maintained.

The emphasis of traditional Chinese medicine is on the prevention of disease. Every morning in China today, one can observe hundreds of ordinary people practising T'ai-chi: exercises designed to encourage the free flow of *chi*. The practitioner of traditional Chinese medicine aims in the first instance to detect subtle changes in the flow of energy before these changes become gross and give rise to disease.

The principal premise of the *Nei Ching* is that health is achieved through a balance between opposing forces, represented by *yin* and *yang*. *Yin*, originally signifying the northern side of the mountain, implies coldness, darkness, passivity, interiority, and the negative. *Yang* the southern side, implies warmth, light, activity, expressivity, and the positive. When either *yin* or *yang* quality predominates, disorders of health result. Thus an organ that is too *yin* is too sluggish, and static, and accumulates waste.

Besides *yin* and *yang*, Chinese medicine employs other polarities by which all diseases and disharmonies can be described. These are known as the eight principles, including empty–full, hot–cold, excess–deficient. They are used to group symptoms. For example, red face, dark urine, fever, and pain increased by warmth, are hot symptoms; while slower movements, slow pulse, pale tongue, thin clear urine, and pain lessened by warmth are symptoms of a cold condition. Such a classification of diseases in itself suggests suitable methods of treatment: for example, if a patient is diagnosed as too hot, treatment will aim to disperse this heat; if too weak, it will aim to build up strength.

Alongside this system of opposing principles stands another tradition known as the theory of the five elements (or five transformations), which like the Greek system distinguishes qualities such as solidity, heat, fluidity, etc., metaphorically described as earth, fire, water, wood, and metal. The relationship between these five elements is subject to certain laws that govern the flow between them; these cyclical laws can be applied to the working of the body, enabling the practitioner to treat disorders.[3]

Another important tenet of traditional Chinese medicine is that it regards man as a 'whole being', i.e. as an indivisible combination of mind/body/spirit, where it is impossible to treat one aspect without affecting the others. The patient is also seen as an inextricable part of the environment. Disease is interpreted either as originating within man himself (internal) or as being derived from environmental factors (external).

The internal causes of disease may be constitutional ('the hereditary energy') or the somatic consequence of unwise actions such as overindulgence, or of an emotional nature. Normally a person's natural emotions dictate an appropriate response to a given situation. However, when such responses become too intense or prolonged, disease may develop; this would be discernible at first as a distortion of the energy balance and eventually as a distortion of the organs themselves. Conversely, if an organ becomes diseased, there will be a corresponding imbalance in the emotion associated with that organ. It is entirely consonant with the holistic view of the patient that emotional problems can be traced to a physical origin and physical symptoms explained as emotionally induced. For example, excessive anger allows the energy to rise up and may cause stiff shoulders, headache, tinnitus, sinusitis, etc., and diseases of the lung may cause periods of deep melancholy, crying, rigid ideas, etc. According to the ancient classics: 'Joy and shock injure the heart, anger injures the liver, worry and overconcentration injure the spleen, grief injures the lungs, fears injure the kidneys'.

The external causes of disease are largely associated with climatic conditions. A healthy constitution should be able to withstand changes in the weather, but in extreme cases or where the person does not take adequate precautions (e.g. by wrapping up in cold winds), certain conditions can enter the body and cause disease, an obvious example being epidemics of colds and 'flu in winter.

Climatic conditions are not the only external causes of disease; poisoning and traumatic experiences are other examples. These categories are not simple or discrete, and in reality disease may be caused by any combination of factors. This considerably complicates the process of diagnosis. In understanding disease the emphasis is not on a germ invading the body but rather on the individual's ability to cope with internal and external factors.[4] Thus, the quality of the patient's *chi* is vital for the prognosis.

The role of traditional Chinese medicine is two-fold: to prevent disease and recognize pre-disease conditions, and to treat disease according to a patient's needs as well as his symptoms. This may involve advising on diet or lifestyle and promoting general health education. Eventually the emphasis shifts from treating a disorder to supporting good health.

Diagnostic and therapeutic practices

The main application of these elaborate theories lies in the techniques of acupuncture. To treat a disorder the practitioner can manipulate the patient's *chi* at certain points along the body in order to balance the subtle energies. Over the surface of the body runs a network of pathways known as meridians; these connect with the inner organs and constitute channels through which energy can pass. For example, the meridian of the colon runs from a nail point on the index finger along the arm and over the shoulder and neck to the nose; from there it follows a deep pathway down to the colon itself (Fig. 6.1). Because the meridian system connects the exterior of the body by pathways to the viscera, external factors can penetrate and produce symptoms such as abdominal pain, migraine, etc. Conversely, diseases of the internal organs will produce superficial symptoms which may appear along the lines of the meridians. Thus, kidney disease can induce back pain, while disease of the gall bladder can bring pain to the shoulder, these being areas through which the respective meridians run.

There are 12 basic meridians which are named after the organs or functions to which they are attached. Six are predominantly *yin*: heart, heart protector, spleen, lungs, kidney, and liver; and 6 are predominantly *yang*: small intestine, triple heater, stomach, colon, bladder, and gall bladder. The *yin* organs are those of storage, while the *yang* organs are regarded as 'hollow' and are organs of activity. Two extra meridians are the Conception Vessel which runs up the centre-front of the body, and the Governor Vessel which runs up the spine and over the head. Emphasis is placed on the relationships between organs; for example, the spleen is included in the digestive function, and the kidneys are regarded as involved in the production of marrow. Traditional Chinese physiology also recognizes two functions which are not included in Western models; the heart protector protects the heart from external pathogenic factors, and the triple heater has connections with all the organs and regulates the body's temperature.

In order to ascertain the nature of a patient's disorder, the

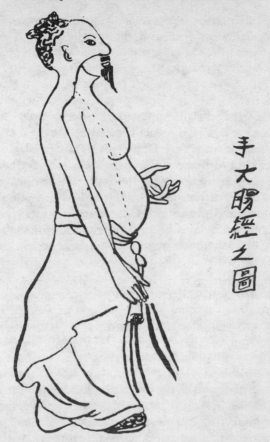

手
大
陽
經
之
圖

Fig. 6.1: Illustration from the ancient classic showing the meridian
pathway of the great intestine (colon).

acupuncturist will employ traditional methods of diagnosis. These
include the observation of significant features of the patient: the
appearance and colour of the face, the sound quality of the voice, the
distinctive odour of the body, the quality and texture of the skin, and
the emotional disposition. The practitioner will also take a full
history from the patient, measure his blood pressure, palpate the
abdomen and take a reading of the pulses. Finally, there is a whole
system of diagnosis based on observation of the colour, shape, coa-
ting, moisture, etc., of the tongue. These techniques of diagnosis all

require an acute perception on the part of the practitioner which is acquired through years of careful training and practical experience.

The technique of reading the pulses has a special importance and calls for further explanation. Chinese medicine recognizes 12 different pulses (as opposed to the single pulse in Western medicine). The 12 pulses correspond to the inner organs and are palpable on the wrists of the left and right hands, 6 being deep and 6 superficial. From reading the pulses the experienced practitioner is able to diagnose illnesses the patient has previously suffered, illness now present, and future illnesses. Refinement of the technique takes many years, and by mastering it the acupuncturist obtains insight into the degree of seriousness of a disorder. For example, a tight pulse can indicate heat, a hasty pulse extreme heat, while a weak pulse reflects an empty condition. In all there are 28 qualities which can be recognized from the pulses. As the *Nei Ching* states

The pulse is the store house of the blood. When the pulse beats are long and the strokes markedly prolonged, then the constitution of the pulse is well regulated.

When the pulse is small and fine, slow and short, like scraping bamboo with a knife, then it indicates that the heart is irritated and painful.

It should be remembered that there is no easy formula in traditional Chinese diagnosis: no patient will fall exactly into a textbook category, and no single diagnostic tool will be absolutely conclusive. An understanding of the subtle permutations of normal physiology and pathology is thus essential for correct treatment. While using the traditional methods of diagnosis (listening, smelling, looking, asking, and touching) the acupuncturist is attempting to analyse the disorder according to the laws of the five elements and eight principles (i.e. interior-exterior, hot-cold, deficiency-excess, *yin-yang*). Thus he is looking for certain signs that indicate that an organ is out of balance.

For example, in terms of the five-element model a disorder in the liver may manifest itself by wood-type characteristics: greenish colour in the face, shouting voice, angry disposition, rancid smell with perhaps symptoms of migraine, anorexia, and insomnia. The pulse may be full, indicating that the energy needs dispersion. In terms of the less diffuse eight principles model, the acupuncturist has to ask if the disorder is *yin*-type or *yang*-type, cold or hot, etc. The patient might then be classified as a liver-*yang*-full, of the wood-type. A symptom such as a headache can arise from any kind of imbalance. It should disappear as a matter of course when treatment is applied according to the patient's general needs and his system is restored to balance.

Once a patient's problems have been diagnosed, treatment normally proceeds by one of two methods; these are respectively the dispersion and the 'tonification' (meaning both stimulation and gathering) of energy in the meridians. Certain conditions require the use of moxa (see p. 126) as well as needle techniques. There are numerous points along each meridian where needles or moxa can be applied. The points are chosen according to their action and relevance to the patient's condition. For example, 'wind gate' on the gall-bladder meridian can be used to dispel the external factor in disease, wind points may also be used for their cooling action, for their action on the *chi*, on the blood, or on the element in need of help.

The *Nei Ching* explains in detail the techniques of inserting, withdrawing and manipulating the needles. To tonify the energy the needle must be inserted at a 45° angle to the required depth, aligned with the flow of the meridian and rotated in a clockwise direction; when the needle is removed the 'hole' is closed by rubbing the skin firmly. Different techniques of tonification are described poetically in the classics, but usually tonification is a quick manipulation to stimulate the energy and takes less than 30 seconds. To disperse the energy the needle is inserted rapidly against the flow of the meridian at 45° and rotated in an anti-clockwise direction; it is left in place until the energy is dispersed. This can take between 10 and 60 minutes and is gauged by reading the pulses and by the flesh 'letting go' of the needle. The needle is withdrawn slowly and the 'hole' left open. The needles enter pathways of energy and naturally no blood is lost during the procedure.

Acupuncture needles are made of stainless steel of varying length, the most commonly used being approximately 12 cm, 25 cm, or 37 cm. The handles are of twisted stainless steel. Each point has its specific depth measurement, which varies with the size of the patient; however, the needle will usually only penetrate a few millimetres beneath the skin. For treating children a special '7 star' needle may be used which pricks the skin superficially by tapping and thus manipulates the energy. Where a patient has a history of hepatitis his needles are isolated and discarded when his course of treatment is completed. Otherwise needles are sterilized between patients and discarded when they become 'tired', i.e. bent or barbed.

The technique of moxibustion involves burning a herb, moxa. The traditional moxa is made from the dry leaf of mugwort (*Artemisia vulgaris*). A small cone of this is placed on the acupuncture point and lit at its apex; this burns down until the patient is able to feel the heat and is removed before it burns the skin. Moxibustion tones and supplements the energy and is useful in the treatment of chronic ailments and pains from cold.

Applications and contra-indications

Acupuncture aims to re-balance vital energy and restore normal functioning to the body–mind. Since energy is partly derived from food, simple dietary changes may be enough to restore balance and eliminate disorders. Acupuncturists will always encourage good diet as this improves the quality and quantity of energy, and thereby aids in the treatment of the disease.

Because traditional Chinese medicine treats the individual as a whole person, including both susceptibilities and symptoms, acupuncture can help most ailments. However, there is no such thing as an instant cure: disease has to work its way out of the body, and a longstanding illness may take considerably longer to do so than one recently contracted. It is unrealistic to expect immediate alleviation of symptoms, whereas it is realistic to expect to feel changes within oneself such as a feeling of general well-being and ability to cope with or shake off the symptoms. The patient's attitude is itself important: even the confirmed sceptic will experience changes, but clearly a positive attitude to health will allow treatment to work more effectively. Acupuncture is generally harmless. In the rare cases where a complication has occurred,[5] this can usually be traced back to a badly trained practitioner.

There are certain situations in which treatment should only be administered by the experienced practitioner, for example in pregnancy, where points which may affect the fetus must not be needled. Cranial points are similarly forbidden in the treatment of infants, although they may be massaged safely and to good effect. Needles should also never be inserted into tumours or glands. If a practitioner suspects certain gross underlying diseases such as cancer, the patient is always referred to his GP for a thorough investigation. In general, patients with advanced or terminal cancer are not suitable for treatment by traditional acupuncture, since their disease is no longer reversible and their energy levels are too depleted. Acupuncture can, however, be of immense value in the relief of pain and in preventing the establishment and spread of certain diseases.

An acupuncturist should always take proper consideration of any other forms of treatment the patient may be undergoing, whether of a conventional nature or otherwise. For example, drugs may mask symptoms and complicate diagnosis, but awareness of their use may guide the practitioner towards the proper course of treatment. Standard practice dictates that treatment should not be given to patients who are intoxicated or in an extreme state of emotional excitement. Although it is not expressly forbidden, it is wise to avoid treatment immediately after a meal. Finally, it is generally considered that a practitioner who is not in good health should not treat patients, a principle which accords with common sense as well as with the well-known proverb: 'physician, heal thyself'.

Theoretically, it should be possible to treat any disease with a reversible physiological process, to treat many psychiatric problems, and to alleviate symptoms in certain other cases such as chronic arthritis. In 1979 the World Health Organization listed 40 major diseases that could find relief by acupuncture treatment. These ranged from diseases of the respiratory tract (common cold, asthma) and of the gastro-intestinal tract (duodenal ulcer, colitis) to addiction,[6] nervous disorders (neuralgia, Bell's palsy, enuresis, sciatica, osteoarthritis, tinnitus),[7] migraine, and period pains. Because traditional Chinese medicine considers the body–mind to be a complete unit, it is able to link physical and mental disorders and to achieve a degree of success with problems such as depression, angina,[8] anorexia, and even toothache, which elude Western medicine. All psycho-physiological problems are particularly suitable for acupuncture treatment.[9]

Research

Acupuncture and related forms of treatment cannot easily be assessed in Western terms. Therapeutic acupuncture utilizes processes which have so far defied measurement by scientific instruments: meridians and the flow of energy along them are examples of this. However, acupuncture has caught the imagination of many

Western scientists[10] and there are now both theories and experimental evidence to explain some aspects of acupuncture, particularly its effect in pain relief.

The 'gate theory of pain', put forward by Melzack and Wall in 1965 states that stimulation of larger nerve fibres (A fibres) can block off pain impulses from the smaller C fibres when the impulses are 'integrated' in the spinal cord and brain.[11] This theory does seem to fit experiments in which electrical impulses can block pain, however it does not explain chronic pain relief nor, of course, therapeutic effects. It is superseded by the finding that after acupuncture treatment, endorphins are released in the brain providing long-term natural pain relief. Other brain messengers, such as serotonin, are also known to be involved which could have a profound effect on well-being. In other words, some of the effects of Chinese medicine could be the result of adjustments to the hormone messengers of the mind and body, which then in turn manipulate or 'balance' organ function.[12]

There has also been some progress in investigating the nature of the meridians and acupuncture points, although we do not know how messages actually get from the needle point to the neuro-modulator-producing tissues of the brain, or what, in fact, meridians are. However, acupuncture points are known to be points of low electrical skin resistance and there are a number of devices available which locate them exactly on that basis.[13] They can be located in animals and even in recently dead bodies. They have been clearly photographed by Kirlian electrophotography[14] and shown to change after acupuncture treatment and during disease. For example, an investigation at the Californian College of Acupuncture has shown that if heart rate is increased or decreased there is a precisely matching change in electrical conductivity at heart acupuncture points, but not at other acupuncture points, nor at random points on the skin.[15] Patients with tuberculosis have low electrical resistance on the lung meridian on the upper arm compared to healthy people.[16] There are also suggestions of a transfer of light in the ultraviolet wavelength between tissues, which might account for meridians.[17] They are certainly not anatomically identifiable[18]—only electromagnetic conduction of some kind could account for the speed of the message transmission along the meridians.

Clinical evaluations of acupuncture are beset with difficulties.[19] Observations without a placebo do not demonstrate anything specific about the treatment. However, if a weak placebo, such as a vague 'pretend acupuncture' is used, a study might only show that real acupuncture, possibly, is a stronger placebo. It is virtually impossible to carry out a true double-blind study as the acupuncturist must know all the time what he is doing. However, there are many studies assessing the value of acupuncture in pain relief, which are well reviewed in a recent paper.[20] In China, the success of acupuncture anaesthesia and analgesia has been clearly demonstrated in exhaustive studies.[21] Acupuncture has a 60–80 per cent success rate in acute and chronic painful conditions, more than placebos of any kind. However, it has not been possible, so far, to prove that acupuncture is better or worse than various kinds of electrical or electro-acupuncture treatments.

There is nevertheless extensive research literature on therapeutic acupuncture.[22] Successes with conditions such as a bronchial asthma,[23] headache,[24] musculoskeletal problems,[25] addictions,[6] kidney stones,[26] migraines, and a variety of other conditions[9] have been reported frequently in China and the Far East, and occasionally in the West. Although impressive, few of these therapeutic studies have been performed under strictly controlled double-blind conditions.

New types of therapy

The influence of the West on Chinese medicine over recent years has led to the modernization of certain techniques and to the introduction of new ideas. Such ideas range from monitoring the pulses and electrical resistance over acupuncture points to a complete system of treatment by needling the ear only. Organs and parts of the body are said to be represented on the ear and by puncturing specific areas on the external ear, disease can be treated in the body. Other forms of ear acupuncture are used in the treatment of pain, obesity, and addictions. In these cases a small staple is inserted into the ear and stimulated by the patient when he/she desires to eat or smoke. Ear acupuncture is not particularly Oriental. It was developed in France by Dr Nogier with new points added pragmatically to the traditional ones. It is symptomatic and relatively easy to learn, thus finding favour with medical doctors in pain and addiction centres in the West.

Electro-acupuncture is a rapidly developing field, as

technologically-minded doctors rise to the occasion. The surface of the body is seen as an electromagnetic map of the interior, with the meridians as the major, though by no means the only, features. The best known system is electro-acupuncture (EAV) developed by Dr Voll. The acupuncture needle is replaced with a stylus carrying a controlled electrical charge at the microvolt level at its tip. The machine is used both to diagnose and treat disease at acupuncture points.[13] Another kind of apparatus is a laser needle, a machine delivering a thin infrared laser beam to the acupuncture points. Laser acupuncture is also becoming more popular in pain clinics. Another new system (MORA) measures the frequencies of the patient's own bio-electricity, then it purifies and amplifies the electromagnetic wave before returning it to the patient via acupuncture points.

Some of the equipment used to deliver electric pulses to the body surface was developed with acupuncture in mind but does not involve acupuncture points at all. Transcutaneous nerve stimulation (TENS) stimulates nerve fibres which block pain messsages. It is used in various kinds of chronic pain, including post-operative, low back, arthritic, or phantom limb pain. It has the advantage that the patient can take it home and use it frequently there, although it is acknowledged to be less effective than acupuncture. The pads deliver a pulse to acupuncture points, points that are tender, or simply areas close to the pain site. Like the other electronic systems, TENS has not been adequately evaluated as yet, and its application involves a certain amount of trial and error.

Other adopted forms of therapy developed over recent years include scalp acupuncture, for treatment in brain damage diseases, and the injection of drugs into acupuncture points for the alleviation of paint in such diseases as arthritis. These new techniques have developed under the influence of Western ideas and technology and contain an allopathic approach to medicine. The acupuncture points are regarded as 'buttons' which help certain symptoms when manipulated. There is little connection to the basic principles of traditional complementary medicine, which usually seek to find and treat the causes of disease.

Obtaining treatment

Acupuncture is now widely available in the UK, but the quality of treatment is variable. When seeking treatment a person should be sure that the practitioner is properly qualified. Besides acupuncturists treating patients according to traditional therapeutic principles, it is possible to receive symptomatic acupuncture, particularly for the relief of pain. Some NHS pain clinics in the UK make use of acupuncture.

During the first visit to a traditional acupuncturist the patient will be given a traditional diagnosis; this may take between an hour and an hour and a half. The course of treatment will vary from person to person and it is generally said that a month of treatment is needed for every year of illness. As a rule the acupuncturist can assess if the patient can be helped by acupuncture after the diagnosis and first few treatments. Once the energy begins to be balanced the patient will experience changes in himself and his symptoms.

To stimulate the energy successfully, the acupuncturist must obtain *dequi* (or needle sensation) which is experienced both by the patient and the practitioner. *Dequi* can be different for each person and the sensation varies from a temporary painful feeling, burning, or prickling sensation to numbness. This sensation can be felt in different parts of the body as the energy travels along the meridian. The effects of a single treatment may be observed immediately or several days later.

Any age group can receive acupuncture, although young children, in whom energy levels fluctuate rapidly, should be treated only by an experienced practitioner. Acupuncture is primarily a preventive medicine. The subtle system of diagnosis allows for the correction of minor disturbances in patients who have no obvious illness but feel a little below average; if treated at this stage, the later development of obvious disease can be prevented. Because of seasonal variations in the activity of different organs different imbalances are more evident and more readily treated in particular seasons. Thus, a change of season is usually the best time at which to make an evaluation of an individual's condition with a view to deciding whether treatment is required.

In ancient China the physician gave his patient seasonal examinations to maintain his health, and was only paid while his patients were well! The wise physician would only accept as patients those who paid heed to the Laws of Nature. Such laws are still applicable today; they include sensible eating habits, exercise, and rest, the avoidance of toxins and self-abuse, and learning to live in harmony with the environment.[27] Such natural laws are basic to traditional Chinese medicine.

References

1. Needham, J. and Gwei-Djen, I. (1980). *Celestial Lancets: A history and rationale of acupuncture and moxa.* Cambridge University Press. Gwei-Djen, L. and Needham, J. (1980). Pains and Needles. *New Scientist,* **87,** 860–5.

2. Pálos, Stephan (1982). *The Chinese art of healing.* Bantam Books, New York. Kaptchuk, T. (1984). *The web that has no weaver.* Hutchinson, London.

3. Pokert, Manfred (1974). *The theoretical foundation of Chinese medicine: Systems of correspondence.* MIT Press, Cambridge, Mass.

4. Plummer, J.P. (1981). Acupuncture and homeostasis: Physiological, physical (postural) and psychological. *American Journal of Chinese Medicine,* **9,** 1–14.

5. Carron, H., Epstein, B.S., and Grand, B. (1978). Complications of acupuncture. *Journal of the American Medical Association,* **228,** 1552–4.

6. Smith, M.O. (1979). Acupuncture and natural healing in drug detoxification. *American Journal of Acupuncture,* **2,** 97. Clement-Jones, V., McLoughlin, L., Lowry, P., Besser, G.M., Rees, L., Wen, H.L. (1979). Acupuncture in heroin addicts: Changes in met-enkephalin and β-endorphin in blood and cerebrospinal fluid. *Lancet,* **ii,** 380–2.

7. Chen, C.H. (1979). The neurophysiological mechanism of acupuncture treatment in psychiatric illness: An autonomic-humoral theory. *American Journal of Chinese Medicine,* **1,** 183–7. Liu, X. (1981). Psychiatry in traditional Chinese medicine. *British Journal of Psychiatry,* **138,** 429–33.

8. Chen, G.S. (1977). Treatment of angina pectoris with acupuncture. *American Journal of Acupuncture,* **5,** 341–6.

9. Mann, F. (1974). *The treatment of disease by acupuncture. Part 1: Function of acupuncture points. Part 2: Treatment of disease.* (3rd edn), Heinemann Medical Books, London.

10. Wei, L.Y. (1979). Scientific advance in acupuncture. *American Journal of Chinese Medicine,* **7,** 53–75; a very good summary of current world acupuncture research, containing hundreds of reports, is: People's Medical Publishing House (1979) *National Symposium of Acupuncture, Moxibustion and Acupuncture Anesthaesia,* World Books, Peking.

11. Melzack, R. and Wall, P. (1965). Pain mechanisms: A new theory. *Science,* **150,** 69–83.

12. Malizia E., Andreucci, G., Paolucci, D., Crescenzi, F., Fabbri, A., and Fraioli, F. (1979). Electroacupuncture and peripheral β-endorphin and ACTH levels. *Lancet,* **ii,** 535–6. Liao, Y., Seto, K., Saito, H., Fujita, M., and Kawakami, M. (1980). Effects of acupuncture on andreno-cortical hormone production. *American Journal of Chinese Medicine,* **8,** 160–6. Editorial (1981). How does acupuncture work? *British Medical Journal,* **283,** 746–8. Fulder, S.J. (1981). Ginseng and the hypothalamic-pituitary control of stress. *American Journal of Chinese Medicine,* **9,** 112–8.

13. Bergsman, O. and Woolley-Hart, A. (1973). Differences in electrical skin conductivity between acupuncture points and adjacent skin areas. *American Journal of Acupuncture,* **1,** 27–32. Voll, R. (1975). Twenty years of acupuncture diagnosis. *American Journal of Acupuncture,* **3,** 7–17.

14. Moss, L. and Wei, L.Y. (1975). Brain response and Kirlian photography of the cat under acupuncture. *American Journal of Acupuncture,* **3,** 215–223.

15. Rosenblatt, S. (1980). The electrodermal characteristics of acupuncture points. *American Journal of Acupuncture,* **10,** 131–7.

16. Seisawa, K. (1978). An approach on meridians and acupuncture points in modern medicine. *Journal of Comprehensive Rehabilitation,* **11,** 789.

17. Hill, S. and Playfair, G. (1979). *The cycles of heaven.* Pan, London.

18. Monteiro-Riviere, N.A., Hwang, Y.C., and Stromberg, M.W. (1981). Light microscopic morphology of low resistance skin points in the Guinea pig. *American Journal of Chinese Medicine,* **9,** 155–63.

19. Vincent, C.A. and Richardson, P.H. (1986). The evaluation of therapeutic acupuncture: Concepts and methods. *Pain,* **24,** 1–13.

20. Jenerick, H.P. (ed.) (1973). *Proceedings of the National Institute of Health Acupuncture Research Conference.* Bethesda, Maryland. Department of Health, Education and Welfare (NIH), Publication No. 74–165. Richardson, P.H. and Vincent, C.A. (1986). Acupuncture for the treatment of pain: A review of evaluative research. *Pain,* **24,** 15–40.

21. Peking Children's Hospital (1975). A clinical analysis of 1474 operations under acupuncture anaesthesia among children. *Chinese Medical Journal,* **1,** 369–74.

22. Turban, E. and Urlich, S. (1978). The evaluation of therapeutic acupuncture. *Social Science and Medicine,* **12,** 39–44.

23. Aldridge, D. and Pietroni, P.C. (1987). Clinical assessment of acupuncture in asthma therapy: a discussion paper. *Journal of the Royal Society of Medicine,* **80,** 222–4. Jobst, K.A., Chen, J.H.,

McPherson, K., Arrowsmith, J., Brown, V., Efthimiou, J., Fletcher, H., Maciocia, G., Mole, P., Shifrin, K., Lane, D.J. (1986). Controlled trial of acupuncture for disabling breathlessness. *Lancet,* **2,** 1416–9. Fung, K.P., Chow, O.K.W., and So, S.Y. (1986). Attenuation of exercise-induced asthma by acupuncture. *Lancet,* **2,** 1419–22.

24. Dowson, D.I., Lewith, G.T., and Machin, D. (1985). The effects of acupuncture versus placebo in the treatment of headache. *Pain,* **21,** 35–42.

25. Peng, A.T., Behar, S., and Yue, S.J. (1987). Long term therapeutic effect of electro-acupuncture for neck and shoulder pain—a double blind study. *Acupuncture and Electrotherapeutics Research,* **12,** 37–44. Ozer, F.T. and Coan, P.L. (1980). The acupuncture treatment of low back pain: a randomized controlled study. *American Journal of Chinese Medicine,* **8,** 181–9.

26. *Anon.* (1976). Clinical and experimental studies on general attack therapy of ureteral stones. *Chinese Medical Journal,* **2,** 25–32.

27. Ionescu-Tirgoviste, C. (1980). Proper nutrition in the concept of traditional Chinese medicine. *American Journal of Acupuncture,* **8,** 205–13.

7

Alexander and Feldenkrais Techniques

Alexander Technique

Background

Born in Australia in 1869, F.M. Alexander found his promising career as a young Shakespearean actor beset by vocal troubles. Finding no assistance from medical practitioners he concluded that the problem lay within. So began years of painstaking self-observation and experimentation. During this time he noticed that while reciting he tended to stiffen his neck and pull his head back and down, thereby depressing his vocal cords and shortening his spine. The correct posture, he found, could only be achieved by consciously allowing the head to assume its correct orientation in relation to the neck and torso. Of course the new posture was easily lost as force of habit made him revert to his usual stance. However he realized that if he did not compel himself to reach the end result directly, but attended only to the means for achieving it, he could break his habitual pattern.

His own success encouraged him to teach his discoveries to other actors. When he saw improvements in voice, in other functions, and in health, he concluded he had come across a fundamental approach to improving the use of the human organism as a whole. Encouraged by doctors, he came to London at the turn of the century and taught his technique both in England and America until 1955.

Concepts and research

It is often held that man is still not perfectly adapted to the upright posture. However, it can be readily demonstrated in Alexander work that there can be perfect balance and poise with the minimum degree of tension. The way we use our body is faulty, not the mechanism itself: 'Mis-use' is one of the major factors in 'dis-ease'. This concept is largely unacknowledged in medicine and the effects of misuse can be more insidious even than nutritional factors.

Dr Wilfred Barlow,[1] a student of Alexander Technique, has investigated postural defects as an indication of misuse. Surveys of college students showed substantial defects in most of them. He then compared the efficiency of standard methods of postural re-education (admonishments to correct particular faults) with Alexander re-education, and found that the conventional approach produced deterioration, whereas the Alexander pupils improved markedly during their course. Nikko Tinbergen,[2] on being awarded the Nobel Prize for Physiology and Medicine in 1973, devoted half of his oration to the Alexander Technique, which he described as one of the true epics of medical research and practice. He recommended it for autism and stress diseases. Professor Tinbergen, an ethologist, assumed that a precise assessment of improvement in posture would be a sufficient demonstration of the value of the Technique. However in practice it has proved difficult to assess posture objectively.

Frank Pierce-Jones,[3] recognizing these limitations, proposed that the movement pattern itself should be the criterion of effectiveness of Alexander Technique. By means of multiple-image photography he was able to record the trajectory followed by the head during movement. He recorded a greater area underneath the trajectory in an Alexander-guided movement, compared with 'normal', showing greater efficiency of use.

The instruction

Alexander lessons powerfully confirm the need and possibility of changing one's habitual pattern of movement and bearing. They are a technique of re-education. In individual lessons, the pupil is made aware of what he is doing, and how this interferes with the head-neck-torso relationship in rest and activity. The teacher conveys through his hands the fact and sense of a new manner of use, and the pupil is encouraged to think with the teacher so that he learns increasingly to create this improved co-ordination for himself. There is an experience of lengthening, expansion, and ease in movement, although it almost certainly feels strange at first. A slight touch may be all that is necessary to allow an effortless change from sitting to standing, such is the extraordinary freedom and lightness when the head is allowed to lead the body.

The teacher is careful about correcting specific defects and postural faults. These usually arise out of poor general conditions which must be put in order first. Alexander deprecated breathing exercises, relaxation (collapse!), and other specific 'cures'. He was very concerned about the integrity of the psychophysical organism and therefore did not give 'treatment' or promise instant relief.

The range and application of the Alexander Technique is as wide as human activity itself; indeed John Dewey, the American educational philosopher, thought it bore the same relation to education as education does to living. It has great potential in all manner of psychosomatic and mechanical disorders, particularly back and neck problems, and in rehabilitation following accidents or injury.

Experience has shown that it is almost impossible for the individual by himself to break through the circle of habitual doing, and unreliable postural awareness. In a few lessons from a competent teacher the pupil can cover the same ground that Alexander took years to establish. Many come to lessons after years of chronic pain to find its cause. Ideally one should learn how to *prevent* the distorting effects of the conflicting demands of modern civilization from an early age.

Feldenkrais Technique

Like F. Mathias Alexander, Moshe Feldenkrais is a founder of a technique for restoring full efficiency and function of the body. He synthesized this technique from Eastern and Western body concepts, combining some aspects of the Alexander Technique with knowledge of Oriental body training in the martial arts—he was a Judo teacher for 30 years. The result is a sophisticated and well thought out series of exercises which facilitate awareness of the body in movement.[4] Habitual movements are reduced to their component parts, games are played with gravity, new types and ranges of movement are explored, and the body is retaught its basic language of natural, pleasurable, and instinctive action. Its focus on gradually training awareness and sensitivity puts the Feldenkrais Technique in the same class as Alexander Technique, although it differs in its concentration on the body in motion rather than the body in space. In that sense one might liken it to a Western T'ai-chi. The teaching includes, for example, new perceptions of walking, crawling, the natural movements of babies, the consciousness of breathing while moving, self-image, the way the head, eye, pelvis, spine, and limbs move in relation to each other and so on. It has a directly therapeutic side in which the therapists re-train patients with musculoskeletal or neurological problems, particularly the ubiquitous bad back. Although popular in the US, there are few practitioners in the UK.

References

1. Alexander, F.M. (1985). *The use of the self.* Gollancz, London.
2. Barlow, W. (1982). *The Alexander principle.* Gollanz, London.
3. Tinbergen, N. (1974). Ethology and stress diseases. *Science*, **185**, 20–7.
4. Jones F.P. (1976). *Body awareness in action: A Study of the Alexander Technique.* Wildwood Press, London.
5. Feldenkrais, F. (1972). *Awareness through movement: health exercises for personal growth.* Harper & Row, New York.

8

Anthroposophical medicine

Background

Anthroposophical medicine constitutes an extension of medical thought and practice based on and inspired by the work of Rudolf Steiner (1861–1925). Steiner first created a philosophical basis for what he later termed anthroposophy in *The philosophy of freedom* (1894),[1] his fundamental work on the theory of knowledge. He went on to elaborate a description of the nature of man as a being of soul and spirit, as well as body,[2] and to outline the method and discipline which this research involves. At the same time he worked towards a renewal of the arts, including a new art of movement, eurythmy, which he later also developed for therapy.

After the First World War, the implications of anthroposophy for practical life and work began to be more widely recognized. Steiner was approached by people in various vocations seeking a new basis for their work. These included physicians, teachers of normal and handicapped children, farmers, scientists, and architects. In 1923, 15 months before his death, Rudolf Steiner founded the School of Spiritual Science, which had the task of providing the training and social framework for continued research and its application in cultural, economic, and social life. The School is divided into sections, each responsible for one field of practical work, e.g. a Natural Science Section, a Medical Section, etc. It is based at the Goetheanum in Dornach near Basle, Switzerland, which is also the centre of the worldwide Anthroposophical Society, founded at the same time for the furtherance of this work.

It was only in the latter years of Rudolf Steiner's life that his work took him into the field of medicine. He was not himself a medical practitioner, but worked with doctors who saw that anthroposophy could have a real contribution to make in the sphere of medicine. Amongst the doctors who worked with Rudolf Steiner was the Dutch physician Dr Ita Wegman. Their close collaboration led to the founding of a clinic in Arlesheim, Switzerland.

Anthroposophical work in Germany was suppressed by the Nazis, but after World War II further specialized clinics and general hospitals were founded. At present, anthroposophical medical work is most widely developed in Germany, The Netherlands, and Switzerland, where there are two general hospitals and eight specialized hospitals using these methods. In addition there are many hundreds of general practitioners and specialists. These hospitals are fully recognized and funded by state and private medical insurance schemes, as are most of the individual practitioners. In the two West German district general hospitals anthroposophical work is fully integrated with general surgery, accident and emergency services, intensive care, obstetrics and gynaecology, paediatrics, general medicine, and psychiatry. By comparison, in the English-speaking world the number of practitioners and the range of services and institutions is still very limited. In the UK, individual practitioners work both within the National Health Service and privately. A number of anthroposophical doctors offer their services as medical consultants to Rudolf Steiner Schools for normal, maladjusted, and mentally-handicapped children. There is a residential therapeutic centre in Worcestershire where more intensive anthroposophical medical treatment is offered.[3]

Anthroposophical medicine is one aspect of a wider movement responsible for innovative work in education, agriculture, the arts, social development, and finance. Best known are the Waldorf Schools (some 200 world-wide, including 12 in the UK) and the homes and schools for children and adults in need of special care, including the Camphill Villages and communities.

Fundamental concepts

In order to understand anthroposophical medicine, its relationship with conventional medicine must be considered. The latter is based on physical experiment and observation guided by hypotheses. Only hypotheses about tangible and measurable phenomena are admitted as legitimate. The underlying assumption is either that other kinds of (immaterial) realities do not exist, or that they are not accessible to investigation. The consequence is that all living, emotional, and mental phenomena must ultimately be reduced to physical events.

Steiner's challenge was not to the *spirit* of science, which he vigorously upheld, but to the self-imposed limitations of its practice. He contended:

1. The phenomena of life, of feeling, of consciousness, are not explained by reductionism which simply diverts attention from our actual experiences of them.

2. While physical perception is by definition confined to physical realities, disciplined thought is not so confined (if it were, a great deal of higher mathematics would not exist).

3. Other forms of perception can be developed which reveal other levels of reality. These may also be permeated by disciplined thought. It is then apparent that we do not, in fact, yet have an adequate science of life, sentience, or consciousness.

4. The outline of a science of life can be grasped conceptually irrespective of whether the appropriate modes of 'supersensible' perception are available to a particular individual.

Such insights can then show us many apparently familiar experiences in nature and in human life in a new light, thus allowing the systematic development of new approaches in therapy, education, agriculture, etc.

This is not the place to explore these contentions in depth. They are elaborated in the extensive anthroposophical literature, notably in Steiner's own 20 books and 6000 published lectures. They are, nevertheless, the foundations for an approach to therapy, which aims to be not an alternative to, but an *extension* of, scientific medicine.

Health and disease

To define the human being as a 'naked ape', E.F. Schumacher once remarked, is like defining a dog as 'a barking plant or a running cabbage'. A proper understanding must include a relationship to the mineral, plant, and animal kingdoms of nature, but must also acknowledge our uniqueness—notably a capacity to understand nature and change it.

Anthroposophical medicine is founded on a recognition of four distinct aspects of the human being, as outlined by Steiner: the physical body (shared with all other kingdoms of nature); the life or 'etheric' body (shared with plants and animals), which is the force that establishes and sustains life similar to the Chinese 'ch'i' and Indian 'prana'; the sentient or 'astral' body (shared with animals) which is the soul aspect; and the 'I', the human intelligent self. The last three principles are each to be understood as a net of forces or energies different from each other and from those constituting the physical body. While inter-related, none is reducible to the laws of another. It is in terms of these four sets of activities, and their particular modes of inter-relation in a sick person, that the doctor seeks to understand an illness.

Life depends on maintaining a dynamic balance within the contrasting metabolic processes of catabolism (breaking down and using energy) and anabolism (building up and storing energy). Anatomically, this polarity is manifest in the contrast of nerves indicating nervous activity, and blood indicating nutritive processes; psychologically, in the contrast of waking and sleeping. For example the 'I' and 'sentient body' are to be conceived as working from 'outside' the physical and life bodies in sleep, and from 'inside' when we are awake. Degenerative and sclerotic illnesses may be pictured as a consequence of excessive activity of the 'I' and the sentient organizations working destructively on the physical body. Inflammatory conditions and mental illnesses manifesting as manic and schizophrenic symptoms may be pictured as an excessive activity of the life forces and physical bodies.

The physical bearers of the day-time consciousness which come to dominate the life of the organism are the nerves, the senses, and the skin. While extending throughout the body their activity is particularly centred in the head. The physical bearers of the restorative and nutritive functions, in contrast, are the metabolic organs (e.g. the liver, digestive organs generally, and the muscles), centred particularly in the abdominal region and the limbs. Between the activities of these two polar systems lies the rhythmic organization, centred in the region of the chest and expressing its functions through the heart, the lungs, and the circulatory and respiratory systems as a whole. Within this rhythmic system the contrasting nerves and senses on the one hand, and the metabolic functions on the other, interpenetrate, producing all bodily rhythms. This system is of particular importance to the physician in that pathological processes within any region of the body may first show themselves as disturbances of rhythms, for example, in the pulse and respiration.

Such a picture of human physiology represents a radical departure from the generally accepted view that all functions of the mind and soul are centred in the brain. Although the conscious functions of thought and perception are centred in the nervous system, these represent only a part of our inner life. Steiner recognized explicitly what we often apprehend intuitively, that the life of feelings and emotions is centred physiologically in the rhythmic system, and the will in the system of metabolism and limbs. (To say that someone has 'no stomach for a fight' then ceases to be a mere figure of speech.)

In human beings, the realm of 'instinct' includes the unconscious working of the 'I', which guides individual destiny. Steiner was concerned that modern medicine should begin to include some awareness of this realm in its work. The outward expressions of this deeply hidden activity are found in individual biographies or in important illnesses or 'accidents', which may be recognizable not simply as unfortunate events requiring suppression or elimination, but as landmarks in personal development.

This picture of illness gives the anthroposophical physician and his patient the task of uncovering any potential meaning and purpose of an illness while using treatments to promote healing.

Diagnostic and therapeutic practices

Diagnostic procedures include conventional history taking, physical examination, and appropriate laboratory and radiographic investigations. In addition, special attention may be given to forming a picture of the patient's biography and social context, including a search for underlying patterns which may be seen in the light of an anthroposophical understanding of the phases of development.[4] It may also be important to observe some or all of the following signs: characteristic body shape and formation, tissue fluid distribution in skin and soft tissue, muscle tension, distribution of body warmth (the special field of observation for the masseur), posture, movements and gestures (the special province of the eurythmist), modes of artistic expression (e.g. too much or too little form), awareness of colour (the field of the artistic therapist), social behaviour (e.g. outgoing, inward-looking). A central motif underlying these phenomena is then sought. This represents a 'qualitative diagnosis', which includes but transcends the conventional medical diagnosis. It may be described in terms of the four-fold picture of the human being as outlined above. Such a procedure represents the 'ideal case' which may be realized in a residential clinical setting. An ordinary medical consultation will normally only include some of these aspects.

Anthroposophically developed medicines may be prescribed in addition to some of the following: special diets, massage, hydrotherapy, therapeutic eurythmy, and artistic therapies such as painting, drawing, modelling, music, and speech formation. These therapies can be composed into an integrated therapeutic programme.

Medicines

Most medicines used in the practice of anthroposophical medicine are derived from natural sources—mineral, plant, and animal.[5] They may be used at homeopathic potencies or in material dosages. The anthroposophical approach sees the essential nature of a potential medicinal substance in terms of the forces and processes which have produced it. In order to derive a medicine from a plant source, for example, the plant itself must first be studied in connection to its unique form, its particular life-cycle and the way it relates to its environment. Its one-sidedness or peculiarities are noted. A qualitative picture of the plant may then be built up which includes its life in time as well as its form in space.

The influence of a medicine on the human organism is not seen as being limited to chemical processes and reactions, but may directly stimulate more subtle processes and bring about changes in life energy. It may have a facilitating or 'catalytic' effect. For example, through an appreciation of the relationship between silica and nerve-sense processes on the one hand, and between iron and sulphur and metabolic processes on the other, a preparation containing these substances has been formulated for the prophylaxis and treatment of migraine. Pharmaceutical laboratories which had started in order to meet the requirements of the first doctors working with this approach developed into an international pharmaceutical manufacturing company, Weleda. Later the Wala company was founded, and pioneered new methods to prepare biologically stable products without the use of preservatives such as alcohol.

Following up Rudolf Steiner's suggestion that misletoe (*Viscum album*) should be developed as a treatment for cancer, several cancer research institutes were founded which have developed medicinal preparations for this illness.[6] The best known is Iscador. Other medicines have been developed from similar considerations, including medicines used in the treatment of psychiatric illness, based on Steiner's indication that many such illnesses stem from disturbances in the functioning of internal organs.

Physical treatments

Out of an understanding of the life body and its activity in the tissue fluids and the fluid organization as a whole, a special method of rhythmical massage was developed by Dr Margarethe Hauschke[7] and Dr Ita Wegman. A method of hydrotherapy using plant oils finely dispersed in water—oil dispersion baths—has also been developed. These baths allow the warming, stimulating, or relaxing effects of various oils on the skin to be enhanced.

The arts and therapy

In contemporary society many illnesses and problems arise from the individual's estrangement from his own creative capacities. Fundamental healing may only be achieved through their rediscovery and development. Steiner's work has encouraged the development of a number of artistic therapies which may restore deformations within man's four-fold organization as described above and therefore have a central role to play in the practice of anthroposophical medicine.

Therapeutic eurythmy

Eurythmy, an art of movement created by Steiner, has been called 'visible speech' and 'visible music'. The performing eurythmist seeks to make the whole human organism an instrument for realising the movements out of which music and speech are born. In this sense, eurythmy can awaken us to a fuller consciousness of what we already know. As speakers, we use both physical movements and inner movements of feeling and consciousness to utter language. For example, the vowel 'ah' cannot be spoken with the mouth closed; the sound 't' cannot be spoken without involving the tongue and teeth in particular movements. At the same time, each physical sound embodies a characteristic quality of experience, which gives poets their working material. The eurythmist must transform all this into an exact discipline of movement, just as a musician learns to play his instrument so that it renders faithfully the music he wishes to be heard.

In an artistic performance the movements of eurythmy flow quickly into one another, shaping a continuous stream of movement. In therapeutic eurythmy, individual movements connected, for example, with single vowels or consonants are isolated and intensified through rhythmic repetition so that they can work back on the person performing them. The exercises may aim to change the way a patient relates to the world, to help him concentrate, to free him from crippling emotional responses, etc., or they may aim to influence the physical organism itself through posture and movement; these may even bring changes in the function and structure of specific organs. For example, the person who finds his environment frightening may keep his neck muscles tense, his shoulders hunched, and his breathing shallow. He can then be given eurythmy exercises in which he first experiences more consciously the contracted posture he habitually adopts and the cramped feelings that tend to accompany it. Such an exercise would involve an almost uncomfortable crossing of the arms and legs, and gives rise to an experience of being locked in oneself. This might be followed by an exercise of stretching the arms out in a gesture of wonder. The aim is not just to do the movements but to be open to the type of feeling that can accompany the gestures. In alternating two such exercises not only a physical but also an 'emotional' breathing is encouraged.

Therapeutic eurythmists work with medical doctors. The doctor may prescribe certain exercises for a patient, or doctor and eurythmist may collaborate in a search for exercises suitable for him. However, in the final analysis, given this help from doctor and eurythmist, it is the patient's own activity which has healing value for him.

Art therapies

Therapeutic work in painting, drawing, modelling, sculpture, speech, and music has also been developed from Steiner's indications. Each therapy draws upon different qualities and faculties within the individual, as each art has a different form and rhythm, and works in a different medium. Within any one medium, there is a wide choice of techniques and themes. It rests with the therapist and doctor to determine which can be most helpful in a particular case. For example, in drawing, a particular rhythmic diagonal shading may be used therapeutically. Acquiring this discipline and using it in drawing exercises to balance extreme polarities of darkness and light may be particularly helpful in cases of anxiety, obsessions, and complexes, helping to strengthen and direct the will, and promote clarity in thinking.

Painting therapy centres in the use of colours, to which we respond with our emotions. These, in turn, influence the breathing and circulatory rhythms and consequently the individual's sense of well-being. Water colour paints are used for their luminosity and for the experience of freedom and fluidity of the watery medium itself. Again, a first step will often be to acquire a technique of long, continuous brush strokes, which create a mood of quiet and relaxation. The therapist will then begin to work with specific colour combinations and particular themes. Some individuals needing to come out of themselves and find confidence in their surroundings may be helped through painting clear forms and images. Others, suffering from sclerotic or cancerous conditions, may benefit from more spontaneous exercises, exploring light and dark and movements in pure colours without the use of forms or hard contours.

Modelling and sculpture, using clay, beeswax and/or plasticine, offer other possibilities. The senses of touch, movement, and balance are awakened in coming to grips with three-dimensional forms. It is particularly valuable to engage in exercises of metamorphosis, transforming one form into another, or making sequences of related forms. These can strengthen imaginative mobility, flexibility and the capacity for change in other aspects of life. Sculpture therapy can be valuable in many psychiatric and psychosomatic disturbances which involve a loss of orientation in space, giddiness, vagueness, disconnected thinking, lack of concentration, and nervousness.

Applications

Although anthroposophical treatment has helped many patients who have not felt helped by conventional medicine, its importance lies less in the statistics of its 'cures' than in the qualities of the healing processes it facilitates, and in its comprehensive approach to the sick human being. However 'human' its practitioners, the positivistic basis of conventional medicine tends to see the patient as an object and illness as an unfortunate breakdown of his physical mechanism. In anthroposophically based medicine, there is a basis for considering the patient as a developing individual with a meaningful biography, and his illness as a difficult but potentially important episode in his life. This can mean that in some cases, a patient may be challenged to endure certain symptoms longer than if they were treated conventionally, so that a more fundamental improvement, rather than symptomatic relief, may be achieved. However, surgery and other conventional treatments may equally well be prescribed where appropriate. Steiner's insistence that all doctors seeking to extend medicine along anthroposophical lines must be fully qualified in the conventional sense widens rather than narrows the scope of their work.

This means that, in principle, an anthroposophical physician can be consulted about any medical problem. While anthroposophical medicine can contribute to the treatment of most illnesses, it has a special value where conventional medicine has little to offer. For example psychosomatic illness and functional disorders cannot be adequately understood, let alone treated, by a medicine based essentially on a physio-chemical model, whose rational *materia medica* for such conditions is limited to sedatives, anti-depressants, or other symptomatic treatments. Similarly, in treating cancer, conventional medicine must rely on surgery and on destructive treatments which weaken the patient's vitality and general resistance. Here the anthroposophical approach, while not offering miracle cures, has a special contribution to make with specific medicines and other therapies which enhance the patient's vitality and resistance.

Research and development

Steiner saw clearly that science embodies, in effect, a schooling. However, its nature and scope are confined by history and convention to a limited framework, which excludes in advance a full exploration of the phenomena of life, sentience and human self-awareness. He saw within all human beings the potential for a much wider and deeper schooling. In this context, it becomes natural for a physician in anthroposophical medicine to feel responsible for training his own faculties of perception, thinking, and feeling, and to see the care of each patient as calling for continuous research.

Various individuals and groups have also pursued more general lines of research: the Gustav Carus Institute near Pforzheim in West

Germany has made significant contributions to the assessment of medicinal plants and their relations to pathological processes.[8] More conventional methods have been used to document the results of the use of mistletoe preparations in the treatment of cancer.[6] In the Department of Clinical Pharmacology at Herdecke Hospital a critical examination of the problems both of animal experiments and of clinical trials to demonstrate the efficacy of medicaments has been undertaken, and various studies published in medical journals.[9] These demonstrate clearly the very limited value of these trials. Recently, Herdecke has made an extensive study of the considerable ethical problems inherent in such trials arising from the inevitable conflict of interest between giving the best available treatment to each patient, and running the trial so that statistically significant results are obtained.[10]

Types of therapy and availability

A list of practitioners available for consultation is published by the Anthroposophical Medical Association. The length of treatment and the number of consultations depends entirely on the individual case and may vary from one or two consultations to a prolonged course of treatment over many months. The Park Attwood Therapeutic Centre usually suggests a minimum of three weeks' residential treatment to ensure noticeable results.

The cost of treatment depends on the situation. Patients on the list of an anthroposophical NHS general practitioner receive his advice free of charge and can obtain the medicines he prescribes on NHS prescriptions. They will be expected to make some financial contribution if a course of treatment with a specialist anthroposophical therapist is prescribed. A modest fee is normally charged for private consultations with such general practitioners if the patient is not on their NHS list and most private practitioners also charge a modest fee. In recent years patients in various localities have set up funds to support the services of an anthroposophical doctor outside the NHS. The Park Attwood Therapeutic Centre, although independent of the NHS, does not charge fees. Instead, patients are informed of the average costs per patient per week and asked to make a responsible contribution, based on their own financial circumstances in relation to Park Attwood's needs.

References

1. Steiner (1979a). *The philosophy of freedom*. Rudolf Steiner Press, London.
2. Steiner (1979b). *Occult Science—An Outline*. Rudolf Steiner Press, London.
3. Park Attwood Therapeutic Centre, Trimpley, Bewdley, Worcs. DY12 1RE; Tel: (02997) 444.
4. Lievegoed, B. (1982). *Phases—Crisis and development in the individual*. Rudolf Steiner Press, London.
5. Pelikan, W. (1978). *Healing plants*. Rudolf Steiner Press, London.
6. Khwaja, T.A., Dias, C.E., Pentecost, S. (1980). Recent Studies on the anticancer activities of mistletoe and its alkaloids, *Oncology*, **43**, 42-50. Twentyman, L.R. (1953). Observations on the Medical Treatment of Cancer. *British Homeopathic Journal*, **43**, 89; Fellmer, K.E. (1968). A clinical trial of Iscador. *British Homeopathic Journal*, **57**, 43; Morris-Owen, R.M. (1969). On the action of Iscador—A stimulus for reaction to neoplasia?. *British Homeopathic Journal*, **58**, 17; Nienhaus, J., Stoll, M. and Vester, F. (1969). Thymus stimulation and cancer prophylaxis by viscum proteins. *Experientia*, **26**, 5 (1971). Leroi, A. and Heisel, L. (1971) Iscador therapy of breast cancer. *British Homeopathic Journal*, **60**, 52; Leroi, A. (1978). Viscum album therapy of cancer. *British Homeopathic Journal*, **67**, 167. Bloksma, N., van Dijk, H., Korst, P., and Williers, J.M. (1979). Cellular and humoral adjuvant activity of a mistletoe extract. *Immunobiology*, **156**, 309-19.
7. Hauschke, M. (1979). *Rhythmical massage*. Rudolf Steiner Press, London.
8. *Mitteilungen des Carl Gustav Carus Institutes Nos. 1–38*, Carl Gustav Carus Institut, Am Eichof, D-7532 Niefern-Oeschelbronn, West Germany.
9. Burkhardt, R. and Kienle, G. (1980). Controlled clinical trials and drug regulations, a report of recent developments in the Federal Republic of Germany. *Controlled clinical trials*, **1**, 151-64. Elsevier, North Holland, New York.
10. Burkhardt, R. and Kienle, G. (1978). Controlled clinical trials and medical ethics. *Lancet*, **1**, 1356-9.

9

Chiropractic

Background

Bonesetting in the nineteenth century enjoyed extensive public support. The bonesetter's methods of treating strains, sprains, fractures, and other musculoskeletal problems were gentle and instinctive. They were methods that people could understand. Bonesetters provided stiff competition to surgeons whose techniques for stretching and reducing joints were both violent and mystifying. Surgeons and physicians in turn avoided any form of manipulation which they regarded as unscientific, although some distinguished physicians successfully employed manipulation in their practices.

Osteopathy and then chiropractic evolved in the US during the latter part of the nineteenth century; both were derived from charismatic and observant lay bonesetters. Chiropractic—from the Greek *keir* (hand) and *praktikos* (practice)—was developed by D.D. Palmer in 1895. Palmer was a grocer who also worked as an osteopath and healer. He realized the potential of spinal adjustments when he cured one patient who had been deaf for 17 years, and another who had a history of heart disease, solely by adjusting vertebra in the neck region. He was so impressed by these achievements that he announced the end of his quest for the basis of disease: it lay in the spine. Misaligned or maladjusted ('subluxed') vertebrae restricted nerves; the interference with the proper flow of nervous impulses prevented the 'innate intelligence' (Palmer's phrase for vital force or *vix medicatrix naturae*) from passing through the body. 'A subluxed vertebra is the cause of 95 per cent of all disease', stated Palmer. 'Luxated bones press against nerves. By their displacement they elongate the pathway of the nerve . . . modified impulses cause functions to be performed abnormally.' It followed that treatment of all diseases could be effected exclusively by manipulation of the vertebra to realign the joints.

To some extent Palmer's concern with the spine and the nervous system reflected current medical preoccupations. Earlier in the nineteenth century physicians had made extensive use of spinal treatments with leeches, cauteries, and so on, in attempts to treat disease in organs on parallel body segments. During Palmer's time the nerves were still a focus of scientific investigation. However, Palmer's insistence that virtually all known diseases could be cured by spinal treatments was anathema to the medical establishment, which became implacably opposed to his views. Medical opposition, especially in the US, has continued to this day although modern chiropractors no longer hold Palmer's extreme views.

Concepts

The British Chiropractors Association defines chiropractic as:

. . . an independent branch of medicine concerned with the diagnosis and treatment of mechanical disorders of joints, particularly spinal joints, and their effects on the nervous system. Diagnosis includes the use of X-rays and treatment is done mostly by hand without the use of drugs or surgery.

Chiropractors are therefore spinal specialists who hold that most of the problems relating to the spine stem from misalignments, maladjustments, and excessive strain placed on intervertebral and other joints. They call these problems *subluxations*, or small displacements. When used by doctors this term implies a small physical dislocation. However in chiropractic it is broadened to mean a functional as well as structural defect: 'the alteration of the normal dynamics, anatomical or physiological relationships of contiguous articular structures'. A subluxation may be manifested in physical displacement, or local, or radiating pain; there may be muscle spasm as a result of strain on the joint capsule; restriction or excessive movement of the joint, swelling, or weakening of more distant muscle groups.

Subluxations can be caused by many adverse influences such as strains, accidents, stresses, or innate skeletal distortions. Poor posture is often to blame, particularly where it places uneven or excessive loads on the back joints of the vertebrae. Chiropractors insist, as do many medical authorities, that however caused, defects in the joints will not be restricted to the spine itself, but will affect surrounding muscles, nerves, ligaments, and biochemical function, with which the joints are in intimate relation.

There have been several unsuccessful attempts to understand the subluxation in terms of our current knowledge of the biomechanics of the spine and the functions of the contiguous tissues, particularly where no physical displacements occur or are seen on X-rays. Possible suggestions include a reversible distortion of the cartilage, distension or squeezing of the joint capsule, or stretching of ligaments, all of which could produce the observable symptoms of a subluxation (tenderness, restricted movement, etc.), partly through reflexes triggered off by the nerves around the joint. It is, however, still an under-researched subject. 'The area of spinal mechanics and its implications in neurophysiology has not been explored by orthodox medical science. Chiropractic theories are only just beginning to evolve on a scientific basis from new discoveries and new scientists in the field', wrote the New Zealand Government Commission of Inquiry on chiropractic.[1]

The subluxation may also extend its influence beyond the spine to affect organs and tissues within the relevant body segment. Palmer envisaged this occurring by compression of the nerves as they emerge from the foramina to enervate the viscera. In the light of modern science it is possible to suggest other mechanisms, 15 of which were presented by one senior chiropractic researcher at a US Department of Health Education and Welfare conference on research into chiropractic.[2] For example, persistent irritation of nerves could interfere with the transmission of impulses or the flow of materials along the nerve.

The basis for the clinical observations of both chiropractors and osteopaths is that certain diseases can occasionally clear up after spinal manipulations, although osteopaths differ in seeking a vascular rather than nervous explanation. Thus dizziness, migraine, or lack of co-ordination can sometimes be traced back to a subluxation at the first cervical vertebra in the neck, while heart conditions or thoracic pain may be associated with a subluxation at the second thoracic vertebra. The subluxations are more likely to contribute towards these conditions than actually to cause them. This aspect of chiropractic philosophy has engendered considerable and violent dispute in the past. However, there is evidence for the interdependence between the functions of the spine and viscera.[3] (See also Chapter 19.) Kunert, an eminent authority in this field stated:[4]

We have no evidence that lesions of the spinal column can cause genuine organic diseases. They are, however, perfectly capable of simulating, accentuating or making a major contribution to such disorders. There can, in fact, be no doubt that the state of the spinal column does have a bearing on the functional status of the internal organs.

Practice

There are several aspects to a chiropractic diagnosis. It begins with a full personal history which would include traumas and injuries going back to childhood, as well as personal health habits. Many chiropractors also use X-rays, in which the spine is photographed segmentally or in its entirety. The use of X-rays is based on the belief that although functional and soft tissue (including intervertebral disc) displacements or damage do not show up, they may be detectable by a careful examination of the alignment of surrounding bony structures. The X-rays also give a powerful indication of the effect of posture on the spine, of any actual displacements of bones, and of medical conditions, such as osteoporosis or cancer, which would modify or prevent manipulative treatment. Palpation of the vertebral column before, during, and after movements is invariably used in diagnosis. For example, the practitioner may feel the play or movements of the vertebra as the patient is passively bent from side to side with his weight supported by the chiropractor. Leg raising and positioning tests are often used to assess pain and the alignment of the pelvis with the vertebral column. Chiropractors also examine posture, measure lengths of the extremities, assess muscle function, and carry out standard neurological and other basic medical tests.

Chiropractic diagnosis aims to discover whether the patient's complaint, usually joint pain, originates from systemic or underlying disease, or from a non-pathological mechanical disorder. The former is referred to orthodox medicine, the latter further investigated for its suitability for treatment by chiropractic. The treatment strategy varies according to whether the complaint is a painful lesion or strain, a disc problem, sciatica, an arthritic condition, and so on. Its main aims will be to restore the proper motion of the joints, to correct distortions or subluxations, to improve posture, and to remove the irritations, interference, or painful stimulation to nerves.

Manipulation is the standard procedure unless contra-indicated. This is accomplished by sudden short thrusts which prevent patient muscular resistance. The manipulation is carried out with considerable precision and control. Indeed, much of the art of chiropractic treatment is in the design and careful execution of manipulations, which are therefore of considerably greater sophistication and power than the manipulation sometimes available from physiotherapists or physicians. For example, a specially built couch is used to position the patient accurately so that each manipulation is most effective.

Other techniques are often used in conjunction with manipulation, in particular soft tissue techniques. These may take the form of sustained pressure on ligaments, or a massage of muscles, in order, for example, to relieve muscle spasm and pain, and prepare the joint for manipulation. Supportive measures are sometimes provided. Occasionally heat treatment or electrogalvanic apparatus is used, and a few chiropractors will also employ a variety of dietary and remedial treatments. Prophylactic advice is often given concerning ergonomics and correct physical activity.

Research

The possibilities for research have been severely restricted in the past by the unwillingness of medical researchers to explore chiropractic. The situation is now changing and much more research is beginning and expected. One boost to research was the US Department of Health, Education and Welfare conference in 1975 on the basis of spinal manipulation.[2] Another has been the formation of the Society for Back Pain Research. However, so far little is known about spinal biomechanics and neurophysiology. Studies such as that of Crelin, which failed to find anatomical peculiarities in cadavers at the site of supposed subluxations, only emphasize how little we know even of the way to approach the problems.[5] For that reason study is recognized as quite inappropriate to detect dynamic and functional disturbances at the site of joints.

There have, however, been a number of serious studies of the success of manipulation in general and chiropractic in particular for various kinds of back problems (see also Chapter 19, p. 235). As far as simple manipulation (which is not chiropractic) is concerned, trials have shown that manipulation is better than 'pretend' treatments without manipulation,[6] and that manipulation is also better than the usual medical treatment of back pain.[7] (The usual medical treatment, known as 'conservative' treatment, treats the pain symptoms, and ensures rest and immobility of the joint, in some ways a technique diametrically opposed to that of manipulation.)

Medical trials of specific chiropractic manipulation versus other kinds of treatment have rarely been carried out. However, one notable study appeared in the *Lancet* in 1974.[8] In this study patients who were treated by both doctors and chiropractors for back problems were selected from Compensation Board records, interviewed and examined. Steps were taken to ensure that the two groups of patients were comparable. It turned out that chiropractors were somewhat better at restoring function to patients than physicians. Chiropractors saw their patients more frequently and over a shorter period than doctors. More recent clinical studies confirm this report.[9]

Workmen's Compensation Commissions have provided a golden opportunity to compare the efficiency of chiropractic and medical treatment in general terms. For example, the medical director of the Oregon Workmen's Compensation Board found that 82 per cent of the claimants with certain injuries treated by chiropractors could return to work within one week, twice as many as those with similar injuries who were treated by doctors.[10] Other boards in Kansas, Iowa, and Florida confirm that chiropractors have their patients back to work much sooner, with less suffering. Their treatment is also much cheaper overall.

These comparative studies have related purely to musculoskeletal problems. However, a group at the University of New South Wales has made a bold attempt to assess the value of chiropractic in the treatment of migraine.[11] In this highly sophisticated trial migraine patients were selected on the basis of their expectation of treatments as well as other factors, and were well matched. It turned out that the patients who had been treated with manipulation by chiropractors or other specialists were significantly improved when compared to patients who were simply helped, by non-specialists, to move their neck and shoulders. Chiropractors were better able to reduce their patients' pain than other specialists, whether or not the others also used manipulation. The trial supports the use of chiropractic in the treatment of migraine.

Uses and risks

Most common musculoskeletal problems are treatable by

chiropractic. These include arthritic and rheumatic conditions which may respond well to manipulation, for the extent of joint deterioration (spondylitis) may not be as irreversible as has been supposed. Sciatica, lumbago, neuralgia, slipped disc, non-specific back pain, strains, dislocations, and so on are the major cases seen by chiropractors. (About 32 million working days are lost every year in the UK because of these conditions.)[12] However, some musculoskeletal conditions, in particular systemic rheumatism, gout, osteoarthritic hips, bone malignancy, infections, and prolapsed (i.e. ruptured) spinal discs, are referred elsewhere for treatment, usually to doctors or conventional medical specialists.

Only some 10 per cent of chiropractic cases are seen for an organic disease (see Chapter 2, p. 33). Chest pain, migraine and headache, asthma, digestive disorders, and neurological disorders are organic conditions most frequently treated, and sometimes respond well. In some cases the patient and even the patient's doctor will assume an organic disease which is, in reality, pain radiating out from a subluxed vertebra; these cases respond well to chiropractic treatment.

Chiropractic manipulation is extremely safe and in sensitive cases pressure techniques are used. The risks of treatment are minimal, and very rare. Some cases have been reported,[13] but their frequency is less than virtually all known medical treatments.

The chiropractic treatment available in the UK is predominantly from graduates of the Anglo-European College of Chiropractic, although those qualified before 1969 will have been trained in the US. There is also a small group which treats the whole spine (rather than simply the subluxations) at every session, using massage and gentle manipulation to adjust its overall alignment.

References

1. *Report of the commission of inquiry* (1979). Chiropractic in New Zealand. New Zealand Government Printer.
2. National Institute of Neurological Communicable Disorders and Stroke (1975). *The research status of spinal manipulative therapy*, Department of Health, Education and Welfare, NIH, Washington D.C.
3. Kunert, W. (1963). *The vertebral column, automonic nervous system and internal organs*. Enke, Stuttgart.

4. Kunert, W. (1965). 'Functional disorders of internal organs due to vertebral lesions.' In *CIBA Symposium*, **13**, 85–110.
5. Crelin, E.S. (1973). 'A scientific test of chiropractic theory.' *American Scientist*, **61**, 574–81.
6. Glover, J., Morris, J., and Khosla, T. (1974). 'Back pain: A randomised clinical trial of rotational manipulation of the trunk'. *British Journal of Industrial Medicine*, **31**, 59–64.
7. Fisk, J.W. (1971). 'Manipulation in general practice.' *New Zealand Medical Journal*, **74**, 172–5. Mierau, D., Cassidy, J.D., McGregor M., and Kirkaldy-Willis, W.H. (1987). A comparison of the effectiveness of spinal manipulative therapy for low back patients with and without spondylolisthesis. *Journal of Manipulative and Physiological Therapeutics*, **10**, 49–55.
8. Kane, R.L., Olsen, D., Legmaster, C., Woolley, F.R., and Fisher, F. D. (1974). 'Manipulating the patient, a comparison of effectiveness of physician and chiropractic care.' *Lancet*, **i**, 1333–6.
9. Meade, T.W., Browne, W., Mellows, S., Townsend, J., and Webb, J. (1986). Comparison of chiropractic and hospital outpatient management of low back pain: a feasibility study. *European Journal of Chiropractic*, **34**, 172–81. Kukurin, G.W. (1986). Medical and independent studies on the evaluation of chiropractic therapeutics. *Digest of Chiropractic Economics*, **29**, 67–9. Bronfort, G. (1986). Chiropractic treatment of low back pain: a prospective survey. *European Journal of Chiropractic*, **34**, 182–211. Sheladia, V.L. and Johnston, D.A. (1986). Efficacy of various chiropractic treatments, age distribution, and incidence of accident- and non-accident-caused low back pain in male and female patients. *Journal of Manipulative and Physiological Therapeutics*, **9**, 243–7.
10. Martin, R.A. (1975). A study of time loss back claims: Workmen's Compensation Boards (Medical Director's Report, State of Oregon). *Archives of the California Chiropractor's Association*, **4**, 83–97.
11. Parker, G.B., Tupling, H., and Pryor, D.S. (1978). A controlled trial of cervical manipulation for migraine. *Australia and New Zealand Journal of Medicine*, **8**, 589–93.
12. Brompton, S. Back pain. *The Times*, 4 June 1987.
13. Mueller, S. and Sachs, A.L. (1976). Brain stem dysfunction related to cervical manipulation. *Neurology*, **26**, 247. Terrett, A.G.J. (1987). Vascular accidents from cervical spine manipulation. Report on 107 cases. *Journal of Australian Chiropractor's Association*, **17**, 15–24.

10

Creative and sensory therapies

Creative therapies

The creative therapies, that is art and music therapy, are unusual in that they integrate mind, body, and spirit with treatment given by complementary medicine yet are also an accepted part of conventional medicine. These therapies are supplementary to conventional psychiatry and psychology but as psychiatrists refer patients for the creative therapies, therapists find their humanistic approach to be sometimes in conflict with medical practice. For example, should an art therapist willingly accept a doctor's request to use the paintings of a patient as a guide for his drug treatment? The major use of creative therapy is in rehabilitation of the mentally ill, although often it is found to be successful in the rehabilitation of the chronically ill and the aged.[1] Music therapy is used as an aid to socialization and expression,[2] and can help the infirm to keep moving, listening, and thinking.[3]

Creative therapies are to a large extent beyond the scope of this book, because their concern is with mental rather than physical handicap, and they are part of, rather than complementary to, conventional medicine. Nevertheless they are of interest because of their emphasis on *wholeness*.[4] They use the same media but an entirely different philosophy to anthroposophical medicine. An indication of their rationale can be gained from the following quotations:

We act as a bridge, not only between a client's inner and outer world, while he may not yet be able to do so for himself, but also between himself and his outer social world . . . a connecting link but not a betraying one.

The art therapy department in a psychiatric hospital is often an asylum within an asylum . . . It provides people with space to express inconvenient or unspeakable feelings. The relationship between an Art Therapist and the hospital that employs him is often abrasive. It can scarcely be otherwise since . . . the pictures often get worse as the patient gets 'better'.[5]

Colour and sound therapies

As the creative therapies are on the fringe of conventional medicine so colour and sound therapies are on the fringe of complementary medicine. They are of an ancient vintage: colour and sound were used in therapy by the Greeks, and are still used by traditional Ayurvedic Indian practitioners.

The theory behind these therapies is uncertain: it is a mixture of psychological, sensory and parapsychological. On the psychological level it is well known that colours affect mood quite profoundly; blue is appealing, and relaxing, red alarming and arousing. There are published studies showing how contemplation of blue light will lower blood pressure while red light will raise it.[6] Our language is full of colour-mood connections, such as 'green with jealousy' or 'yellow' as fear.

Yet the theory of colour therapy goes beyond this. It conceives of colour as containing energy of a particular vibrational character which can complement or interfere with the energy of the function of the body. It sees the body, or its organs, in illness as lacking one or other colour types, and aims to harmonize and balance body energy by the application of missing colours.[7] In diagnosis it reads the colours of the skin or perhaps of the aura, to assess which is missing.

Colours are given by means of food of particular colours, liquids that have been bathed in coloured lights or sunlight, the environment and clothes, or special colour-emitting lamps. In India gems are used to focus coloured light on specific parts of the body. Meditation on different colours, as in Kabbalistic practice, is a common aspect of the therapy.

Sound therapy is also taken at a number of different levels. On the one hand practitioners point to the well known prosaic action of sound on the human organism—the effect of ultrasonics or the power of music. On the other hand there is the possibly greater power of sound at a more subtle level, for example the mantric seed syllables used in meditation.

In a similar manner to colour therapists, sound therapists believe each tissue resonates at a particular frequency and the frequency is changed by illness. Therapists treat illness by applying what they believe is a vibration of exactly the correct frequency to the outside of the body so that the vibrations penetrate to the desired spot. The mix of frequencies is specific to the organ and its condition.

Sound therapy is most frequently used in rheumatic complaints which seem to respond to the vibrations. Colour therapists, on the other hand, state that they can treat almost any disease. In recent years electronic apparatus has been developed both for the practitioner, and for the patient's use at home. For example, there are sophisticated units which 'inject' colour into acupuncture points as part of electro-acupuncture treatment. Hand-held ultrasound generators are becoming popular. This, while not exactly sound therapy, does employ sound waves in an unconventional manner. There is recent evidence that ultrasound, locally applied, brings long-term pain relief in cases such as tennis elbow.[8] However, there is as yet little accumulated experience or exploration of these therapies.

References

1. Richardson, T. (1981). 'Moulding the character.' *Nursing Times*, 77, 474–5.
2. Halpern, S. and Savary, S. (1985). *Sound health: music and sounds that make us whole*. Harper & Row, New York. Alvin, J. (1976). *Music therapy for the handicapped child*. Oxford University Press.
3. Alvin, J. (1985). *Music therapy*. Hutchinson, London.
4. Kliphuis, M.A.R. (1978). Concepts for a general methodology of creative process therapy. *Confinia Psychiatria*, 21, 99–104.
5. Gulliver, P. and Holton, R. In *Ideas in art therapy* (eds D. Waller and A. Gilroy). British Association of Art Therapists (n.d.), London.
6. Birren, F. (1950). *Colour pscyhology and colour therapy: A factual study of the influence of colour on human life*. McGraw-Hill, New York. Ott, John N. (1973). *Health and light: The effects of natural and artificial light on man and other living things*. Devin-Adair, Old Greenwich, Connecticut.
7. Clark, Linda A. (1975). *Ancient art of colour therapy*. Devin-Adair, Old Greenwich, Connecticut.
8. Binder, A., Hodge, G., Greenwood, A.M., Hazleman, B.L., and Thomas, D.P.P. (1985). Is therapeutic ultrasound effective in treating soft tissue lesions? *British Medical Journal*, 290, 512–4.

11

Ethnic medicine

Ayurveda, along with its offshoots, Unani and Siddha, is at least as sophisticated as Far Eastern medicine. It is less popular in the West because it does not have a specific exportable skill, such as acupuncture. Its tenets are also published in Sanskrit. However, there are practitioners in the UK who serve the Asian community, and a wider interest in Ayurveda is developing in the therapeutic community. A number of Western practitioners have now undergone the gruelling and lengthy Ayurvedic training in India.

Ayurveda, or the 'Science of Life', is a section in the last of the Vedas, the *Atherva veda*, written in 2000 BC. However, the main Ayurvedic texts are the *Susruta samhita* and *Charaka samhita*, dating back to the fifth and second centuries BC respectively. It is virtually impossible to give any notion of the thoroughness and erudition of these texts. They set up several branches of medicine and present a practical teaching that covers every aspect of living in great detail. There are ancient texts on surgery which, for example, describe primitive proctoscopes and endoscopes, several different kinds of suturing, and how agents are carried by bodily contact, inhalation, and other channels to cause postoperative infections.[1] These texts were written 2500 years before Semmelweis was persecuted for suggesting that surgeons should wash their hands before operations. Indeed the *Charaka samhita* lists 20 kinds of *krimies* or microscopic pathogenic organisms (in addition to beneficial ones), and describes the body as composed of cells, and was written about 2000 years before the invention of the microscope.

Like other traditional systems, the essence of Ayurveda is balance between all the constituents, qualities, and energies within and without. There are five basic elements (*doshas*): earth (solid components of body, compactness, structure); water (fluids, soft material, cohesiveness); fire (digestion, metabolism, heat, adaptation); air (sensation, nervous system, animation) and ether (networks, connections, channels). Earth and water are usually combined to give *kapha* (mucus, structural element), fire is *pitta*, and *vathia* is air and ether combined as wind or activity. Like Chinese philosophy there are also basic energetic qualities, the *gunas*, namely *sattva* (unifying, wise), *rajas* (active, creating, somewhat like *yang*), and *tamas* (passive resisting, somewhat like *yin*). There are other anatomical and constitutional classifications.

Foods, climates, and all environmental influences and cycles contain the *doshas* and *gunas* to varying degrees. People too are constitutionally of one type or another, and the essence of Ayurvedic self-care knowledge is continually to balance these forces. Dr Chandra Sharma, a doctor in the UK, described how his mother would examine the climate, the state of health and activity of the family, their digestive energies, their moods and so on, and then cook a meal as a prescription for the occasion. The complexity of Indian curries is partly due to the requirements for balancing components, such as the water-generating nature of coriander to balance the heating quality of chilli.

Ayurvedic diagnosis includes some 32 pulse qualities identifying the condition of the viscera, as well as voice, face, iris, urine, sweat, diagnosis, and detailed personal history including astrological aspects. Complex prescriptions are designed according to the kinds of disease, the patient type, the anatomical site of the condition, the dominance of *dosha* or *guna*, the stage of the disease, the season, the age of the patient and so on. Each is formulated from the 8000 medicines recorded in Ayurveda. Unani medicine uses somewhat similar materials based on a philosophy which owes as much to Greek and Arab sources as the Vedas. Siddha medicine is a variant which has particularly adopted the use of minerals. Typical examples of herbs include *Piper longum* (pippali) used particularly in liver disorders, *Conifer mukul* resin (gogul) in atherosclerosis, *Emblica officinalis* (amalki) in duodenal ulcers and digestive problems. There are various non-medicinal treatments within Indian traditional medicine such as massages, diets, special exercises, yogic breathing techniques, surgery, blood-letting, urine treatment, yogic purification, and cleansing procedures.

A very great deal of research is carried out on Indian traditional medicine, although little of it ever reaches the West. A feeling for the research can be gleaned from the *Journal of Research in Indian Medicine*.[2] Much of it is very intriguing. For example when the author explored Ayurveda in India he was shown data indicating that certain remedies could induce muscles to regenerate (Western medical authorities state that this cannot be done).

The Ayurvedic and Unani practitioners in the UK are commonly known as *hakims* or *vaids*. They treat largely according to traditional principles, although they will be more westernized than many. They will have up to 1000 remedies at their disposal. Even so, they can have difficulty in obtaining the best quality materials and also in authenticating plants. There has been a trend towards using ready-made patent mixtures, which deviates from the Ayurvedic tradition of remedies designed and mixed for each patient. One or two of these mixtures, prescribed perhaps by the less qualified of the practitioners, have been found to contain unwholesome amounts of heavy metals. Therefore only properly qualified practitioners should be consulted. However, Indian traditional medicine's usefulness in areas such as rheumatism, arthritis, asthma, metabolic problems, cancer diseases, wound repair, digestive complaints, kidney and gall stones, tuberculosis, senility, and many other conditions should encourage more Westerners to try Ayurveda.[3]

References

1. Singh, L.M., Deshpande, P.J., and Thakral, K.K. (1970). Sushruta's contribution to the fundamentals of surgery. In *Advances in research in Indian medicine* (ed. K.N. Udupa). College of Medical Sciences, Benares Hindu University.
2. Varma, M.D., Singh, R.H., and Udupa, K.N. (1973). Physiological endocrine and metabolic studies on the effect of Rasayan therapy in aged persons. *Journal of Research in Indian Medicine*, **8**, 1-10.
3. Aslam, M., Bano, H., and Vohora, S.B. (1981). Sartan (cancer) and its treatment in Unani medicine. *American Journal of Chinese Medicine*, **9**, 95-107.
4. Collins, J. The *Guardian*, 25 May, 1981.
5. Bannerman, R.H., Burton, J., and Wen-Chieh, C. (1983). *Traditional medicine and health care coverage*. World Health Organization, Geneva.

12

Healing

Background

Spiritual healing can be described as the re-creation of the flow of life energy between body, soul, and consciousness so that the whole person may return to balance and harmony. Healing can be given by anybody who restores energy and attitude in another person. However, it usually implies an active transmission of therapeutic energy by a healer, or group of healers, to a patient.

Healing involves experiences that are sublime yet awe-inspiring. They do not lend themselves to easy interpretation, and are difficult to grasp by people who do not themselves share these altered states of consciousness. Analyses of healing reflect as much the mind of the commentator as the phenomenon he is describing. Thus some people see it anthropologically as beneficial social ritual, others as a form of hypnosis; some try and subvert it to rational physiological explanations,[1] while others visualize it as a miracle of divine intervention. Today, in our post-atomic era, there is a current of explanation which makes use of the notion of 'energy'. This may be a helpful model, yet it is still a gross concept describing subtle and inexplicable processes.

The primitive roots of healing are in shamanism and magic. Elaborate rituals are used to create attunement between the shaman, his guiding influences or spirits, and the patient. The shaman enters a trance state by means of drugs, breathing, dancing, or music. Power is invoked by supplication, and then focused towards the patient.[2]

The magical nature of healing has, since medieval times, strained its relationship with organized religion in the West, although not in the East. While the great spiritual teachers could usually heal, the religious institutions that bear their names have kept this activity at arm's length. The 'gifts of the Spirit' in Corinthians, 12, was confused with the Old Testament warning that 'Thou shalt not confer with familiar spirits', so that all true intuitive communication was considered heretical. While it is possible to accept that some individuals have exercised their powers in a negative way, most healing has been beneficial to the recipients. Nevertheless, healing groups within Christianity (e.g. Christian Scientists, Pentecostalists), Islam (e.g. Sufis), and Judaism (e.g. Hasidim) are still on the fringe.

Fundamental concepts

It is useful to distinguish faith healing from psychic or spiritual healing.[3] The first involves an interaction between the psyche and physiology of the patient, and is essentially a marshalling of the will and energy of the patient to release his self-healing capacities. It is based on trust in the ability, authority, and personality of the healer, or direct hypnosis. This sort of healing is also involved in the placebo effect. It operates through the power of suggestion. Its mechanisms are discussed in Chapter 15.

The second type of healing concerns us here. This is the transmission of some form of energy, as yet unknown, from the healer to the patient. The energies involved are similar to those manifest in other paranormal phenomena, particularly psychokinesis. In this kind of healing, energy acts directly on the patient's body and spirit, and although the receptivity of the patient and a belief in healing is useful, it is not necessary. Indeed, as seen in the section on research, this kind of energy can heal animals and affect isolated cells and tissues. Of course, there is a good deal of overlap between faith and psychic healing; a healer may transmit energy through touch, for example, and healing may occur also through the patient's faith in this act as a symbol.

Psychic healing is predominantly a gift or a 'grace'. It comes to some people naturally when they have attained a refined and pure state of consciousness. Contemplatives and ascetics see the arrival of healing abilities as one of the *siddhis* or psychic powers indicating progress on the spiritual path. Occasionally people discover that they have this gift without self-development. For example, two well-known contemporary healers, Oscar Estebany and Bruce McManaway, both discovered it while fighting in the army. Perhaps the stress and demand of battle crystallized this potential within them.

Healing is also taught. This teaching used to be part of an initiation given by word of mouth to those who had reached the required stage in their overall spiritual development. The secret doctrine was considered to be of such potency that years of patient study and devotion were necessary in order to prepare for the privilege of service to mankind. Today there is a tendency to teach healing as an uncovering, expressing a form of energy that exists to some extent in most of us though obscured by thought forms and conditioning.

One general prerequisite for healing is a strong desire to do so. As one well known healer put it:

the healing gift is born of the feelings of inner compassion and sympathy for the sick. This is expressed through a deep inner yearning to help take away pain, suffering and sickness . . . It follows that many nurses and doctors possess the healing potential even though they may not be aware of it.[4]

The healer is a channel, and the desire to offer healing enables him to open the mind towards the receipt of these energies and their controlling influences. As the healer becomes more receptive, so the purity of his channel is increased. Pure white light is often seen as a tangible representation of the divine energy and all healers wish to be able to convey this. White light is of course made up of all colours, each at a correct and balanced level. However, the healer who has not progressed very far will block much of the healing spectrum because of his own impurity.

Healers have different beliefs concerning the source of this channel of energy. Many healers talk of discarnate entities which they allow to work through them whilst others prefer to feel that all healing comes from their own being. One group links with the source of light, whilst others focus on God. Those that make use of discarnate entities sometimes recognize them to have been doctors or healers when alive. They state that it is reasonable that someone who has spent his earthly life in helping others should wish to continue to do so after death. The effectiveness of that help will be in accord with the knowledge and understanding of the intelligence directing it.

There may be two levels to a healer's energy. On one level it reaches a patient's physical body. This is sometimes known as magnetic healing[5] and it can be done by many people, the mother for her child, a visitor to the sick, or the doctor or nurse for their patient. It is a more physical energy which, when given, will often leave the healer feeling sapped or exhausted. The healer has effectively given out some of his own energies and unless certain simple techniques are used for their replacement, he may suffer. The second level is at the energy prototype of the physical body (sometimes known as the etheric). This contains all the disharmony of the inherited character, the anxiety of negative thoughts and situations, as well as the flow of life energy. Healing of the etheric stems from the souls of the patient and the healer and may well not be felt by either healer or patient. However, it may be possible for an intuitive healer to 'watch' the energies being transferred by means of clairvoyant sight. This is seen as changing colours radiating towards the patient and harmonizing tones.[6] The greater the self-purification of the healer the more refined and powerful are the energies which he can transmit.

Despite a vast literature on healing energy in particular and psychic energy in general, very little is actually known concerning what it is or how it affects the body. Reich's 'orgone energy', Hall's 'animal magnetism', Herder's 'universal force', von Reichenbach's 'odic force', not to mention the Eastern concepts of *prana, ch'i, shen*, and so on, are all descriptive systems depicting the same vital energy. Yet it is seen by its effects; its nature is a mystery. This remains the case despite some fascinating studies. For example, during healing the hands of a healer emit flares visible in Kirlian photographs, with simultaneous changes in the photograph of the recipient,[7] a healed person sometimes experiences considerable heat; psychic phenomena are prevented in a positively charged ionic atmosphere.[8] Modern physics has been encouraging in its revelation that not only is energy an emanation of matter, but matter itself is actually a form of energy. It is then suggested that the state of energy permeating our physical body will inevitably affect its organization and renewal. However, this raises other imponderables.

Diagnosis and treatment

Since disease or disharmony is caused by incorrect flow of life energy it follows that the deficiency must be isolated before a cure can be found. Diagnosis in psychic healing is therefore a two-stage process; first locating the physical seat of the problem, the disease, and then determining its origin in the etheric. It is felt that the physiological processes and cellular replication give off radiations which can be 'seen' through a sixth sense. Disharmonies are reflected in this aura. Therefore those who are sensitive and experienced can spot diseases through the aura at their very earliest stages.

The use of parapsychological faculties in diagnosis has certainly increased since the time of Edgar Cayce whose phenomenal abilities astounded the world but who was regarded as something of a freak. Now a large number of therapists and trainee therapists are learning to develop this insight. The more relaxed climate of opinion towards the supernatural helps them to keep an assured and balanced mind, an essential prerequisite to the development and use of these faculties. The technique may vary from observation of the colours of an aura or corona around individuals, to visualizing patches of light or shade on their bodies, or to sensing heat or tingling from diseased areas.

Just as there are different channels whereby the healer gains access to his energy, there are different practices whereby this energy is transferred on to the patient. Many healers lay their hands on a person or on a diseased part. This is particularly the case with therapists, such as osteopaths or nurses who have used hands to ease discomfort manually and then discovered a healing ability which is effective with the hand above as well as on the body.[9] The hands may also be used to 'stroke' the space around a person in a form of psychic massage. However, in all cases the hands are only focusing instruments for the healer's energy. Many healers heal without hands, and without even the presence of the patient. This is known as absent healing, and is carried out by many of the healing groups in the UK.

The most common form of healing is prayer. This can be done either through a direct request for divine intervention to bring about some change, or by the focusing of creative thought which surrounds the patient with the energies needed to assist in reharmonization. Personal prayer is a powerful and effective method, especially when it is accompanied by the recognition that some change in attitude and lifestyle may well be necessary to re-create balance and harmony. It can take time to work because the body may well be already depleted of energy and unable to respond quickly enough for the patient to feel the difference. Thus he may become dispirited and wonder if the effort is worthwhile.

Perhaps the best method of healing is the use of the technique of visualization of the problem, together with the provision of those energies which will bring about a change. This can be effective when used to help a patient who does not know that it is happening but a speedier result will be achieved if co-operation is possible. If the patient knows that healing will be transmitted at a certain time of the day, he can then relax, open his mind and visualize the energies surrounding and healing. This disciplined schedule and the knowledge that someone is helping can be very effective.

The visualization method can be illustrated by an incident related by the well-known healer Mathew Manning.[10] He described a vision he had while treating an autistic child. He felt himself travelling through her mind which appeared to him as a vast dark network. He moved about it as an aircraft moved over a dark city at night. As he moved he saw areas light up. The process continued until there was a sudden almost audible explosion of light at which point the girl's eyes focused for the first time.

Healers generally fall into two main classes. The vast majority are those who have developed their abilities and use them to provide a service to the public whilst continuing with a full time occupation. The strain required to do this is sometimes considerable. These healers do not charge fees for they believe that 'you cannot serve God and Mammon'. Furthermore, a stated fee might well prevent someone receiving healing because of restricted means. The second class of healer is the one who has had outstanding success and the demand for help has meant that healing has become a full-time occupation. As healers in this category rely on fees from patients they are obliged to state the minimum which they require. Some organizations run a referral service to both full- and part-time healers.

Healing is often combined with counselling. This enables the patients to look at their own attitudes in depth and discover unhelpful traits which they can then put right for themselves. Thus the thought processes are realigned towards harmony and the reactions are modified accordingly, so that after healing the physical body is not left in a stressed condition under which the disease will return.

Research

While there are a great many anecdotal reports of healing,[11] there have never been any significant controlled trials. Besides all the usual problems in applying double-blind methodology to complementary therapies, there is the problem that other explanations could usually be found for any definitive therapeutic result after healing.

There is a new research programme, announced by the Confederation of Healing Organizations in 1986, to spend £0.5 million on such research over the next few years. Patients at the Leeds Royal Infirmary with rheumatoid arthritis will receive conventional treatment alone, or combined with healing or simple counselling. Their long-term progress will be monitored. Another study will assess if healing will halt the normally irreversible clouding of the lens in cataracts.

Laboratory studies have been more successful. This is despite the fact that laboratory conditions are not ideal for most healers. In order to work effectively, the healer must maintain concentration on the patient whilst channelling the energies required. This is best done in an atmosphere of peace and tranquillity. The presence of people emitting destructive thoughts or even those who simply question the validity of the experiment can bring about failure.

A classical series of experiments carried out at McGill University in the 1960s showed that wounded mice healed much faster when a healer held his hands over them for 15 minutes twice a day. The controls in this case were a group of wounded mice who were similarly treated by a person who was not a healer, and an untreated group.[12] Similar kinds of experiments have shown that the growth of plants or fungi can be significantly affected by healing.[12,13]

Human cells cultured in the laboratory have been used in such studies. In one case a healer induced cancer cells to drop off the glass tube to which they had adhered but this did not happen when the tube was handled without 'switching on' the healing intention. In another case Mathew Manning was able to prolong the life of red blood cells within a weak salt solution (in which they normally burst) by up to four times. The chance of this happening normally was, according to the experimenters, about 100 000 to 1.[14] Experiments have been carried out with pure enzymes (biological catalysts) in the test tube. Under controlled conditions, a healer was asked to hold flasks of the enzyme trypsin. Other flasks of similar enzymes were either left untouched or exposed to a strong electromagnetic field. Time and again the effect of the healer's hands was found to be similar to that of the magnetic field. The activity of the enzymes was increased although the healer was not emanating any measurable electromagnetic energy.[15]

There have also been failures. Many noted healers 'dry up' in a laboratory setting, and others fail for reasons that are quite inexplicable to them. Mathew Manning, in reviewing his past record of 32 psychic experiments, stated that 17 were deemed successful by the experimenters. These were invariably with animals or biological materials, rarely with physical targets such as electrical gadgetry. He argues that naïve or sceptical experimenters almost never obtain significant results in their controlled experiments. The identical tightly controlled experiment performed within a positive milieu will generate positive results. 'The experimenter,' he concludes, 'has to conduct his tasks not as an Inquisitor, but as a partner.'[14]

It is also necessary for the experimenter to use his insight in order to disentangle a complex interaction within healing situations. For example, consider the phenomena of psychic surgery. In Brazil and the Philippines healers have traditionally used a technique in which they appear to extract diseased tissue, kidney stones, or tumours from patients who are then remarkably cured.[16] However, when the tissue is analysed, it has been found to be derived from an animal and not from the patient at all, a discovery that has been used in attempts to discredit these healers.[17] More dogged investigators have learnt that the healers do not really claim to have extracted the tissue, but use it for the display and theatre that attunes the patient to the healer. For as Westerners believe in surgery, the healer appears to accomplish it for their benefit. It certainly isn't all trickery. Lyall Watson reports that after submitting to 'a psychic injection' blood appeared on his arm under several layers of plastic sheet which was not punctured.[18] These controversies do not disprove the healers' undoubted powers.

Another fruitful line of research has been the analysis of brain wave patterns. Max Cade has demonstrated with electroencephalographic brain wave monitoring devices that healers, clairvoyants, and yogis show similar brain wave patterns when utilizing their concentrative abilities. The brain wave patterns of patients alter simultaneously with the receipt of healing. An experiment has been undertaken to show the power of distant or absent healing. In this case the patient was not told when the healer intended to begin and since healer and patient were many miles apart there was no possibility of collusion. Within a few minutes of the healer commencing work the patient's brain wave pattern changed and he went into a state of relaxation.[19]

Uses and risks

Healing is potentially applicable to any kind of condition; however, it is especially useful in the treatment of chronic conditions where the patient has insufficient energy and vitality for his own natural immune and self-healing abilities to operate. It is also very useful in a preventive role, restoring wholeness and resistance in an individual who is at risk, before a full blown disease develops.[20]

The famous miraculous instant cures of long-term and otherwise incurable diseases are a rarity in healing. Often a patient may lose his pain immediately and seem to be better—the 'throwing away of crutches'. However, the condition is still there and the symptoms soon return. Healing is, rather, a gradual process of removal of the problem and repair of the energies, which may take a considerable time. In addition, since patients may have incurred their disease through in some way living contrary to basic laws of natural good health, changes may be needed in their attitudes and lifestyle before the problem can be permanently overcome.

Healers report cases where cancer sufferers have overcome the disease with their help. The majority of cancer cases do not consider healing until they have been told that their situation is terminal. At this stage, the physical body will often be weakened but it is never too late to begin work.[21] Where the disease does not regress the healer is very often capable of relieving the pain and distress.[22]

There are no direct risks involved. Occasionally there may be a transient worsening of the symptoms after healing. This is usually a good sign, indicating that the body is throwing off the condition. The only risk is that, as with other therapies, a patient may delay other treatment that he needs while he is being healed. For this reason, if a patient has symptoms he should consult a relevant practitioner first as a matter of course. Healing can then be given in addition to or after other kinds of treatment.[23]

References

1. Sargant, W.W. (1973). *The mind possessed: A physiology of possession, mysticism and faith healing*. Heinemann, London.
2. Eliade, M. (1964). *Shamanism: Archaic techniques of ecstasy*. Princeton University Press. Halifax, J. (1982). *Shaman: The Wounded Healer*. Thames and Hudson, London.

3. Calestro, K.M. (1972). Psychotherapy, faith healing and suggestion. *International Journal of Psychiatry*, **10**, 83-113. Haynes, R. (1977). Faith healing and psychic healing. Are they the same? *Parapsychology Review*, July, 10-13.

4. Bloomfield, B. (1984). *The mystique of healing*. Skilton and Shaw, Edinburgh. Edwards, H. (1975). The science of spiritual healing. *Nursing Times*, **71**, 2008-10.

5. De Saussure, R. (1969). The magnetic cure. *British Journal of Medical Psychology*, **42**, 141-63.

6. Regush, N.M. (ed.) (1974). *The human aura*. Berkeley Medallion, New York.

7. Gennaro, L., Guzzon, F., and Marsigli, P. (1987). *Kirlian photography*, East West Publications, London. Moss, T. (1979). *The body electric*. Granada, St Albans.

8. Puharich, G. (1977). *Beyond Telepathy*, Granada, St Albans.

9. Krieger, D. (1976). Therapeutic touch. *Nursing Times*, **72**, 572-4. Davis, G. (1980). The hands of the healer. Has faith a place? *Journal of Medical Ethnics*, **6**, 185-9.

10. Wrekin Trust lecture (1981). Loughborough University.

11. Le Shan, L. (1985). *From Newton to ESP*. Viking, New York. Krippner, S. and Villoldo, A. (1976). *Realms of healing*. Celestial Arts, Millbrae, California.

12. Grad, B. (1965). Some biological effects of laying on of hands—A review of experiments with animals and plants. *Journal of the American Society for Psychical Research*, **59**, 95-126.

13. Barry, J. (1968). General and comparative study of the psychokinetic effect on a fungus culture. *Journal of Parapsychology*, **32**, 237-43.

14. Manning, M. (1979). Why experimenters upset results. *Alpha*, 11, November issue.

15. Smith, M.J. (1972). Paranormal effects on enzyme activity. *Human Dimensions*, **1**, 15-19.

16. Valentine, T. (1975). *Psychic Surgery*. Pocket Books, New York.

17. Granada Television 'World in Action' (4.4.75).

18. Watson, L. (1982). *Supernature*. Hodder & Stoughton, London.

19. Cade, M. and Coxhead, N. (1987). *The awakened mind: biofeedback and heightened states of awareness*. Element Books, Shaftesbury, Dorset.

20. Green, R. (1986). Healing and spirituality. *Practitioner*, **230**, 1087-93.

21. Magaray, C. (1981). Healing and meditation in medical practice. *Medical Journal of Australia*, **338**, 340-1.

22. Cadwell, D. (1986). Healing. *Health Visitor*, **59**, 347.

23. Havilland, D. (1986). Current position of spiritual healing in the United Kingdom. *Holistic Medicine*, **1**, 271-5.

13

Herbalism

Background

The use of plant materials for the treatment of illness is as old as civilization. Records containing lists of plants going back some 5000 years have survived from both ancient Egypt and China, with plants differentiated according to specific disease conditions for which they could be used.

There is certainly no form of human society known which, having access to flora in the locality, does not exhibit a profound understanding of the potential use of these plants. They are used for foods, medicines, and dyestuffs as well as for arrow poisons and antidotes, in religious rituals as hallucinogens, and for cosmetics. Indeed, such understanding seems to match directly the extent to which that society is integrated with its natural surroundings; the onset of civilized developments has often tended to diminish rather than enhance this fund of knowledge.[1]

Herbal knowledge is gathered through trial and error over long periods. Large numbers of plants are collected for various conditions and purposes, from food preparation and household maintenance at the one extreme to ritual practices at the other. Another source of herbal knowledge is intuitive revelations. Healers have often trained for years to amplify their sensitivity, observation, and intuition. They may detect effective substances by trying them out on themselves, or by receiving information while in ceremonial or altered states of consciousness. Most folk cultures will tell how plants appeared to their witch doctor in his dreams and told him of their powers. The Emperor Shen Nung, the 'heavenly husbandman', originator of Chinese herbal medicine, is said to have had a 'grace' which allowed him, on one occasion, to discover 70 new remedies in one single day. It is interesting to speculate that perhaps remedies discovered in this way are mild, adjustive, and preventive, just those remedies which cannot be detected by trying them out on sick people.[2]

From time to time in human history the evolution of a prosperous, creative civilization has been accompanied by attempts to formalize the available health care systems, most notably during the Greek and Islamic eras in the West, and as a continuous process in China and India in the East. However, at the level of village society, even today, primary health care is still largely herbal, and in the hands of an untrained, most often female, member of the group, who has maintained her direct intuitive link with local plants.[3] The herbal practitioner still trusts in experience and intuition rather than in works of scholarship. This has meant that herbal medicine has escaped literate attention and in its essential form has played little part in the social affairs of man in the West.

The use made of plants as medicines has always conformed to the whole view of the human organism in its universe. In China and India the cosmology has emphasized the integration of existence. This has produced vitalistic concepts in which the qualities of herbs are matched to the qualities or disharmonies which have caused disease. For example, according to Chinese medicine, the tastes of plants are an indication of their likely effects on disturbed organ systems. The early traditions of the West, particularly Greece, led to an inclination to see the world analytically, producing a symptomatic cause-and-effect manner of using plants (see p. 13). This way of using plant medicines has tended to dominate in the West and has shaped, during the nineteenth century, the methods of drug use of modern medicine.[1]

During medieval times the use of herbs was laden with superstition, incantation, and ritual. A sick person taking a certain herb might have to walk seven times round a tomb reciting a Latin phrase to ensure efficacy. When European herbals were being written in the sixteenth and seventeenth centuries, a large part of the information came from ancient Greek (Dioscorides and Galen) and Islamic (Avicenna) sources; these were combined with scatterings of folklore to create the patchy accounts for each remedy that have marked popular books on herbalism ever since.[4] Traditional herbalists still practised relatively efficiently at the village level but in urban areas the stage was occupied by practitioners pursuing symptomatic medicine.[5] These found herbal remedies unsuitable for their purposes and turned more and more to inorganic remedies and surgery.

Violent arguments raged between the herbal 'Galenicists' and the 'Chymists'. The power and purity of the Chymists' compounds were so attractive to a rapidly growing technological age that herbal remedies were gradually discredited. With the arrival of scientific medicine this process continued—not because the herbal remedies were demonstrably ineffective, but because they did not fit into the system. 'Many of the plants used as medicines can no longer be considered within the pale of rational therapeutics', explains a pharmacology textbook.[6] The plants were dropped from the pharmacopoeia during the first part of this century despite the fact that plants were and still are used as starting materials for the manufacture of drugs. Of 1.5 billion prescriptions dispensed in the USA annually 25 per cent contained active constituents obtained from plants but only 2.5 per cent contained crude plant material. More serious, the knowledge of how best to use these plants was also threatened with extinction.

The survival of modern herbalism owes a good deal to widespread emigration from Europe to North America in the eighteenth and nineteenth centuries. In this period thousands of emigrants were distributed over the huge continent with a minimum of standard European health care. They brought with them the memories of common herbal treatment in rural areas of their native country and often the actual medicinal plants themselves. They also encountered the considerable medical intelligence of the North American Indian, based very largely on herbs. It was in many other ways of course a destructive meeting, but in medicine the combination of necessity, disenchantment with European sophistication, and a raw enterprise resulted in the brief flowering of many new developments. Osteopathy and chiropractic have survived to this day, but there were also several short-lived schools of herbal medicine. Several times around the turn of the century the new herbal medicine was re-imported back to the UK where it hybridized well with the herbal traditions still surviving there. Today, the largest body of herbal practitioners in the UK sees itself as the heir to the North American experiment.

In the UK medical herbalism has for centuries been practised mainly in country districts and, after the Industrial Revolution, in the new working-class cities. It has survived to the present day and a combination of a successful move to protect the definition 'medical herbalist' under the terms of the 1968 Medicines Act, and the emergence of a new generation of practitioner seeking an alternative to allopathic practice, has now transformed the profession.

Fundamental concepts

Because of the primitive and diffuse origins of herbal medicine, in the West, there has never been any 'school' determining basic philosophy nor even any universally accepted fundamental concepts. Because it has been *the* medical system for most people most of the time, it has tended to be all things to all men. However, the main assumption in herbal medicine is that there is a vitality in the human frame that stands apart from the therapeutic endeavours of the practitioner. This vital force can be seen as a purposeful, self-correcting, resistant force transcending the abrasions of life. For example, the astonishingly exact maintenance of body temperature through a wide range of situations is to the modern herbalist a clear manifestation of an ability that no man-made therapy can augment. The aim of herbal medicine is to support the action of this vital adaptive energy wherever it appears to be weakening.

Modern Western herbalists use much the same terminology and concepts as current orthodoxy but they are interested in detecting and restoring normal function rather than acting to stop a pathology. The symptom is seen as a sign, if read correctly, pointing to the seat of the disorder. For example an infection may point in the first place to 'stagnation' of the affected tissues. Healthy tissues, like running water, cannot suffer colonization by bacteria; such an invasion can only occur in the histological equivalent of the brackish pond. Treatment of infections then demands that the tissue be 'cleansed' and brought back into the vital circulation. Antibiotics would only be necessary in this scheme if the colonization was so excessive that there was real doubt as to the host's ability to overcome it from vital resources, and then appropriate only if underlying stagnation were treated as well. Using antibiotics alone is seen as being as productive as pouring disinfectant into a brackish puddle and pronouncing it 'clean'.

The same concern with underlying causes marks the herbal practitioner's approach to other conditions. A spasmodic condition like asthma or colitis speaks first of an irritant factor combined with a tendency to over-react. An inflammatory condition like skin disease or arthritis speaks of a healthy but insufficient attempt to eliminate toxic accumulations. Similarly, in dealing with migraine or the autoimmune conditions a primary aim is to search for the source of toxicity, perhaps in defective digestive or liver function or in inadequate elimination.

Victorian herbalism divided herbs into classes according to their effect on discrete physiological processes—diuretics to cause urination, alteratives to adjust the metabolism, purgatives to clean out toxic materials from the digestive system, and so on. Modern herbalism is much more sophisticated, but it has developed these adjustive concepts, largely through an awareness of modern medical and biochemical science, rather than displaced them.

What are the essential therapeutic features of the herbal remedy? They can be classified in three ways.[7]

1. Herbal remedies have challenging qualities which tend to provoke a number of protective responses from the body. In particular they make excellent local applications in damage to skin and stomach lining. Mucilaginous components, such as marshmallow root, soothe and provide physical protection and relief from irritation and pain; tannins and other astringent factors, such as witch hazel, form tough antiseptic coats over exposed tissue or mucosal surfaces. Both these properties generate useful reactions in the stomach, reducing spasm and colic. Other herbs trigger helpful physiological reactions. For example the anthraquinone glycosides of senna work by gently irritating the bowels to produce elimination, the acrid glycosides in chilli, ginger, and mustard stimulate the blood vessels to increase the flow through the tissues, and the bitter herbs, such as gentian, stimulate a range of digestive reflexes (flow of bile, movement of gastrointestinal muscles, gastric secretions, appetite, etc.) when held in the mouth. Other examples include the production of expectoration (cough) reflexes or diuresis in the urinary system. These kinds of agents rely on the presence of the reactions in the body which the plant triggers.

2. Herbal remedies can adjust body processes. They exhibit a normalizing, supportive action on organs and tissues, acting almost like foods rather than medicines. For example, the effect of oat extracts on chronically poor vitality, nervous exhaustion, or 'neurasthenia' is likely to be due to the balance of minerals and other nutrients supplied as well as to the dynamic action of saponins and alkaloids; a similar relationship is likely to hold for the dandelion

root and the liver, coltsfoot and the lungs, or couch grass root (*Triticum repens*) and the kidneys. A balanced action can be demonstrated for other remedies. By simultaneously increasing coronary blood flow and yet slowing the heart rate, the hawthorn (*Crataegus oxyacantha*) finds application in cases where the heart is under strain.[7] In another variation, the action of the ginseng root improves the ability of the adrenal cortex to respond optimally to stress. The fruit of the chasteberry tree is thought to influence a wide range of gynaecological problems by acting on the pituitary to 'balance' the secretions of progesterone and oestrogen. In other cases the presence of a number of constituents in the same plant helps to explain paradoxical actions. The isolated cardiac glycosides of the lily-of-the-valley plant are not as effective as those of the foxglove yet in the context of the whole plant it is a most useful and relatively safe cardiac remedy for it has a graded effect and is also a diuretic. In all these cases much of the benefit arises from the whole remedy being used, the many often uncounted constituents having total effects greater than the sum of their parts.

3. In a great number of ways herbal remedies are eliminatory. They are particularly good at improving the action of the eliminatory organs, the bowels, kidneys, lungs, and sweat glands, and at improving circulation ('heat'). This results in increased nourishment as well as drainage, both to tissues at large and to particular organs. Herbal remedies also work at improving the ability of the digestive system to handle and detoxify potentially dangerous substances in the diet and particularly at enhancing the ability of the liver to convert and excrete the whole range of metabolites. The herbalist feels justified in claiming to be able to 'clean out' the body to a degree that other therapies do not attempt to match.

There are also a considerable number of herbs, derived from folk medicine and used today as household remedies, which have effects on specific symptoms outside the above categories. Examples include aloe vera (wound healing, antibacterial, and anti-inflammatory), garlic (antibacterial, antifungal), valerian (sedative), or wormwood (antihelminthic).

Diagnostic and therapeutic practices

The modern Western herbalist most often uses the diagnostic

methods and tools of the good general practitioner in Britain, although he will place more emphasis on finding out why the disease occurred at this particular time. There are also some practitioners who use Chinese diagnostic methods (see Chapter 6) or radionics, iridology, and some intuitive methods. Generally, the herbalist will determine the patient's medical history, the nature of current stresses, dietary habits and lifestyle, and performance of the main functions of the body: digestion, respiratory system, genito-urinary systems, circulation, and nervous and emotional functions. This is combined with such clinical assessments as are considered useful: blood pressure, pulse taking, physical examination, microscopic assessment of urine and blood smears, etc. The terms of the diagnosis may only partly include the name of a disease state or pathology and it usually includes functional terms such as 'vascular spasm', 'hypersensitivity', 'hyperacidity', 'chronic inflammation', 'nervous debility', and so on, the better to reflect the therapeutic direction of the treatment.

Treatment is selected according to what aspect of health is judged most in need of support. An attempt will be made to deduce what is likely to be the 'primary lesion' and this treated first; this might present some difficulties in those advanced pathologies where layers of secondary effects and tissue damage have to be taken into account. Advice is given concerning environmental stresses and diet, the consensus opinion being that where possible diet should be as primitive as is practicable, using whole foods, fresh fruits, and vegetables. Nervous tension, both obvious and otherwise, is treated less by herbal 'tranquillizers' (such as Passiflora) than by use of 'relaxants', such as camomile or hops, that reduce the effect of such tension on the viscera. Where there are debilitated conditions these will be treated with restoratives, trigger remedies may be given to arouse normal function, and temporary protection will be provided where practicable by the use of mucilaginous and other such agents. The overall aim is to lead to sufficient correction of body functions that normal homeostatic regulation may take over; in other words treatment is as short as possible and discontinued as early as conditions allow. Any extended treatment is seen as something of a failure and generally denotes either an advanced pathology or else incorrigible environmental stresses.

For example, in the treatment of rheumatoid arthritis a dietary regime may first be organized, usually with vitamin supplementation and instructions on avoiding certain foods. Internal remedies may include angelica to increase diuresis and sweating and *Apium* where there is depression. *Cimifuga* is used where sciatica and neuralgia exist; this is combined with *Phytolacca dec.* especially where the condition is chronic, and *Galium aparine* which aids in effects on lymph. *Dioscorea vill.* is used for rheumatism and rheumatoid arthritis, acting through the hormones, and *Filipendula* against acidity. External applications of *Symphytum* will reduce inflammation, rosemary is used against pain, and it also, like mint and cayenne pepper, aids the circulation.

Preparations may contain a complex mixture of constituents: a dozen would not be unusual. The remedies will usually be provided by the practitioner rather than through a third party. Sometimes they are provided 'off the shelf' by retail herbalists although this is now rare. They will most often be in the form of tinctures (concentrated extracts of the herbs in water/alcohol solvent) for ease of dispensing. If bulk is not a problem the herbs may be provided in capsule or tablet form. However, these are inappropriate in many cases due to the large quantities of herbs often needed; a tincture remains the most compact way of administering herbs.

Uses and risks

Medical herbalists generally feel confident in treating most conditions that they might encounter.[8] There are one or two legal limitations in the UK, notably venereal disease, and acute and dangerous conditions are referred to casualty wards or doctors. Moreover, most practitioners avoid interfering with vital allopathic treatment already under way, such as insulin, antithrombotic drugs, and so on, because of the risks involved, and in other cases the contribution of other therapies will be accepted. In particular, manipulative work will be referred elsewhere for appropriate treatment, and psychiatric or emotional disorders are often passed on as well. Epilepsy, schizophrenia, and neurological diseases prove particularly resistant to treatment, and no false claims are made when there is other established tissue damage to contend with.

Herbal medicine comes into its own where there are physiological tasks to be done and where there are accumulations to clear. It is thus useful in organic problems of any sort, for chronic infective conditions anywhere in the body, and for restoring debilitated organs or functions. It also has a largely undervalued role in external applications where there is no suitable alternative therapy. There are few risks with herbal treatment provided it is monitored by a competent herbalist. However, as material dosages are used minor side-effects, such as irritations from the stimulating trigger remedies, might occasionally be encountered. Herbs, when used by the herbalist to restore function, do not have the toxic effects of the more pharmacologically incisive conventional drugs.

Research

With the predominance of allopathic medicine in the developed world this century comparatively little active work has been done in researching into the efficacy of plant remedies.[8] A notable exception in the West has been West Germany where plant remedies are widely used by the semi-orthodox Heilpraktikers. There are several German journals reporting on research work into aspects of phytotherapy. In the UK the amount of research is particularly low and is confined to the disciplines of pharmacognosy (the definition and analysis of medicinal plants) and phytochemistry (biochemical analysis of plant function).

In Eastern bloc countries, where the monopoly of the drug companies is less complete, there has been a more appreciative interest in plant-based medicine. Original research work is also frequently reported in China, Japan, and India. There are several specialist journals that report this work[10]. Examples include studies showing that garlic and onion juice are highly effective in reducing cholesterol and lipids in the circulation;[11] that liquorice root is more effective at healing gastric ulcers than any current conventional drug, provided it is taken on an empty stomach;[12] that *Bupleurum* species, used in the Far East for jaundice, can repair damaged liver tissues;[13] that *capsicum* from cayenne pepper has specific stimulatory effects on nerve cells;[14] that a large number of hallucinogenic and traditional ritual remedies—*datura, iboga, yaje, peyote, cannabis, psilocybe, coca*, etc.—have all be shown to contain psychoactive substances of great interest;[15] *Pueraria* root, used traditionally to relieve circulatory problems, has been found to be highly effective in improving cerebral blood supply;[16] thyme is known to be antibacterial;[17] the green-lipped mussel has been shown to be effective in treating arthritis;[18] aloe vera has been demonstrated to improve skin blood supply, reduce inflammation, and hasten wound healing and cell growth;[19] garlic is now well established as an anti-infective agent—the author has á database of some 700 scientific papers on this plant alone.[20]

A steady stream of conventional drugs has been derived from traditional remedies. Recent examples include the anticancer substances *vinblastine* and *vincristine* from periwinkle, the blood pressure lowering and antitussive *reserpine* from the Indian insanity herb, steroid hormones from *Dioscorea*, and an antimigraine remedy from feverfew. It is very clear that published research has only scratched the surface. There are half a million plants on this planet, and only about 5 per cent have been scientifically investigated. Even in these cases they have only been tested against certain diseases. In the US National Cancer Institute plant screening programme some 20 500 species of plant have been investigated against one or two kinds of animal tumours. Professor Farnsworth commented:[21]

This single example clearly points out that in the most extensive pharmacological investigation of plants in the history of the world, only a fraction (1 per cent) of the total available plants have been evaluated for a single type of activity. Thus even plants from this study can be considered 'uninvestigated'.

Researchers can, however, greatly increase the chance of demonstrating medicinal activity in plants by working with the traditional practitioners that use them.[22] There is no lack of opportunity.

Types of therapist

The most common types of herbal therapists now practising in the UK can be classified in five groups:

1. The retail herbalists, still common in the Midlands and North, supplying across-the-counter medicines in a near-symptomatic fashion, and a variable range of professional treatments as well, often through using the same patent medicines. This was the only considerable body of practitioners in this country until recently but is now diminishing in number. Retail herbalists often possess an uncanny knack of hitting the nail on the head but also provide a refuge for incompetent practitioners.

2. The hakims, the name givem to herbal practitioners in Islam and the Indian sub-continent. In Britain these are found entirely in immigrant areas administering the various Indian medical systems to immigrant patients.

3. The Chinese herbalists are both traditional, confined to Chinese centres in the main cities, and, increasingly, modern, where the practitioner is usually a young European who uses herbs in conjunction with an acupuncture practice.

4. The professional medical herbalists, applying Western herbal medicines in the confines of the consulting room. Usually members of the National Institute of Medical Herbalists, these practitioners have increased in number recently. They tend to hold a sophisticated view of their therapy and are the nearest to aligning it with mainstream medical thought; in fact a few are medical practitioners.

5. A miscellaneous group who temper their practice of herbal medicine with other modes of diagnosis or treatment. It is almost impossible to generalize about these. Some use healing, dowsing, radionics, hair analysis, or iris diagnosis; others are also osteopaths or naturopaths or even homeopaths primarily, using herbs as a supporting therapy.

6. Aromatherapists, who use herbs in the form of distilled essential oils.[23] These oils are concentrated, and often used as an adjunct to massage (see Chapter 16). However they are also prescribed internally in doses of a drop or two, for example to relieve symptoms such as intestinal cramps and pain in the case of peppermint oil,[24] or lift mood in the case of basil oil.

References

1. Griggs, B. (1981). *Green pharmacy: A history of herbal medicine.* Jill Norman, London.
2. Fulder, S. (1987). *The Tao of medicine: Ginseng, oriental remedies and the pharmacology of harmony.* Destiny Books, Rochester, Vermont.
3. Bannerman, R.H. Burton, J., and Wen-Chieh, C. (1983), *Traditional medicine and health care coverage.* World Health Organization, Geneva. Doyal, L. (1987). Health, underdevelopment and traditional medicine. *Holistic Medicine,* **2,** 27–40.
4. Culpeper, N. (1979). *Culpeper's complete herbal.* Foulsham, Slough,

Middlesex. Grieve, M. (1982). *A modern herbal*. Peregrine Books, Harmondsworth, Middlesex. This title is the best herbal available. Wren, R.W. (1979). *Potters new cyclopaedia of botanical drugs and preparations*. Health Science Press, Holsworthy.

5. Ruppere, V. (1981). The survival of traditional medicine in lay medical views. *Medical History*, 25, 411–4. See also Vogel, V.J. (1982). *American Indian medicine*. University of Oklahoma Press, Norman. Whorton, J.C. (1987). Traditions of folk medicine in America. *Journal of the American Medical Association*, 257, 1632–5.

6. Melmon, K.L. and Morrelli, H.F. (eds) (1972). *Clinical pharmacology*. Macmillan, New York.

7. Grieve, M. (1982). *A modern herbal*. Peregrine Books, Harmondsworth, Middlesex. Fluck, H. (1976). *Medicinal plants*. Foulsham, Slough, Middlesex.

8. Mills, S. (1986). *The dictionary of modern herbalism: The complete guide to herbs and therapy*. Thorsons, Wellingborough.

9. Wagner, H. and Wolff, P. (1977). *New natural products and plant drugs with pharmacological, biological and therapeutic activity*. Springer-Verlag, Heidelberg. World Health Organization (WHO), (1980). Traditional medicine: A world survey on medicinal plants and herbs. *Journal of Ethnopharmacology*, 2, 1–92. Krieg, M.B. (1965). *Green medicine*. Harrap, London and Toronto.

10. Important journals in English in the field are *Lloydia, Planta Medica, Journal of Ethnopharmacology, Quarterly Journal of Crude Drug Research, Chemical and Pharmaceutical Bulletin, Economy Botany*. Mowrey, D.B. (1986). *The scientific validation of herbal medicine*. Cormorant Books, Leha, Utah. Fulder, S. (1987). *The Tao of medicine: ginseng, oriental remedies and the pharmacology of harmony*. Destiny Books, Rochester, Vermont (Oriental herbs.) Bhatia, S.L. (1972). Research on Indian medicinal plants. *Indian Council of Medical Research Bulletin*, 2(4), 1–6; 2(5), 1–11; 2(6), 1–6. (For Indian research.)

11. Bordia, A., Bausal, H.C., and Arora, S.K. (1975). Effect of essential oils of garlic and onion on alimentary hyperlipaemia. *Atherosclerosis*, 21, 15–9.

12. Chen, K.K. and Mukerji, B. (1965). *Pharmacology of oriental plants*. Pergamon Press, Oxford and New York.

13. Arichi, S., Konishi, H., and Abe H. (1978). Saikosaponins from Bupleurum falcatum and the restoration of function in the carbon tetrachloride damaged liver. *Liver*, 19, 430–5.

14. Nagy, J.I., Vincent, S.R., Staines, W.A., Fibiger, H.C., Reisine, T.D., and Yamamura, H.I. (1980). Neurotoxic action of capsaicin on spinal substance p. neurones. *Brain Research*, 186, 435–4.

15. Schultes, R.E. (1969). Hallucinogens of plant origins. *Science*, **163**, 245–54.
16. Qicheng, F. (1980). Some current study and research approaches relating to the use of plants in traditional Chinese medicine. *Journal of Ethnopharmacology*, **2**, 57–63.
17. Pat'akov, D. and Chl'adek, M. (1974). The antibacterial activity of thyme and wild thyme oils. *Pharmazie*, **29**, 140.
18. Gibson, R.G. and Gibson, S.L.M. (1981). 'Green-lipped Mussel in Arthritis', *Lancet*, **i**, 439.
19. Zawahry, M., Hegazy, M.R., and Helal, M. (1973). Use of aloes in treating leg ulcers and dermatoses. *International Journal of Dermatology*, **12**, 68. Cere, S. *et al.* (1980). The therapeutic efficacy of aloe vera cream in thermal injuries. *Journal of the American Animal Hospital Association*, **16**, 768.
20. Blackwood, J. and Fulder, S. (1986). *Garlic: Nature's original remedy*. Javelin Books, Poole, Dorset.
21. Farnsworth, N.R. and Morris, R.M. (1976). Higher plants—the sleeping giant of drug development. *American Journal of Pharmacology*, **148**, 46–52.
22. Farnsworth, N.R. and Kaas, C.J. (1981). An approach utilising information from traditional medicine to identify tumour inhibiting plants. *Journal of Ethnopharmacology*, **3**, 85–99.
23. Tisserand, R.B. (1985). *The art of aromatherapy*. Daniel, Saffron Walden, Essex.
24. Dew, M., Evans, B.J., Rhodes, J. (1984). Peppermint oil for the irritable bowl syndrome: a multicentre trial. *British Journal of Clinical Practice*, **38**, 11–21.

14

Homeopathy

Background

Homeopathy is a system of treatment developed from the natural law of *similia similibus curantur*—'like is cured by like'. That is, a substance or preparation which can cause groups of symptoms, whether physical, emotional, or behavioural, in the healthy, can cure similar groups of symptoms when they appear as a deviation from normal in the sick. This principle was recognized by both Hippocrates and Paracelsus but was only developed as a practical method of healing by Dr Samuel Hahnemann who published his *Homeopathic Materia Medica* in 1811.[1] Hahnemann first noticed this principle in action in observing the effect of Peruvian bark, the standard treatment for malaria at the time; it produced 'malarial' fevers when he ingested it.

Through careful observation of the effect of remedies upon himself and others over a period of years, Hahnemann was able to define the effect of very many substances. He called this system 'the proving of remedies'. The conditions for this self-testing procedure were stringent. Only healthy and balanced individuals could test the remedies. Any deviations from usual function and patterns of behaviour, however small, were noted. In some cases Hahnemann mentions up to 4000 symptoms.

Although Hahnemann was most successful with his form of selecting remedies, he was aware that in using significant dosages he often added to the symptoms caused by the disease. Because he was always concerned that medicine should cure without harm, he attempted to give small dosages of his remedies to patients. But these had reduced therapeutic effects. It was then that he made a curious and astonishing discovery. When he shook the preparations violently during dilution, he retained their potency despite a considerably reduced dose. This process, described as 'potentization' has become a key element of homeopathy. In some ways it has wrongly eclipsed the other aspects of Hahnemann's system, for 'homeopathy' has crept into common language as a word for a minute dosage.

Hahnemann went on to discover that although the homeopathically indicated remedy cured the patients' acute conditions with ease, it did not seem to stop more than temporarily the degeneration of health we call chronic disease. He spent some 12 years in research and observation to find out why. Finally, he deduced that there were general influences, inherited and acquired, which affect the whole of our health processes. These chronic disease tendencies, which he called 'miasms', are the soil in which the weeds of disease can grow. They are not what we call disease but without them there could be no disease. This theory has provoked controversy among homeopaths and others ever since it was formulated in the *Theory of chronic diseases* published in 1828.[1]

Hahnemann died in 1846, leaving behind a reasonably complete system for curing the sick. Since then, many homeopaths have added to the store of knowledge, not the least of whom was Constantine Hering, who formulated what was known as the Law of Cure, an observation about the progression of symptoms in the disease process and the healing process. He observed that if the patient was being cured then the symptoms moved from the vital internal organs to the less vital organs, and finally to the skin; symptoms also disappeared downwards and in the reverse order of their development. Observation by other homeopaths over the past 120 years has verified this law, which has the value of revealing if the patient is being cured or the condition suppressed.

Fundamental concepts

The therapeutic system known as homeopathy works because of certain generally unacknowledged characteristics of human and other organisms. These characteristics are defined as follows:

1. The organism is in a constant state of self-repair, and all organs and parts are constantly renewing themselves. This means that there is a considerable capacity for overcoming the cause of disease, if that capacity can be stimulated into activity.

2. The cure can only be achieved by the organism through its own devices. This means that the homeopathic definition of cure may be different to more common uses of the word.

3. The organism becomes sensitive to that which will stimulate cure: i.e. that which is *homeopathic* to the patient. The extreme degree of sensitivity of the organism to the unique (homeopathic) stimulant is appreciated by those who are familiar with the amount of dilution involved with most homeopathic remedies.

Homeopathy employs an essentially 'vitalistic' model of the body. As Hahnemann stated:

In the healthy condition of man the spiritual, vital force, the dynamism that animates the material body (organism), rules with unbounded sway and retains all parts of the organism in admirable harmonious vital operation . . . when a person falls ill . . . it is only the vital force, deranged from such an abnormal state, that can furnish the organism with its disagreeable sensations, and incline it to the irregular process we call disease.

Disease therefore occurs when the vital principle is unable to cope with changes occurring to the organism. It becomes overwhelmed, demonstrating that fact by the production of symptoms in the body.

In homeopathy, disease is regarded as a process not a 'thing'. It can be detected as close to its origin as the training and sensitivity of the observer or patient allows. The conventional usage of the word disease describes only the final stage of its development, the pathological stage where the *structure* of the physical body begins to lose its integrity and there is tissue damage. However, there are several other stages previous to this where there is a loss of integrity of *function*. A characteristic of these previous stages is a sense of malaise, of dis-ease, within the person, the 'I don't feel well' stage which may precede development of the pathological stage by days, weeks, months, or even years. These previous stages are accessible to the homeopathic practitioner. Cure can therefore be accomplished farther 'upstream', before a serious condition develops.

The homeopath does not regard the symptoms as being the disease, rather as an expression of the body in its reaction to the underlying problem. He therefore reads the symptom picture of the body in order to define the sort of curative efforts the body is making of itself. He will then work for the remedy that will stimulate self-healing. The correct remedy is the one which produces an identical pattern of symptoms when given to healthy people in material dosages. The art of the homeopath is, to a large extent, the interpretation and matching of the symptom picture of the patient with the correct drug picture of a remedy. For example, arsenic poisoning produces symptoms so close to those of cholera that it is hard to tell them apart without tests. Therefore, highly diluted arsenic trioxide is a remedy for cholera or gastroenteritis. The process is like that of finding two patterns which interlock exactly, or two vibrational frequencies which will resonate together. For that reason a single remedy, the simillimum, the most similar, is sought. A remedy that duplicates three-quarters of the symptoms of the patient, even if combined with another which duplicates the other quarter, will be useless.

The matching of symptoms defines homeopathy: 'the determination as to whether or not a remedy is homeopathic is derived neither from its amount nor from its form, but solely from its relation to the disease' is a classic definition put forward by the German national homeopathic organization in 1836. However, it is based on empirical observation going back to Greek medicine. The reason for it is still mysterious, although a recent bold attempt to derive a 'unified field theory' of homeopathy has suggested that there are archetypes in nature (from which remedies are derived) and human archetypes (expressed as characteristic sets of symptoms). If the archetypes match, they cancel each other out, like the self-annihilation of two equal but opposite vibrations.[2]

Conventional medicine could accept a small segment of homeopathic teaching, largely in the field of immunology. Hahnemann in fact referred to Jenner's cowpox vaccine as homeopathic. There are treatments which are comparable, though unrelated to, homeopathy. Today's 'attenuated' vaccines are viruses which are so highly diluted that they stimulate body defences without producing the disease itself. In pharmacology some metabolic and anticoagulant remedies work on a like cures like principle,[3] and it is very well known that remedies which have toxic effects at higher dosages are stimulatory or beneficial at low dosages. A good example is strychnine, from *Nux vomica*, which is highly toxic but used in both conventional and homeopathic medicine in small doses.

It is this question of dose which has caused the greatest

controversy. Not so much that the patient is sensitive to the minute doses of the exact remedy that will cure him, but that the doses involved are sometimes so minute that it seems inconceivable that any of the original material is left at all. For if something is diluted beyond Avogadro's Constant (6×10^{23}) there should no longer be a single molecule of the original left. Many homeopathic remedies are diluted well above this, and these high dilutions are regarded by experienced homeopaths as their most potent. They are often used in more chronic and difficult conditions. To some extent homeopathy regards this as a conundrum only for scientists, and a reliable everyday reality for practitioners. However, much of the research on homeopathy has been directed towards this 'magic of the minimum dose'.[4] This research tends to show a remarkable phenomenon, that when poisons stimulate biological processes at the lowest invisible dosages, there are 'peaks' and 'troughs' of maximal and minimal activation. Mercuric chloride has been found, for example, to activate an enzyme, diastase, maximally at 10^{-15}, 10^{-25}, 10^{-45}, 10^{-65}, 10^{-75}, and 10^{-110}, and minimally at 10^{-20}, 10^{-55}, 10^{-85}, and 10^{-105}.[5] However this activation only happened with dilutions prepared with vigorous shaking. An ingenious proposal has been put forward by two American physicists, who attempt to explain this not in terms of chemicals but of information. They suggest that a dissolved substance leaves an imprint of itself after high dilution. That is, the energy of shaking aids the substance to act as a template, producing matching configurations within the water, which are then replicated within the body. Homeopathic remedies do not transmit chemicals but information. The homeopathic physician matches 'the pure quantised informational content of particular chemicals to the informational needs of his patient'.[6]

On the other hand physical explanations may be missing the point. These high potencies may be acting at a subtle level on the subtle energy body rather than the physical body. It may be that at high potencies homeopathy takes off into this realm of healing, whether the homeopath recognizes it or not.

Diagnosis and treatment

Diagnosis involves finding out what changes from the normal the patient had experienced. These changes may be registered by the patient or observed by the homeopath and may be physical, sensory, emotional, mental, or even moral. The aim of 'taking the case' is to describe the abnormal, which we call symptoms, as completely as possible. A pain may be noted by the patient, but the homeopath will ask what time of day the pain occurs, whether the pain is intermittent or continuous, how the patient feels under different weather or temperature conditions, and so on. The peculiar or abnormal symptoms (e.g. 'pain in wrists when lying down') are the most important in a hierarchy of significance; how they vary under changing conditions is next. The psychological profile of the patient is also significant, while general habits and preferences such as liking for sweet or sour foods, are added on to give a constitutional picture. There is usually a physical examination.

Diagnosis in homeopathy is expressed not in the name of a disease, nor even in a description of a symptom picture, but in the name of the remedy which corresponds to it. A good description of this is given by Vithoulkas[7] who lists various kinds of influenza experienced during an epidemic (influenza being one of the most straightforward cases). A *Gelsemium semper virens* influenza is characterized by lethargy, dullness with a paradoxical tendency to insomnia, the face is flushed, the lips and skin dusky, there is an unstable heat reaction to the fever, the skin hot and sticky, the lips very dry, there is a throbbing congestive headache with dizziness, and so on. *Bryonia Alba* patients have some of these symptoms, but are also irritable and depressed. During their influenza they experience thirst with generalized aching pain, and they are restless, and always moving about. There are many other types of influenza each with a somewhat different set of symptoms.

In acute cases the remedy may be any one of hundreds and the homeopath is guided to it by the individual version of disease produced by the patient. In chronic cases the remedy will usually be what is called the 'constitutional', since it is indicated by the individuality of the *patient* and not the individuality of the disease. The *constitution* of an individual is more or less fixed and the remedy which stimulates the recuperative ability will usually stay the same throughout life, although with the increased pace, pressure, and complexity of our lives, and the increasing power of symptom-modifying orthodox drugs, the clarity of the constitutional picture is sometimes much obscured. One talks, for example, about a *Nux vomica* type, a *Sulphur* or *Pulsatilla* type. These types arise empirically during provings where it is noticed that certain kinds of constitutions react strongly to certain remedies. However the same remedies can also be used for acute conditions. *Pulsatilla* is often indicated in the symptom grouping of measles. Some remedies are also chosen on the basis of affinity to the affected part. Thus *Sepia* (squid ink) corresponds to the female reproductive organs.

Only one remedy needs to be given at a time, except where the patient has had previous suppressive therapy in which case this is usually treated first. The homeopath will observe the changes in the patient produced by this remedy. A temporary aggravation of the symptoms indicates that a curative process has been stimulated in the body and is a good sign. Similarly, if symptoms move outwards, for example, if skin eruptions occur in an asthma patient, a curative process has been stimulated. When there is no result the homeopath will try to match another remedy, or re-question the patient to establish what symptoms were omitted previously. The more experienced homeopaths use high potencies which are more subtle and yet powerful. However, less experienced homeopaths usually use remedies at a lower potency, such as $6 \times$, which is 1×10^6. First aid remedies available to the public are generally at a low potency. In the cases where several chronic disease tendencies (miasms) are involved then treatment may be prolonged, involving peeling off 'the layers of the onion' one at a time. This process is the re-creation of lost health and not merely a conquering of disease as we normally think of it.

Remedies are prepared by grinding plant materials in alcohol and leaving them for two weeks before filtering to give a 'mother tincture'. This, as with all homeopathic remedies, should be stored away from chemical influences such as strong smells. Minerals and insoluble materials are very finely ground with lactose. Dilutions are then prepared by mixing with solvent and dropping the bottle onto a hard rubber slab or by trituration with more lactose. 1:10 dilutions are described as $1 \times 2 \times \ldots$; 1:100 as 1c, 2c . . .; and 1:1000 as 1M, 2M . . . $\times$ dilutions are meant to be more powerful than c dilutions. The remedies are presented in the homeopathic pharmacopoeia of various countries, which are currently being unified. There are about 3000 remedies: plant, mineral, and occasionally animal. Only some 500 are in regular use.[8]

Research

Homeopathy has been extensively researched for most of this

century, the earlier work being in Germany, and the more recent research coming from the large homeopathic establishment in France, as well as India, the UK, and the US. Most of this research is reported in the national homeopathic journals—virtually none has appeared in conventional medical literature. Research has focused on physical, chemical, and biological, and some animal studies. Clinical studies on man have rarely been carried out because of the difficulties of comparing two totally different therapeutic models.

On the physical level there have been thorough investigations into the physical properties of highly dilute shaken solutions. Techniques such as nuclear magnetic resonance, change in electrical storage capacity, or alterations in the intensity and wavelength of light passed through the solution have all shown certain differences between highly diluted and non-diluted solutions. However, these changes are hard to interpret.[9]

On the chemical side, studies have tended towards the system discussed earlier (p. 192), that is, watching how compounds, particularly salts and metals, inhibit and stimulate biochemical or chemical reactions at progressively greater dilutions. Well-executed studies have found that low doses are often stimulatory. However, the results are hard to duplicate. The absorbance of salts on the glass walls of laboratory apparatus is an ever-present and unknown disturbing factor in these experiments.

Perhaps the most successful homeopathic studies have been with animals or animal cells. Early work had used arsenic, metals, or other poisons which were first given in toxic doses. When this was followed by homeopathic doses of the same material it resulted in an immediate washing out of the poison from the body.[10] Similar 'hair of the dog' research has shown that animals that were made diabetic could be partly cured by homeopathic doses of diabetogenic material and animals poisoned with thujone recovered on being given Thuja 9c.[11] The most interesting research of this kind has been carried out at the National Environmental Research Centre in Plymouth, UK. Dr Stebbing has been investigating in great detail a phenomenon called *hormesis*. That is where minute doses of metals or poisons will stimulate, in a cyclic oscillating pattern, growth of previously poisoned cells or organisms. He has observed stimulatory effects at doses as low as 1 part in 10 million with copper sulphate and other poisons.[12] Biochemically, it is likely that these minute doses of poisons stimulate or induce enzymic repair processes.

As far as clinical research is concerned, there is a very great deal of anecdotal material; the reports of homeopathic treatment of childhood epidemics are particularly striking.[13] Respected physicians have presented countless cases.[14,15] However, controlled clinical double-blind studies are sadly lacking.[14,15] (Clinical trials of homeopathy are fully discussed on p. 21). Despite the methodological problems, serious studies have been carried out which show homeopathy to be at least as effective as, and safer than conventional treatment, in particular in rheumatoid arthritis,[16] but it has not been possible to confirm this finding with osteoarthritis in a short-term double-blind study comparing *Rhus tox* with fenoprofen.[17] In contrast, where the experimental situation is simplified by examining a symptom in volunteers, clear results are obtained. In one case volunteers received identical bruises on both arms, one of which was treated with arnica, and the other with placebo. High potency arnica applied externally helped the bruises disappear more rapidly than placebo.[18] An important recent clinical study of 144 patients also examined homeopathic treatment of a defined set of symptoms, in this case hay fever. High potency (30c) mixed grass pollen was found to be significantly more effective than identical placebo in relief of symptoms.[19]

Uses

In homeopathy it is axiomatic that there are no incurable diseases. There are however 'incurable' people. It is the vitality of the individual which determines what can be expected. A normally serious condition in someone with high recuperative power is not so serious as a normally mild condition in someone of low recuperative power. Therefore patients who respond best are those who have had a simple, ordered, stress-free life, living on wholesome, energy-full foods, and plenty of contact with nature. Where the natural healing resources of the body have been interfered with by destructive habits or by electroconvulsive therapy, cortisone, prolonged drug treatments, radiation, etc., cure is more difficult.

Homeopathy can be successful in all diseases though not all patients. It is especially applicable in acute conditions where the patient does have the vital energy to effect a cure, but relief is needed for distressing symptoms; in chronic cases such as gastric ulcer, digestive problems, gall stones, haemorrhoids, liver complaints, migraines, allergies, skin conditions, angina, psychogenic diseases, and rheumatoid conditions; for convalescents, children, and those who are sensitive to allopathic drugs. Cases which homeopathic practitioners refer to medical or other practitioners include emergencies, musculoskeletal injuries or serious infectious diseases which the patient is failing to overcome, or chronic diseases such as cancer. However, in these cases there may be a role for the adjunctive use of homeopathic remedies.

Risks

Since homeopathy stimulates the organism to the natural activity we call healing, there are no risks involved. There are cases where over-stimulation by too high a potency or too frequent a repetition may take place. This over-stimulation is very rare, and is only possible in cases with severe morbid pathology or in the moribund patient. The means of preparation of the remedies eliminates any risk of toxic side-effects. There is sometimes an initial aggravation, which is short-lived, lasting from a few minutes to a few days, depending on the condition of the patient. Bearing in mind Hering's Law of Cure, 'old' symptoms will sometimes reappear for a short time. By the same laws the externalization of the disease will sometimes produce discharges such as catarrh, diarrhoea, colds, skin eruptions, boils, 'flu-like symptoms, etc. These are also short-lived and are a process of health, not a disease process.

Types of therapy

Homeopaths in general practise according to the rules laid down by Hahnemann: only a single remedy is required; the minimum dose needed to produce reaction, usually a single dose, should be given; both prescriber and patient are to wait until the patient's curative response to the remedy has stopped before another dose is given. Some homeopaths use potentized substances in other ways, namely:

1. Certain remedies specifically for particular diseases.

2. Remedies for parts or organs instead of for the whole patient.

3. Combinations of remedies for specific diseases or even specific symptoms.

The use of such methods of treatment is a modern variant not in accord with Hahnemannian homeopathy. More medically-oriented homeopaths would tend to restrict homeopathy to the kinds of conditions which do not respond to conventional medicine, such as rheumatoid arthritis or allergies. They would not use it in many acute infections or in tuberculosis. The more classical homeopaths will treat a much wider range of problems, without necessarily differentiating them into conventional disease categories. They may also pay attention to diet and general lifestyle.

Simple homeopathy is very widely used in the UK by other practitioners—naturopaths, chiropractors, osteopaths, and therapeutic masseurs—as a supplement to their techniques. It is the most common form of non-medical household first aid.

A variant of homeopathy was developed by a renowned physician and homeopath Dr Edward Bach. He eliminated certain classes of remedies, restricting his sources of homeopathic materials to flowers and twigs. By means of a gentle serial dilution he obtained potentized solutions or extracts which he felt captured the 'essences' of the flowers more effectively than the more violent classical methods of succussion. His remedies are used, on diagnosis, as treatment for subtle psychological roots of disease.[20]

References

1. Hahnemann, S. (1983). *The organon of medicine* 6th edition. (Translated by Kunzli, J., Nande, A., and Pendleton, P.) Gollancz, London. Hahnemann, S. (1981). *The chronic diseases, their peculiar nature and their homeopathic cure.* Jain, New Delhi, India. (translated by Tafel, L. from the 1835 edition.)
2. Whitmore, E. (1981). *Psyche and substance.* North Atlantic Books, Richmond, Cal. (Highly recommended to those interested in the metaphysics of homeopathy.)
3. Guttentag, O.E. (1966). Homeopathy in the light of modern pharmacology. *Journal of Clinical Pharmacological Therapy*, 7, 425–8.
4. Shepherd, D. (1985). *The magic of minimum dose.* Health Science Press, Saffron Walden, Essex.
5. Boyd, W.E. (1954). Biochemical and biophysical evidence of the activity of high potencies. *British Homeopathic Journal*, 44, 7–44.
6. Barnard, G.P. and Stephenson, J.H. (1967). The microdose paradox: a new biophysical concept. *Journal of the American Institute of Homeopathy*, 60, 277–86. (Evidence is presented that many physical characteristics of highly dilute solutions change on shaking.)

7. Vithoulkas, G. (1981). *Homeopathy—medicine of the new man.* Arco Press, New York. (Perhaps the best short introduction available.)

8. Anon. (1981). Homeopathy, a demand for safer alternatives. *Chemist and Druggist,* **215**, 545-51.

9. Wrumser, L. (1967). Evolution of research in homeopathy. *Journal of the American Institute of Homeopathy,* **60**, 68-91. Resh, G. and Gutman, V. (1987). *The scientific foundations of homeopathy,* Bartel and Bartel, Berg Am Starnberger See, West Germany.

10. Hadley, S.J. (1981). An experiment showing an increase with dilution of a physical parameter. *British Homeopathic Journal,* **70**, 129-35. Kollerstrom, J. (1982). Basic scientific research into low dose effect. *British Homeopathic Journal,* **71**, 41.

11. Tetan, J. and Tetan, M. (1960). *Annales Homéopathique Français,* **13**, 669.

12. Stebbing, A.R.D. (1982). Hormesis. The stimulation of growth by low levels of inhibitors. *The Science of the Total Environment,* **2**, 213-34.

13. Mitchell, G.R. (1979). Homeopathic medicine. *British Medical Journal,* **1**, 1354-5.

14. Blackie, M. (1981). *The patient not the cure; the challenge of homeopathy.* Unwin, London. Blackie, M. (1986). *Classical homeopathy.* Beaconsfield Library, Beaconsfield.

15. Pinsent, R.J. (1980). Why not reconsider homeopathy? *Journal of the Royal College of General Practitioners,* **30**, 373.

16. Gibson, S.L.M., McNeill, A.D., Buchanan, W.W. (1980). Homeopathic therapy in rheumatoid arthritis: Evaluation by double-blind clinical therapeutic trial. *British Journal of Clinical Pharmacology,* **9**, 453.

17. Shipley, M., Berry, H., Broster, G., Jenkins, M., Clover, A. and Williams, I. (1983). Controlled trial of homeopathic treatment of osteoarthritis. *Lancet,* **1**, 97-8.

18. Campbell, A. (1978). Two pilot controlled trials of *arnica montana.* *British Homeopathic Journal,* **65**, 8.

19. Reilly, D., Taylor, M., McSharry, C., and Hitchinson, T. (1986). Is homeopathy a placebo response? Controlled trial of homeopathic potency, with pollen in hayfever as model. *Lancet,* **2**, 881-6.

20. Weeks, N. (1979). *Medical discoveries of Edward Bach, Physician.* Keats Publishers, New Canaan, Conneticut.

15

Hypnotherapy

Background

In the course of a trance, a person becomes extraordinarily receptive to suggestion. Primitive healers use this receptivity to implant suggestions for self-cure, and have done so from ancient times. Healing trances include the various kinds of exorcism and convulsive catharsis so frequently recorded in medieval Europe. Hypnosis is also a form of trance but it is passively receptive rather than convulsively explosive. Indeed the word was coined by the Scottish surgeon James Braid since he first erroneously thought of it as an induced sleep.

Franz Anton Mesmer is regarded as the founder of hypnotism. He was a charismatic therapist who successfully treated a large number of people by inducing deep trances. He too discovered that convulsions were not necessary for success. Healing could also be accomplished by means of a deeply relaxed and somnambulistic state. His demonstrations were extraordinary and unequivocal. However, he roused considerable antagonism by wearing flowing robes and using magicotheatrical stage settings. The trance state was anyway in disrepute; scientists saw it as medieval and the Church saw it as a mystical heresy. Despite frequent convincing demonstrations of therapeutic successes, conventional medicine retained its hostility to hypnosis even when new neurophysiological theories were developed by James Braid. During the last century hypnosis was quite widely used in France for neuroses, 'hysterical' (i.e. psychosomatic), and mental disorders. However, in the UK medical opinion insisted that hypnotic phenomena were mimicry, the hypnotic state was one of collusion, and the mind could not influence organic diseases.

During the 1950s doctors began to accept that certain restricted conditions of the body could be generated by the psyche. These psychogenic or psychosomatic conditions were at first regarded as peripheral illnesses that were hard to treat and risky to explore. However, it gradually became clear that the mind had great powers over health or illness. Experiments were carried out in which hypnosis was shown to relieve skin disease and cause warts to disappear. A British Medical Association committee eventually approved it for certain psychogenic and behavioural problems.[1]

Concepts and theory

Hypnosis can be loosely defined as 'a state of mind in which suggestions are not only more readily accepted than in the waking state, but are also acted upon much more powerfully'.[2] However, the boundaries of the hypnotic state are much wider than this. Indeed, any state in which (a) the cognitive controls over the mind are loosened or dissociated; and (b) the person is not asleep and can receive and act on messages, is a hypnotic or partly hypnotic state. While the hypnotic state can be brought on by a repetitive inductive process of one sort or another, it can also occur spontaneously, for example in situations of great fear, tension, space disorientation, starvation, sleeplessness, or when confronted with repeated stimuli such as evenly spaced trees while driving down a road. In fact, it may be that accidental self-hypnosis is an unwitting cause of illness. Debilitating anxieties may be produced in people if they accept suggestions about themselves such as 'I am a failure' while in states of heightened emotion or confusion. 'If the mind is concentrated as the result of any incident or idea of sufficient emotional importance then it is in a condition of hypnosis. Any idea which is then introduced will act in the same way as a hypnotic command.'[3]

Extraordinary potentialities are available to a person in the hypnotic state; feats of strength or of memory, the belief in illusory ideas and perceptions (demonstrated in stage hypnosis by, for example, making the hypnotized individual climb an imaginary barrier), the relinquishing of will and ego, the control over involuntary body processes, and the cure of diseases. In curative hypnosis, a therapist induces a hypnotic state as a means of passing by the conscious mind, and not an end in itself.

Hypnosis usually begins by lulling and distracting the conscious mind through repetitive sensations. Parallel commands to follow the hypnotist's instructions are given. The individual is, at least at the beginning, quite aware of the proceedings, and where instructions are given, feels that they will happen to him rather than by him. The electroencephalogram gives a reading halfway between sleeping and waking, the person relaxes more deeply and muscular action of all kinds, including speech and facial expression, tends to cease. Eventually catalepsy—rigid holding of position—occurs. This is often demonstrated in stage hypnosis by the hypnotist supporting a person solely by chairs under the head and feet.

Many subdivisions of trance states have been proposed, although none can claim to be more than cuts in a length of string. Therapists often find it useful to distinguish three levels:

1. *Light trance*: the eyes are closed, the person deeply relaxed, general psychological and ego-strengthening suggestions are accepted.

2. *Medium trance*: the person is fully hypnotized, physiological processes slow down, the person will be partially insensible to pain, allergic reactions will cease and it is in this state that most therapy is effected.

3. *Deep trance*: the person is in a somnambulist state, in which eyes can be open, but total anaesthesia is possible, along with special powers, age regression, removal of warts, and some of the 'virtuoso' manifestations of hypnosis.

It is said that 9 out of 10 people can be hypnotized by any skilled hypnotist, while the other 10 per cent can be hypnotized by finding a method particular to them. However, only 10 per cent of the population can readily enter deep trance states. In some cases this may be because an individual experiences flashbacks or realizations which act as a barrier to entry into deeper states, in other cases it may be a general lack of concentrative ability. Deeper states sometimes become possible to these patients after repeated entry into lighter trances with the therapist assisting in overcoming barriers on the way. In general, the best subjects are those who can be easily absorbed in what they are doing, while the worst are those with restless, active, questioning, and analytical minds. Often women are more easily hypnotized than men.

The question of susceptibility to hypnosis has been a prime research consideration for a number of years. Various scales, particularly the Stamford Hypnotic Suggestibility Scales, have been designed to measure hypnotizability and then applied to studies in which hypnotherapy occurs. Two bodies of opinion have arisen from these studies. One states that an individual's suggestibility is the major factor in healing and the particular method of inducing the state of heightened suggestibility is not relevant: that is, a suggestible person will tend to be healed whether hypnosis or some other form of implanting suggestions, such as guided imagery, is used. This downgrades the value of the hypnotic state as such.[4] The opposite view holds that the hypnotic state is one in which a person is maximally disposed to absorb effective therapeutic suggestions, that it is necessary for therapy, and that clinical successes can be obtained with everybody whatever their level of suggestibility.[5] There are many studies which will support both views. For example, it is known that hypnotizability is a stable personality trait which is correlated with suggestibility of people when awake. The occasional dramatic cures of migraine, warts, and allergies are related to hypnotizability. On the other hand, alleviations are produced under stringent experimental conditions in people of different hypnotic susceptibilities, provided the hypnotherapist uses appropriate methods. In the end the hypnotizability question is not very relevant in a clinical situation where the will and co-operation of the patient, the rapport with the therapist, the expectations on both sides, the type of method used, the focus attained in each session, the adjunctive use of drugs or other treatments, and other factors will all influence the outcome with each patient whatever his innate suggestibility.

It is important to realize that the effectiveness of hypnosis as a therapy lies in the extent to which a patient retains a suggestion in his waking state. The hypnotic state is used as a vehicle to implant a post-hypnotic suggestion. The simple post-hypnotic suggestion of the stage hypnotist, such as 'when the clock strikes you will stand up and blow your nose' will usually work after a single session because there are no contrary habits or psychological formations. However, in therapy the hypnotist is at the very least attempting to alter ingrained patterns of behaviour, and often he is attempting to root out destructive mental conditionings, moods, and neuroses, replacing them with positive self-esteem, new awareness, and capacities. The post-hypnotic suggestions here have to be inserted gradually, strengthened and maintained by the patient as well as the therapist.

Use is often made in therapy of autohypnosis where the therapist trains the patient to hypnotize himself, using the hypnotic state to introduce instructions which will make this easier. In this way the patient can continually reinforce the therapist's suggestions. For example, autohypnosis can be invaluable for relief of pain since the patient can instruct himself to reduce pain whenever attacks occur. Naturally the question arises as to how a person can use his conscious mind to by-pass his conscious mind. In fact for autohypnosis the person must enter an in-between state of relaxed uncritical awareness called the 'hypnoidal' state. In this bridging situation it is possible to formulate instructions and insert suggestions, including those of the manner of waking from self-hypnosis.

Method

The induction of hypnosis follows a basic pattern. The therapist will talk in a slow, relaxing, controlled, and confident way, drawing the patient's mind into a concentrated and detached state. This may involve depiction of an image, such as a walk down a country lane, or successions of colours, or repetition of a monotonous series of statements. Visual concentration can also be trapped and held by means of lights or wheels, a pendulum, or a pencil held at the upper limit of vision. The therapist then encourages heaviness and closing of eyes, followed by other simple test instructions, such as raising an arm. At this stage, usually after about 15 minutes, the person is already in a light trance. Deeper levels are attained by the therapist counting the patient from 1 to 10, or asking the patient to imagine descent in a lift. The patient is continually exhorted to let everything go bar the instructions of the therapist, and it is at this stage that some trust in the therapist will assist the patient to surrender and go deeper. The whole process can happen very much more quickly in people already 'primed' by states of shock, injury, or distress. This is of considerable use to army medical hypnotists who can often hypnotize wounded soldiers more or less by the pass of a hand. Milton Erikson pioneered a subtle method in which hypnosis is introduced during an apparently normal conversation. In all cases the hypnotist will usually plant a post-hypnotic suggestion which enables the subject to enter a trance much more quickly on subsequent occasions.

Some hypnotists then simply plant the suggestion that the symptom is going—'your migraine is going'—combined with general suggestions of positivity, health, and self-confidence. This may sometimes work, but is generally frowned upon. As the symptoms are usually manifestations of a deeper disturbance at the psychological or physical level, the hypnotist ought to work psychotherapeutically. This is certainly true when hypnotherapy is used to treat chronic pain which, if it is to be of long-term use, must involve a re-education of the patient so as to change his attitude to his suffering. Pain-blocking suggestions are given, for example that another feeling, say tingling, is substituted for the pain, or that the patient alters the meaning of and tolerance to, his pain. However these should usually be combined with work which bares the inner fear, anxiety, guilt, anger, or feelings of hopelessness of the patient. These can then be gradually replaced by positive suggestions such as that the patient is after all glad and successful in that he is alive, that he should have confidence and be aware of the transience of his pain, or that he has suffered enough. It is necessary to teach the patient self-hypnosis so that the therapy can be incorporated into daily life.

Hypnosis can be valuable in psychotherapy because it facilitates the considerable recall of past events. Therefore the hypnotherapist can get to the roots of a destructive behaviour pattern such as overeating or a psychosomatic condition such as asthma much more quickly than with lengthy verbal fencing with the conscious mind. Old experiences are dredged up, relived, and cathartically removed. The patient can go right back to childhood and beyond. In deep hypnosis patients can experience their birth, and sometimes even talk with the voice of their own childhood.

A very useful uncovering technique is that of ideomotor questioning, developed by Le Cron.[6] Patients are asked to respond to questions by movements, such as a raised finger, rather than words. Therapists who use it find that it allows greater access to hidden subconscious material than if the patient had to use verbal processes in order to answer the questions. Ideomotor questioning is also of great value in communicating with patients who are unconscious, say after an accident.

A summary of a thorough hypnotherapeutic course of treatments might go through the following stages:[3]

1. History taking and general diagnosis.

2. Training of the patient to develop his ability to relax, to go deeper into hypnosis to develop re-induction of hypnosis when the therapist suggests it, and to hypnotize himself.

3. A diagnostic exploration under hypnosis in which the patient is questioned so as to dig up deeply rooted causes of his current condition.

4. Analytic procedures to relieve, expose, and remove the emotional content from early experiences.

5. A final synthesis phase to check the level of insight gained, and to re-educate and encourage the patient.

Research

There is now a great deal of published research on the possibilities of hypnosis and its relationship with other states of mind.[7] However, very little is known of the mechanism by which hypnotic suggestions cause the cure or regression of disease. One pioneering study was begun in the UK by Black, who reported his ability to relieve asthma and allergic conditions by hypnosis in the 1950s. He went on from there to show that after a cure of allergy the patient's hypersensitive skin reactions to challenge by antigens had stopped even though the patient still had circulating antibodies to this antigen. Black concluded that hypnosis had prevented the uncomfortable inflammatory results (liberation of histamine) of challenge by antigen but not the underlying immunological situation.[8] Several kinds of controlled experiments have now been able to demonstrate that under hypnosis subjects can control the blood supply, sensitivity to damage or burning, and pain tolerance in their limbs.[9]

This led to research in which other psychological strategies of controlling pain or blood supply were compared with hypnosis. In general, hypnosis has been found more effective than biofeedback in enabling a subject to control the blood supply to his limbs, although it has the disadvantage that someone else has to be there; biofeedback is a self-learned procedure.[10] An interesting controlled experiment compared hypnosis, acupuncture at true loci, and acupuncture at false loci, with drugs—namely morphine, a benzodiazepine tranquillizer, aspirin, and placebo—for the relief of experimentally induced pain. Each procedure was carried out at its optimum time before the administration of the pain. Results of pain ratings show that hypnosis was much better than any of the other procedures ($P < 0.001$). Acupuncture (at appropriate loci only) was next best and shared second place with morphine.[11]

Very often hypnotic induction itself is not necessary to gain control of involuntary processes, but can be substituted by visualization or states of deep relaxation and meditation in which suggestions can be harmoniously received and absorbed. For example, in one study students were told that they were being touched by poison ivy leaves although the leaves were actually harmless. More of the subjects produced contact dermatitis in the local area as a result of prior non-hypnotic relaxation than prior hypnosis. Two groups of women were then hypnotized and given suggestions for breast enlargement. The group which practised autosuggestion, did better than the group with hypnosis alone. In all these cases the authors showed that the blood supply was increased at the site of these effects.[12]

Clinical research is still in its infancy. However, it is now focusing on the use of hypnosis to reduce symptoms during painful medical procedures and in pain associated with serious conditions such as cancer. Newton reports a long-term evaluation of the use of hypnosis in 283 cancer patients. He found improvements in their general condition. They lived significantly longer than expected for their condition.[13] There have been several controlled studies showing that hypnosis can reduce the nausea and discomfort during chemotherapy,[14] as well as reduce pain, bleeding, and stress.[15] Hypnosis is moving away from 'wart-magic' towards a more truly complementary role.

Uses and risks

The public generally associates hypnosis with the cure of obsessive habits, in particular, smoking and over-eating. Indeed, together with sexual problems, these are the stock in trade cases of lay hypnotherapists. However, many more problems, including phobias, allergies, amnesia, gastric ulcer, stress, asthma, anxiety, inhibitions, insomnia, menstrual disorders, migraine, psoriasis, eczema, tremor, warts, and pain, are treated. Hypnosis can be used in any situation where a particular mental stance will promote healing or relieve discomfort. This includes a newer but increasingly important application—the relief of the suffering and depression of people in the terminal stages of their illness, or undergoing severe medical treatment. It is becoming much more frequently used to prepare patients for surgery and to reduce the side-effects of chemotherapy and radiotherapy. Most large hospitals will have at least one member of the medical staff who can use hypnotic techniques. In these cases hypnosis can not only reduce symptoms, but also anxiety and fear. In terminal illnesses hypnosis can prepare the patient for the possibility of dying, improve the quality of life, and aid in the relationship with those looking after the patient.[16]

Expectations of success vary enormously. Hypnotherapists generally feel that anxiety, phobias, and habitual behaviours respond best. Asthma, allergies, and psychosomatic conditions respond well but take time. Pain treatment can often be very successful. For example, one British consultant reports that 90 per cent of minor fractures can be reduced in a casualty department without anaesthesia if hypnosis is used.[17] A similar success can be achieved when hypnosis is used during childbirth.

Hypnosis is generally very safe. Attempts by its opponents to demonstrate its harm have been continually thwarted by lack of any evidence. However, there are three kinds of possible risks. The first is through the careless use of post-hypnotic suggestion without proper familiarity with the case. A few cases where death occurred as an indirect result of the use of hypnosis have been reported. For example, a woman was told that she would have no fear of crossing a road, and she was promptly run over.

A second kind of risk is that by superficial removal of symptoms or uncovering of unconscious traumas a more serious condition, physical or psychological, is precipitated. Although this is unlikely, it is recommended that all hypnotists have some training in psychotherapy so as to be able to respond appropriately to any problems which surface during hypnosis. In actual fact, where controlled studies have been carried out, the experimental hypnotized group have shown fewer side-effects than the control group within daily life. For example, one study compared hypnosis of a student population, to experiences such as two days of college life, examinations, or verbal learning. The hypnotized students reported more relaxation, less anxiety, and more pleasure than the groups in college life. Indeed, the deeper they went into hypnosis the better they felt afterwards.[18]

The third kind of risk is that of manipulation by the hypnotist. This is more relevant to stage hypnosis than clinical hypnosis. There is a dispute as to whether a hypnotist can make people do things fundamentally against their will. He probably can, provided he has time gradually to establish his control and bring the subject into deep hypnosis. There is usually no time for this in stage performances.

Obtaining treatment

There is a variety of approaches in hypnotism, used by both medical and lay hypnotherapists. It is better to go to hypnotherapists who are fully qualified, who do not advertise that they can aid in overcoming smoking or over-eating, and who use a psychotherapeutic approach to treatment.

References

1. Asher, R. (1956). Respectable Hypnosis. *British Medical Journal*, **1**, 309–13.
2. Hartland, John (1971). *Medical and dental hypnosis*. Ballière and Tindall, London. Udolf, R. (1986). *Handbook of hypnosis for professionals*. Van Nostrand, New York.
3. Hartman, B.J. (1977). The treatment of psychogenic heart syndrome by hypnotherapy. *Journal of the National Medical Association*, **69**, 63–5.
4. Hilgard, E.R. and Hilgard, J.R. (1984). *Hypnosis in the relief of pain*. William Kaufmann, Los Altos, California. Diamon, M. (1977). Issues and methods for modifying responsivity to hypnosis. *Annals of the New York Academy of Sciences*, **296**, 119 28.
5. Barber, T.X., Spanos, N.P., and Chaves, J.F. (1986). *Hypnosis, imagination and human potentialities*. Pergamon Press, Oxford and New York. Bowers, K.S. and Kelly, P. (1979). Stress, disease, psychotherapy and hypnosis. *Journal of Abnormal Psychology*, **88**, 490–505.
6. Le Cron, L.M. (1954). A hypnotic technique for uncovering unconscious material. *Journal of Clinical and Experimental Hypnosis*, **2**, 76–9.
7. Burrows, G.D. and Dennerstein, L. (eds) (1980). *Handbook of hypnosis and psychosomatic medicine*. Elsevier, North-Holland, Amsterdam.
8. Black, S. (1963). Inhibition of immediate-type hypersensitivity response by direct suggestion under hypnosis. *British Medical Journal*, **1**, 925–9.
9. Chapman, L.F., Goodell, H., and Wolff, H.G. (1959). Changes in tissue vulnerability induced during hypnotic suggestion. *Journal of Psychosomatic Research*, **4**, 99–105. Maslach, C., Marshall, G., and

Zimbardo, P.G. (1972). Hypnotic control of peripheral skin temperature: A case report. *Psychophysiology*, **9**, 600–5.

10. Barabsz, A.K. and McGeorge, C.M. (1978). Biofeedback, mediated biofeedback and hypnosis in peripheral vasodilator training. *American Journal of Clinical Hypnosis*, **21**, 28–37.

11. Stern, J.A., Brown, M., Ulett, G.H., and Stetten, I. (1977). A comparison of hypnosis, acupuncture, morphine, valium, aspirin and placebo in the management of experimentally induced pain. *Annals of the New York Academy of Sciences*, **296**, 175–93.

12. Conway, A.V. (1986). Cancer and the mind; a role for hypnosis. *Holistic Medicine*, **1**, 43–55. Barber, T.X. (1978). Hypnosis, suggestion and psychosomatic phenomena, a new look from the standpoint of recent experimental studies. *American Journal of Clinical Hypnosis*, **21**, 13–27.

13. Newton, B. (1982). The use of hypnosis in the treatment of cancer patients. *American Journal of Clinical Hypnosis*, **25**, 104–13.

14. Zeltzer, L. and LeBaron, S. (1982). Hypnosis and non-hypnotic techniques for reduction of pain and anxiety during painful procedures in children and adolescents with cancer. *Journal of Paediatrics*, **101**, 1032–5. Redd, W.H., Rosenberger, P.H., and Hendler, C.S. (1983). Controlling chemotherapy side effects. *American Journal of Clinical Hypnosis*, **25**, 161–72.

15. Ament, P. (1982). Concepts in the use of hypnosis for pain relief in cancer. *Journal of Medicine*, **13**, 233–40. Hildgard, J.R. and LeBaron, S. (1982). Relief of anxiety and pain in children and adolescents with cancer: Quantitative measures and clinical observations. *International Journal of Clinical and Experimental Hypnosis*, **30**, 417–42. Rosenberg, S.W. (1983). Hypnosis in cancer care: Imagery to enhance the control of physiological and psychological 'side effects' of cancer therapy. *American Journal of Clinical Hypnosis*, **25**, 122–7. Kohen, D. (1986). Applications of relaxation mental imagery (self hypnosis) in paediatric emergencies. *International Journal of Clinical and Experimental Hypnosis*, **34**, 283–94.

16. Dempster, C.R., Batson, P., and Whalen, B.Y. (1976). Supportive hypnotherapy during the radical treatment of malignancies. *International Journal of Clinical and Experimental Hypnosis*, **24**, 1–9.

17. Jameson, R.M. (1963). Hypnosis for minor surgical procedures. *British Journal of Anaesthesia*, **35**, 269–71.

18. Coe, W.C. and Ryken, K. (1979). Hypnosis and risks to human subjects. *American Psychologist*, **34**, 673–81.

16

Manual therapies

Remedial massage

Although remedial massage has its own techniques and disciplines, it is based on the strongly human instinct to hold or rub a place which hurts. Thus the simplest form of massage may well go back to primitive man. As a minor and instinctive form of therapy, the history of its usage is largely unwritten. We do not know of its systematic use until spas and watering-places became popular during the last century and massage was used in conjunction with hydrotherapy.[1]

Interest in massage is currently undergoing something of a revival. Its value has been newly recognized and re-assessed, and the instinct to use the hands as instruments to assist healing has been formalized into set patterns and types of movement to bring about a desired effect.[2]

Massage is applied to the soft tissues of the body—the muscles and ligaments—but this has a resulting beneficial effect on the nervous and circulatory systems. Techniques are designed to relax, or strengthen and stimulate; both may happen at the same time. Massage eases tensions and knotted tissue, increases the circulation of the blood, and stimulates the lymphatic system, which helps to eliminate waste material. Massage helps to break down adhesions and restore strength and mobility after injury. It is obviously useful in maintaining muscular tone and blood circulation for people confined to bed or wheelchairs for long periods of time. Massage is often used in conjunction with osteopathy or chiropractic in re-establishing and maintaining the postural integrity of the body. In addition, massage also has an undoubted psychological effect, inducing a sense of ease and well-being.

The most commonly used form of massage treatment is Swedish massage, which may be broken down into four main movements.

1. *Effleurage*: a stroking movement which soothes the patient and relaxes the superficial muscles in preparation for stronger movements. Effleurage may be stimulating if used vigorously.

2. *Pettrisage*: involves kneading, rolling, and squeezing the tissues, much as one kneads bread.

3. *Friction*: used deeply with small circular movements against the bone, with the intention of releasing specific areas of tension and blockage.

4. *Tapotement*: movements are stimulating and designed to tone and strengthen the muscles. Cupping, hacking, flicking, and clapping should be followed by further effleurage movements.

In recent years the basic forms of massage have been extended and added to by a number of special techniques. For example, aromatherapy uses those essential oils and plant essences with specific healing properties which are absorbed by the skin. For example, rosemary oil is frequently used to increase peripheral micro-circulation. The perfume of these oils may well work on the emotional and mental levels as well as assisting in physical healing.[3] Polarity therapy, developed by Dr Randolph Stone, involves concentrated pressure on specific body points in order to re-align posture, and encourage the flow of energy ('ch'i' or 'prana') around the body.[4] Reflexology, structural integration, shiatzu, and kinesiology, are described later in the chapter. These extensions to basic massage recognize the psychological and emotional aspects of being, and aim to restore well-being on all levels.[5]

Massage has a wide area of application but there are a number of contra-indications. Massage should not be used in the acute inflammatory stage of arthritis, or any other condition where there is high temperature or inflammation, although its use may be very helpful once the inflammation has dispersed. Restoring strength and mobility after a sprain, or in fibrositis, are obvious examples. Massage should not be used in serious heart disease, or in phlebitis, where a blood clot might be disturbed. Neither should massage treatment be given where there is an infective skin condition.

Massage is used to good effect in health hydros but is little used in hospitals, perhaps because it is time consuming and does not fit well into overworked hospital regimes.

Reflexology

Reflexology is a form of ancient Chinese medicine involving treatment by massage of pressure points in the feet. Research has shown that reflexology was also known to some primitive African tribes, the Red Indians, and the early Egyptians. It was rediscovered in the early 1920s by an American ear, nose, and throat consultant, Dr William Fitzgerald, who found that by applying pressure to a certain area of the foot he was able to anaesthetize the ear; this enabled him to perform minor ear operations. His findings attracted the attention of other medical practitioners and the main pioneer in the field was a nurse, Eunice Ingham, who toured the US lecturing, treating, and training students. One of her students was the late Doreen Bayly who returned to England and introduced the method there in the early 1960s.[6]

There are reflexes in the feet for all parts of the body and these are arranged in such a way as to form a map of the body in the feet. The right foot represents the right side of the body and the left foot represents the left side of the body. The reflexes are found mainly on the soles of the feet but also on the top and sides of the feet. An imaginary line drawn across halfway down the foot corresponds to the waistline in the body. Hence, the big toes represent the head and brain, the little toes represent the sinuses, and the heart reflex is found only in the left foot above the waistline. By massaging a specific area of the foot, an effect can be brought about in a part of the body or a zone quite distant from the foot. By working on these reflexes, the circulation of blood to the corresponding part of the body is improved and a reduction in the nervous tension in the area occurs. This can be of considerable benefit since many disorders are due to tension in parts of the body. It is also able to stimulate the healing forces present in the body and thus increase the body's ability to heal itself.[7]

Similar reflexes are found in the hands. However, the feet are normally used for treatment since the reflex areas are larger and the feet are more sensitive to massage since they are protected in socks and shoes. The hands, though, can be most useful for self-treatment. Another set of reflexes, called cross reflexes, are also employed by the reflexologist; these are links between the shoulder and hip, elbow and knee, and wrist and ankle on the same side of the body. It has been found that a tender area in, for example, the hip will have a similar tender area in the shoulder.

When giving reflexology treatment, the hands, and particularly the thumbs, are used. The thumb is bent and the side and end of the thumb pressed firmly onto the reflex point. To release the pressure, the thumb is pulled back with a slight circular movement. To move from one reflex to the next, a forward creeping movement is used so that the thumbs are kept in contact with the foot as much as possible. Each reflex is about the size of a pin's head so the massage must be precise. If the area being worked on is out of balance, a tenderness will be felt in the foot. This tenderness can be likened to a piece of glass being pressed into the foot; it can feel extremely sharp and often the practitioner may be accused of sticking his finger-nail into the foot. The degree of tenderness felt will depend on how out of balance the corresponding part of the body is and the method can therefore be used as a means of diagnosis. At some of the reflexes, it is sometimes possible to feel little granules beneath the skin. Reflexologists regard these granules as crystalline deposits around nerve endings which cause a blockage around the nerves, thus reducing the normal stimulation of glands and organs. By massaging the areas, these granules can be dispersed so that they are re-absorbed by the circulatory system and excreted from the body. In different cases, different amounts of pressure are required; although there will probably be tender areas in the feet, the pressure should not be such that it causes agony to the patient since this will not allow him to relax.

During a treatment, all the reflexes in both feet are massaged so that the body is treated as a whole. Each treatment lasts about three-quarters to one hour. Areas which appear tender are given massage and normally these areas will become less tender after a few minutes. However, it is not possible to remove all tender areas with one treatment. It is difficult to predict how many treatments are required to correct the imbalances but, in general, results should become evident after about three treatments and a course of six to eight treatments is usually recommended. Those conditions of long standing will probably require more treatments than those of a shorter duration. Children, in particular, seem to respond to the treatment quickly.

A wide range of disorders can be treated using reflexology and it is fair to say that most conditions will benefit to some extent from a course of treatment. Conditions such as migraine, sinus trouble, back problems, poor peripheral circulation, and stiffness and tension can all be helped.[8]

Following treatment, no unpleasant side-effects are experienced. Some people feel revitalized and have a sense of well-being, whilst others may feel tired. In some cases, a form of healing crisis, such as a cold, worsening of a skin rash or the need to pass water more frequently, may occur. All of these reactions are, however, short-term effects as the body fights to rid itself of toxins. As well as being used to treat disorders, reflexology treatment at regular intervals can help maintain the body in a state of good health. It is always advisable to receive treatment from a trained practitioner. There are certain instances, including heart trouble, thrombosis, shingles, or pregnancy, when treatment should not be given or when extra care is required.

A recent development in reflexology—metamorphic therapy —makes use of the Oriental principle that segments of the feet correspond to pre-birth stages. Massage by means of a vibratory motion, along a line stretching from the big toe to the heel, on the inner side of the feet, is intended to work on problems developed by the patient during gestation. Foot, hand, and head massage are also practised in order to promote atrophied or unbalanced abilities.

Structural integration—rolfing

In common with most specific manual therapies structural integration was developed by one inspired teacher, Ida Rolf. She treated people by a special deep form of massage for 30 years before her technique gained recognition and acclaim. It is based on the premise that the shape and contour of our body is a dramatization of our experience. Life events and stresses impose distortions on the body which, over time, are set into the connective tissues. For example, a head forward posture, associated with states such as agitation or timidity, could encourage an opposite bend in the spine and hunched shoulders to re-create an upright posture. However, this misalignment is only maintained as a result of expenditure of energy, continuous muscular tension, and eventually stresses locked into the structure of the body.[9]

Rolfing is a deep and powerful massage designed to soften the collagenous fascias of the body. The masseur applies his weight through fingers, knuckles, and often elbows, reaching into body areas to loosen and realign the musculature and its supports. The standard treatment consists of 10 one hour sessions, each of which is devoted to one particular body area. The final sessions reintegrate the newly flexible tissues. It is a drastic and painful treatment. Yet people emerge from it measurably taller, as from Alexander Training. Posture, chronic musculoskeletal pains and tensions, voice, sensitivity, breath control, attitude to self, and mood can all be affected by this massage. However for a more permanent beneficial effect rolfing should be combined with self-care. It should not, however, be used in cases of organic disease.

Shiatzu—Japanese pressure point massage

Shiatzu is a massage technique which combines massage with finger pressure to acupuncture points and meridians. In Oriental medicine fingers were and are often used instead of acupuncture needles, for example in young children where very mild treatment is indicated, when an individual wishes to treat himself, or for use in emergencies such as snakebite, haemorrhage, or shock where no acupuncturist is to hand. Oriental medicine acknowledges that deep pressure applied to certain points will have a similar effect to puncture with needles, although it is milder and less tightly controlled and the points may differ from the needle points. Because it does not need as much precision and knowledge as acupuncture, and is even safer, it has been taken up as a family and folk self-treatment method, especially in Japan. There are still tens of thousands of shiatzu practitioners in Japan. Some of them are blind, for it used to be one of the classical professions of the blind.

Shiatzu has specific and general applications. It is used in the treatment of specific chronic diseases. The shiatzu practitioner may sometimes diagnose visually in the same way as an acupuncturist and he may be especially expert at interpreting the feel of the body, the painful, hot or knotted areas. Treatment is then given on several points on the required meridians, as well as by general kneading massage, in order to promote the flows of energy in the required directions. It is particularly effective in the long-term treatment of rheumatic, sexual, and circulatory problems. However, there are not many people in the West who have sufficient training in shiatzu to use it as a specific therapy in this way. Instead, many people are finding that points can be used for self-treatment and first aid in daily life. For example, a point on the eyebrows can give relief from head-aches, other points on the face will anesthetize the gums in dentistry, certain points will affect a mood and energy, others, such as the 'revival' point on the perineum, can be used in emergency.[10]

The general use of shiatzu is in whole-body prevention and self-care. A shiatzu massage of this kind will cover all the meridians, paying particular attention to those meridians which need (or 'ask for') attention. The masseur works in a particular sequence, moving down the meridians and opening them to greater flow of energy on the way.[11] It is also an intuitive practice in which the touch of the masseur transmits his healing energy. For this reason shiatzu practitioners must keep themselves in properly balanced health. A kind of do-it-yourself shiatzu, combined with Japanese limbering and toni-fying exercises, forms a health practice called Do-In.

Applied kinesiology

Applied kinesiology (AK) was created in 1965 through the efforts of Dr George Goodheart, a respected chiropractor. He discovered that the kinesiological tests used to determine relative muscle strength and tone over the range of movement of the joints could also give qualitative information about the functions of body organs—the liver, kidneys, small intestines, etc. Using knowledge of chiro-practic, of the trigger or reflex points on the body, and of acupuncture meridians and their relationship to organs and muscle groups, he developed a relatively complete diagnosis and treatment system.[12] Its theoretical basis rests on the assumption that muscle weakness is the result of the functional state of the nervous system, expressed in the muscle-nerve connections (motor neurone facilitation). The organs express their function via nerves to specific muscle groups.

It is used to detect incorrect joint function, spinal lesions, muscle weakness, organic dysfunction, psychological effects on the function of the body as a whole, nutritional needs, and allergies. These last two factors have aroused considerable interest within the health care professions, and some controversy.[13]

A simple muscle test, for example, involves the practitioner applying a downward pressure on the patient's extended right arm while the patient is sitting. If the patient's arm 'locks' in that position it indicates a general strength of the group of muscles in the shoulder; if the arm does not lock and feels 'spongy' then a weakness is indicated. Individual muscles can then be isolated by placing the arm into different positions and re-testing, so giving an accurate picture of the weakened muscles.

Different muscle groups can be tested to diagnose different kinds of organic dysfunction or even dietary deficiency. The precise location of muscle weakness also aids in the traditional chiropractic or osteopathic diagnosis. Treatment of the weakened muscle is secondary to treatment of any underlying problem revealed by AK. However, working on the appropriate reflexes and meridians with finger-pressure strengthens the weak muscles and restores structural balance.

Although a good deal of controversy still surrounds the use of AK in nutritional diagnosis, it is now extensively used in American dental practice and in international sports medicine, as well as in chiropractic and osteopathic practices in Europe, the US, Australia, and New Zealand.

Spinal touch treatment

The recognition of the effects of stress on the body is at the core of spinal touch treatment. The constant bombardment of pressures, problems, illness, inadequate nutrition (not forgetting gravity), puts our bodies under constant stress. Stress is a positive factor in growth and development. However, when pushed beyond natural 'elastic limits', stress becomes strain. Muscles left in a condition of strain for a prolonged period of time will cause body distortion. This can reduce vitality because of an over-accumulation of fatigue poisons such as lactic acid.

Treatment begins with a complete plumb-line analysis of the patient to determine how far his posture has deviated from the norm, the most crucial point of reference being the lumbosacral joint—the centre of gravity of the body, and the point to which all stresses in the body are directed. The differences are noted, and the patient then relaxes in a prone (face-down) position on the treatment table and the practitioner begins treatment (lasting between 10 and 15 minutes) using a very light touch on a number of contact points on the gluteal muscles, along the spine, neck and shoulders, base of skull, and abdomen. Touching these key areas redirects the body's energy, causing the muscles to relax and gently pulling the spine into its more natural position.[14]

Manual therapies 219

Several treatments are required to relax the tissues to the point where the body maintains the correct postural balance, although relief of symptoms and the restoration of proper functioning may take place after the first treatment. Therapists also use kinesiological muscle testing for nutritional needs.

References

1. Kohnlechner, K. (1979). *Handbuch der Naturheilkunde* (2 Volumes). Wilhelm Heyne Verlag, Munich.
2. Downing, George (1972). *The massage book*. Random House, New York. Hofer, Jack (1976). *Total massage*. Grosset and Dunlap, New York. Cohen, N. (1987). Massage is the message. *Nursing Times*, 83, 19–20.
3. Tisserand, R.B. (1985). *The art of aromatherapy*. Daniel, Saffron Waldon, Essex.
4. Stone, R. (1978). *Health building*. Parameter Press, Orange County, California.
5. Downing, George (1974). *Massage and meditation*. Random House, New York. McKechnie, A.A., Wilson, F., Watson, N., and Scott, D. (1983). Anxiety states: a preliminary report on the value of connective tissue massage, *Journal of Psychosomatic Research*, 27, 125–9.
6. Bayly, D. (1982). *Reflexology today*. Thorsons, Wellingborough.
7. Kaye, A. and Matchan, D.C. (1985). *Reflexology: Techniques of foot massage for health and fitness*. Thorsons, Wellingborough.
8. Kunz, K. and Kunz, B. (1985). *Complete guide to foot reflexology*. Thorsons, Wellingborough.
9. Rolf, I. (1977). *Rolfing—The integration of human structures*. Dennis Landmann, Santa Monica, California.
10. Bahr, F. (1982). *The acupressure health book*. Unwin, London. Blate, M. (1982). *The natural healers acupressure handbook: G-J fingertip technique*. Routledge and Kegan Paul, London.
11. Namikoshi, Tokujiro (1977). *Shiatzu therapy, theory and practice*. Wehmann Brothers, New Jersey. Ohashi, Watani (1978). *Do-it-yourself shiatsu: How to perform the ancient Japanese art of 'acupuncture without needles'*. Unwin, London.
12. Birdwhistell, R.L. (1970). *Kinesics and context: Essays on body motion communication*. University of Pennsylvania Press, Philadelphia.
13. Scopp. *et al.* (1985). An experimental evaluation of kinesiology in allergy and deficiency disease diagnosis. *Journal of Orthomolecular Psychiatry*, 7, 137–8.
14. Thie, J. and Marks, M. (1973). *Touch for health*. De Vorss Press, Santa Monica, California.

17

Mind–Body therapies

The mind in disease

Apart from obvious mental diseases, medicine has more or less ignored the mind as a cause of sickness ever since therapeutics ousted magic. However, in the last 20 years research on the subject has forced the medical establishment to adjust its attitudes.[1] It was Hans Selye who first showed that animals under experimental stress developed some of those diseases so common today: indigestion and gastric ulcer, heart problems, and disturbance of the immune defensive systems of the body. He incorporated classical 'fight or flight' physiology in a new model which suggested how psychological disease caused physical disease.[2]

Much of human physiology is designed to maintain a balanced, calm, clement, and constant inner environment. As soon as threat or change is perceived by our senses and interpreted by our minds, physiology adopts a defensive posture to maintain this 'balance that results from the continual and delicate compensation by the most sensitive of scales'.[3] The physiology of the mobilization of body defences is now very well understood. It involves the sympathetic nervous system and adrenaline and steroid hormones of the adrenal glands under the hormonal and nervous direction of the lower brain, the hypothalamus and pituitary glands. The cascade of defence reactions is profound, arousing the mind, altering muscle action, blood circulation, heart action, metabolism, breath, and digestion. The emotions can be visualized as ancient internal mechanisms for marshalling these forces.

These body responses are however a two-edged sword. For when challenges or over-arousal persist, described as a state of stress, continued defensive readiness produces a profound deterioration in health. For example, there is clear evidence that stress or anxiety can undermine the immune system, and thus lower resistance to almost any disease.[4]

There is also a good deal of research which demonstrates that the stress hormones of people who do not 'switch off' properly get used to a round-the-clock mobilization, leading directly to tiredness, irritability, insomnia, and then on to serious psychosomatic disease.[3,5,6] Anxiety, tension, over-stimulation, clock-watching, restlessness, ambition, guilt, fear, and so on are all psychological postures which cause persistent stress reactions.

The diseases that result occur frequently. This does not only mean those diseases which have always been known to be psychosomatic (i.e. directly related to stress and mental processes), such as indigestion, gastric ulcer, migraine, high blood pressure, disturbances of heart function, asthma, and obesity, but also many very serious and widespread diseases which have previously been thought of as having exclusively an external 'accidental' origin, such as cancer, atherosclerosis, rheumatic conditions, and chronic infections. This is not to say that diet and environment do not contribute, but that personality, stress, and mental attributes also have an influence. The psychogenic contribution to cardiovascular disease is now thoroughly accepted by the medical world.[7,8] It is also accepted that the mind has an effect on the origin and development as well as the regression of cancer,[9,10] and some evidence as to how it does this is emerging from the fledgling science of psychoneuroendocrinology. Depression and anxiety causes hormonal disturbances, particularly of corticosteroids. This in turn reduces or exhausts the thymus and the circulating lymphocytes which normally weed out nascent tumour cells.[11]

There have been other findings relating to the mind's connection with health. The placebo response, that is healing occurring solely as result of belief in the treatment, is now better understood and utilized in treatment.[12,13] Research has linked it to changes in brain neuropeptides. It is these same substances which are associated with acupuncture effects, the relief of pain, and the control of stress in the body.[14]

It is not surprising that some authorities consider these brain substances to be a third nervous system bridging mind and body, with powerful controls over states of energy, health, and constitution.[15] Nevertheless, this is only a beginning. Most complementary practitioners, and anyone who holds a more subtle expansive view of man, can only state that *all* disease has a psychological as well as physical, environmental, social, and sometimes even spiritual dimension. This is the assumption underlying all traditional medical systems.

The mind in treatment

There are a considerable number of different psychotherapeutic or psychosomatic methods now available within complementary medicine for preventing and treating disease. These include meditation (especially visualization), relaxation, bioenergetics, prayer and faith, stress management regimes, yoga, concentrative breathing exercises, polarity therapy, autogenic therapy, and biofeedback. They all have certain features in common. First, they may begin with therapy but they all move on to growth, self-awareness, and personal development. To a greater or lesser extent these are therapies for the healthy as well as the sick. Secondly, they all attempt to elicit self-healing capacities. In each case they do so by giving them room to work, usually by removing or neutralizing attachments, emotions, anxieties, and destructive thought processes that lead to negative physiological reactions such as stress or negative behaviour patterns such as compulsions. Thirdly, these methods are largely non-specific, that is they do not apply specifically to a certain set of symptoms discovered by a therapist as a result of diagnosis. Fourthly, the therapist is normally an instructor or even priest, and the patient a trainee. The trainee must work on himself, largely by himself. The prognosis or outcome is as much his responsibility as anyone else's.[1,16]

There are few precautions or side-effects with these methods, providing they are competently taught and executed. Perhaps the only real danger is that a person with a serious organic condition may not receive appropriate complementary or conventional treatment if he chooses a psychological therapy in the absence of a proper diagnosis. Therefore, anyone who is ill, or suspects disease, ought to have a diagnosis by a doctor or complementary practitioner, and make arrangements for his condition to be monitored. Then psychological methods can be used as an adjunctive, or where appropriate, sole treatment. Other problems might arise where the trainee dabbles and muddles different methods, where failure leads to psychological problems, where the method dredges up material from deep within the mind which neither the trainee nor an inexperienced trainer can handle, and so on. These risks are endemic to any psychotherapeutic undertaking.

The many body-oriented psychotherapies as well as yoga therapy, T'ai-chi, bioenergetics (Reichian psychotherapy), and so on, are, for reasons mentioned in the *Preface (p. viii)*, outside the scope of this book. However the Bibliography lists interesting further reading and the books by Matson, Rowan, Assagioli, and Dychtwald are particularly recommended.[17] The body-orientated psychotherapies are also described in the American holistic medicine books listed in the general section of the Bibliography. The organizations concerned can be found through these books or magazines.[18]

Relaxation, autogenic therapy, and biofeedback are discussed below since they are systems which are fully available and taught in a therapeutic setting in the UK. Hypnotherapy has close connections to autogenic therapy, which is a type of hypnotic meditation. Hypnotic induction also utilizes standard relaxation techniques. However, this is described in fuller detail in Chapter 15.

Relaxation techniques

Relaxation is surprisingly difficult to achieve for people who are not naturally relaxed. Lying down is easy but a very great deal of tension will still remain in the body unless the mind too can be stilled. People 'relax' in front of the television but the postures they take, and the tiredness they feel afterwards, demonstrates the opposite; that their physiology continues its state of sympathetic activation and arousal. True relaxation implies a profound shift in many physiological systems, the mind barely ticking over, a deep surrendering of the body to its supports and a slow and regular breath.

Relaxation methods are progressive. First, a setting is arranged so as to induce calm and contentment. Harsh surroundings, such as fluorescent lights, are to be avoided. The setting should establish cues that tend to remind a trainee of previous occasions of deep relaxation. After preparatory introduction and information, the trainee is sometimes taken through limbering, loosening, and stretching exercises to encourage subsequent rest.

The trainee is usually helped towards a comfortable posture, often lying corpse-like on the floor with hands outwards. Instructions are gradually introduced to relax parts of the body in turn, eventually ending with the instructions to the mind to 'let go'.

There may follow sessions of guided imagery, colours, or reflections on pleasurable and absorbing memories.[19] There may be music, or there may be occasional reminders to concentrate on breathing sensations. The breath is often used as a bridge to reach an individual's calm, confident centre, unavailable through his web of discursive thoughts.[20] Relaxation programmes may also be combined with sessions in which people learn to control stressful influences. Useful rule-of-thumb techniques are taught, for example to shift to abdominal breathing when situations get tense.

It is obvious that there is a great deal of overlap between relaxation, meditation in its beginning stages, yoga relaxation, and so on.[21] In fact, in terms of physiology, deep relaxation produces the same alteration in skin resistance, brain waves, breath patterns, and other measures of arousal, as transcendental meditation.[22] The quietening down of the sympathetic nervous system is striking and similar in all of these techniques.[23] A recent survey of the world medical and scientific literature on meditation and other self-control strategies came to the conclusion that various kinds of meditation, relaxation methods, yoga and biofeedback were equivalent from the point of view of health benefits.[24]

This does not mean that meditation is 'no more than' these other self-regulation methods, for obviously it goes very much further, indeed it is the logical conclusion of all these methods. However, the differences relate to the self-transforming experiences undergone by the meditator, not the reduction of stress and removal of psychogenic diseases.

Relaxation methods are demonstrably effective in stress control, asthma,[25,26] the side-effects of cancer treatment,[27] chronic pain,[28] high blood pressure,[29] anxiety, and so on.

For example, Dr Chandra Patel has reported several controlled studies in which patients who are at risk of developing heart problems were taught relaxation, with the result that many of their predisposing signs, such as high blood pressure, were reduced. The improvements in cardiovascular health persisted over several years compared to a control group.[30] Through the additional use of visualization as a therapy, which is the intense concentration on specific images, then a further range of health benefits, particularly the regression of cancer, may be possible in some people, given aptitude and will.[31,32,33]

As with meditation, relaxation will give an opportunity for

thoughts and materials which have been suppressed by cerebral censorship to well up. There is therefore a possibility of increased anxiety, restlessness, and withdrawal in some sensitive or disturbed people. This could hardly be described as a side-effect, but it is important to be aware of it. In addition, relaxation techniques may be inappropriate where they are used as avoidance, or where a person is of a disposition that requires arousal and alertness rather than the opposite.

Biofeedback

The learning of all human abilities requires feedback. When a child learns to speak there is a constant two-way flow of attempts and corrections which are gradually refined down to a communicable tongue. This feedback is an unconscious strategy; however, there are many cases where feedback programmes are designed to supplement or replace those naturally available to man, for example in teaching a deaf person to speak or in teaching the use of limbs in the disabled. Biofeedback is the use of programmes of this kind, not to replace but to extend control into areas not normally manipulable by the will. That is, to control so-called 'involuntary' mental and physical processes.

The origins of biofeedback are found in the psychological experiments demonstrating basic conditioning or learning procedures that have occupied a good deal of experimental psychology for many years. Conditioning is a learning procedure by which some aspect of normal voluntary behaviour is elicited by rewards, a classic being good behaviour for ice-cream. However, researchers such as Kemmel and Miller demonstrated that responses that are normally automatic, or involuntary, such as heart rate, blood pressure, peristalsis of the intestines, blood flow in vessels, or skin temperature, could also be learnt by animals in the laboratory by rewarding them appropriately.[34,35]

It was not long before people hooked themselves up to the plethora of medical machinery used by doctors and researchers to monitor automatic physiological processes: the electroencephalograph (EEG) to measure brain waves, the electromyograph (EMG) to measure muscular activity, blood pressure and heart rate recorders, the electrical skin resistance meter (ESR), and so on. Not only could people learn to control their responses fairly quickly, but clear health benefits ensued. When muscle tension was reduced, the whole body became relaxed; headaches, stress, and anxiety were reduced too when finger temperature was increased people lost their tensions, relieved their migraines, improved their circulation, and could sleep better at night.

In fact, in order to learn a specific ability, biofeedback trainees must enter a state of relaxed awareness. Physiological changes, such as a reduction in skin resistance and a redistribution of blood supply to the periphery of the body, ensue, and all these are superimposed on the original ability. It follows that biofeedback is as good as other procedures in relieving stress-related conditions,[21] such as anxiety, insomnia, high blood pressure, tachycardia, and tension headaches. However, in addition there are certain areas where it excels, for it can bring internal processes under more specific control than is possible by other relaxation methods. For example, learning to raise finger temperature or lower forehead temperature has shown excellent results in the treatment of migraine.[36] A Birmingham clinic found that some 80 per cent of migraine patients improved with this method. The same method is perhaps the best available for the treatment of Raynaud's disease, trench foot, and some other problems arising from inadequate circulation in the small blood vessels of the limbs.[37] It has been used very successfully in increasing blood pressure in those confined to wheelchairs, in re-training incontinent people, and in restoring function to specific damaged muscles.

In practice a trainee must learn the signal language of the equipment he is using, while in a normal aroused state. He then endeavours to alter the meter, tone, or light by any means at his disposal in a state of relaxation. Gradually, he learns to alter the readings of the instrument above his own, now familiar, baseline. Eventually he becomes used to the state of mind which he has empirically found to be successful, and can then dispense with the feedback. The last stage is perhaps the most difficult. For many biofeedback practitioners have found that their subjects learn quickly and can re-create the desired state easily when hooked up to the machinery in a therapeutic setting. However, when the subject goes home the ability is gradually lost. Daily life, of course, tends to distract from entry into states where automatic functions are controllable. There are several possible strategies that avoid this. Training should be extended, should include sessions with the machine switched off, should alter the response upwards and downwards, and should use responses relating directly to the condition, i.e. resistance of the air passages for an asthma patient rather than a more unconnected response such as heart rate.[38] Nevertheless, the fall-off has limited the use of biofeedback in controlling high blood pressure, where biofeedback ought to have a vital role to play. Success seems possible only where biofeedback is combined with other methods.[39]

Biofeedback is in the unique position of being a science-based therapeutic procedure, with some 2500 papers to its credit, at the same time as an exciting self-development tool. 'Clinical biofeedback based on scientific principles and basic science has emerged and it will form an important part of the new discipline of behavioural medicine', states one authority.[40] Yet the same procedure, when used with equipment to monitor brain waves, can be used as a stepping stone to explore altered states of consciousness.[41]

In the UK, biofeedback is taught more as a self-monitoring procedure than a self-training one. That is, in contrast to the American school, trainees are instructed to regard the biofeedback tools as a check on progress in reaching desired psychophysical states. This helps to avoid dependence on the instrumentation.

Autogenic therapy

Johannes Schultz was a German psychiatrist and neurologist, working in Berlin in the 1930s. He was perhaps one of the first to develop practical self-help strategies incorporating scientific discoveries on the physiology of arousal and relaxation. This arose out of his use of hypnosis, for he observed how those entering the hypnotic state became relaxed and passively aware. He reasoned that if people could be taught to enter this state at will, the recuperative and health benefits of hypnosis would become generally available. He constructed an exact system which is something like a mixture of progressive relaxation, self-hypnosis, and meditative affirmations. The essence of the technique is passive (i.e. relaxed and unconcerned) attention to various parts of the body. There are several stages to the method.

The first stage is autogenic training itself. The practitioner or instructor, after taking a personal and medical history, will instruct the trainee in an appropriate relaxed posture, and the technique of passive awareness of parts of the body. Then he gives the trainee an exercise. The first one involves passively attending to the right arm while holding the thought that 'my right arm is heavy'. The heaviness is then extended to the other limbs. The second exercise suggests warmth in the extremities, the third calms the heartbeat, the fourth calms and regularizes the breath, the fifth warms the solar plexus, and the sixth cools the forehead. The trainee goes through the training gradually, keeping a record, with the instructor checking and guiding along the way.

Neither the trainee nor the trainer will direct the technique towards the cure of a specific illness, for it is felt that the innate *vix medicatrix naturae* is sufficiently powerful to achieve a cure once it is unleashed by a receptive state. Schultz records many cures in thousands of well-documented case studies, particularly from peptic ulcer, indigestion, circulatory problems, heart arrhythmias and angina, obsessive behaviours, sexual problems, diabetic pathologies, asthma, migraine, and anxiety.[42] The conditions treated are similar to those treated by hypnosis, with which autogenic therapy has much in common. It also, naturally, has a strong preventive role. There are, as yet, far fewer research studies on autogenic therapy than on hypnosis or biofeedback, partly because success takes a considerable time, and because the trainee integrates the practice into his daily life from which it is hard to extricate it for research purposes. Yet one or two studies have appeared,[43] along with many anecdotal clinical reports.

Like the other mind-body therapies, autogenic training is also the springboard for further work into growth, self-fulfilment and extending capabilities. The next stage after autogenic training is autogenic modification, which amplifies the training and directs it to develop specific areas. For example, 'my lower abdomen is warm' will be used to stimulate the colon, 'my sinuses are cool and my chest is warm' will be used in the case of asthma sufferers. There are also behaviour control and development formulae, which can be used by athletes or performers to remove fears and blocks and develop their powers. Another stage beyond this is autogenic neutralization which focuses on psychological postures and problems in the same state of passive acceptance. The next stage is autogenic meditation which makes use of visualizations, contemplation of ideas, and contact with deeper levels of a person's being. These more advanced procedures are available to trainees with a good grounding in the basic autogenic training.

The Bates method of eyesight training

William Bates was a highly respected eye doctor in New York. During the course of his long career, in which he examined some 30 000 eyes, he came to the conclusion that defects in vision are not irreversible, as is the current medical view. The accommodation of the eye to distance is controlled by muscles which pull the lens. Bates reasoned that many of the defects in vision were due to tensions and poor function in these muscles. He developed a system of re-training of these muscles which obeys the same general principles as those described in other sections of this chapter. That is, the use of the mind and relaxation techniques gradually to relax and re-align muscles and alter customary habits.

One of his great successes was the restoration of full sight to a virtually blind Aldous Huxley who then wrote:

I have been treated by men of the highest eminence in their profession; but never once did they so much as faintly hint that there may be a mental side to vision, or that there may be wrong ways, unnatural and abnormal modes of visual functioning as well as natural and normal ones . . . My own case is in no way unique. Thousands of other sufferers from defects of vision have benefited by following the simple rules of that Art of Seeing which we owe to Bates and his followers.[44]

The method has several components. A basic relaxation method known as palming involves shutting all light out with the hands, followed by a deep progressive relaxation of the body. In the dark, the mind's eye is sharpened and perceptions are focused. For example, an object is imagined to be moving from the observer without losing its clarity. Another exercise involves swinging rhythmically from side to side, with the eyes focused in the distance but moving, relaxedly, with the head. The sun is also used, as a centre of light which is contemplated with eyes shut in order to regenerate and renew the tissues. An eye chart records progress, and is used in exercises of relaxed seeing, without staring and without strain.

Some Bates practitioners explore the psychological dimensions of the defective vision in the same way as those working with posture explore and release locked-up early experiences that led to the locked-in tensions. Short- and long-sightedness as well as astigmatism and squint can all be treated in this way. However, as it is an instructional technique, the treatment depends on the patient's will and persistence. There are very few Bates practitioners in the United Kingdom, most practise in America.

References

1. Monro, R., Trevelyan, J.E., and West, R. (1987). *Mind-body therapies: A select bibliography of books in English.* Mansell, London. Pelletier, K. (1977). *Mind as healer, mind as slayer: A holistic approach to preventing stress disorders.* Delacorte, New York. Tanner, O. (1977). *Stress.* Time-Life International, The Netherlands. Krakowski, A.J. and Chase, P.K. (1983). *Psychosomatic medicine: theoretical, clinical and transcultural aspects.* Plenum, New York.

2. Selye, Hans (1976). *The stress of life.* McGraw-Hill, New York.

3. Cannon, W.B. (1939). *The wisdom of the body.* Norton, New York.

4. Stein, M., Schiavi, R.C., and Camerino, M. (1976). Influence of brain and behaviour on the immune system. *Science,* **191,** 435–40. Editorial (1987). Depression, stress and immunity, *Lancet,* **2,** 1467–8.

5. Frankenhauser, M. (1977). *Journal of Psychosomatic Research,* **21,** 313–21.

6. Johansson, G. (1976). *Biological Psychology,* **4,** 157–72.

7. Friedman, M. and Rosenman, R. (1974). *Type A behaviour and your heart.* Fawcett, New York.

8. Wright, I.S. (1975). Cardiovascular diseases: Role of psychogenic and behaviour patterns in development and aggravation. *New York State Journal of Medicine,* **75,** 2128–32.

9. Riley, V. (1975). *Science,* **189,** 465–7.

10. Achterberg, J., Simonton, C., and Mathews-Simonton, S. (1976). *Stress, psychological factors, and cancer.* New Medicine Press, Fort Worth.

11. Riley, V. (1981). Psychoneuroendocrine influences on immunocompetence and neoplasia. *Science,* **212,** 1100–9. Sklar, S.L. and Anisman, H. (1981). Stress and cancer. *Psychology Bulletin,* **89,** 369–406. Bower, B. (1985). Severe depression depresses immunity. *Science News,* **127,** 100.

12. Raskova, H. and Elis, J. (1978). The role of the placebo in therapeutics. *Impact of Science on Society,* **28,** 57.

13. Shapiro, A.K. (1964). Factors contributing to the placebo effect: Their implications for psychotherapy. *American Journal of Psychotherapy,* **18,** 73–88.

14. Ernst, M. and Lee, M.H. (1987). Influence of naloxone on electroacupuncture analgesia using experimental dental pain test. Review of possible mechanisms of action. *Acupuncture and Electrotherapeutic Research,* **12,** 5–22.

15. de Wied, D. and Jolles, J. (1976). Hormonal influences on motivational learning and memory processes. In: *Hormones, behaviour and psychopathology*. Raven Press, New York.

16. Garfield, S., Bergin, A.E. (1986). *Psychotherapy and behaviour change*. Wiley, Chichester.

17. Brown, M. (1973). The new body psychotherapies. *Psychotherapy: Theory, Research and Practice*, **10**, 98–116.

18. See, for example, Human Potential Resources, 35 Station Road, London NW4.

19. Morse, D.R., Martin, J.S., Furst, M.L., Dubin, L.L., (1977). A physiological and subjective evaluation of meditation, hypnosis and relaxation. *Psychosomatic Medicine*, **39**, 304–24.

20. Geba, Bruno (1974). *Breathe away your tension: An introduction to gestalt body awareness therapy*. Random House, New York.

21. Benson, H. (1976). *The relaxation response*. Morrow, New York. Silver, B.V. and Blanchard, E.B. (1978). Biofeedback and relaxation training in the treatment of psychophysiological disorders; or are the machines really necessary? *Journal of Behavioural Medicine*, **1**, 217–19.

22. Thomas, D. and Abbas, K.A. (1978). Comparison of transcendental meditation and progressive relaxation in reducing anxiety. *British Medical Journal*, **4**, 1749.

23. Hoffman, J.W., Benson, H., Arns, P.A., Stainbrook, G.L., Landsberg, L., Young, J.B., and Gill, A. (1982). Reduced sympathetic nervous system. Responsibility associated with the relaxation response. *Science*, **215**, 190–2.

24. Shapiro, D.M. (1982). Overview: Clinical and physiological comparison of meditation with other self-control strategies. *American Journal of Psychiatry*, **139**, 267–74.

25. Erskine, M.J. and Schonell, M. (1981). Relaxation therapy in asthma: critical review. *Psychosomatic Medicine*, **43**, 365–72.

26. Saxena, R.P. and Saxena, U. (1978). Psychotherapeutic approach in the treatment of asthma. *Journal of Chronic Disease and Therapeutic Research*, **1**, 25.

27. Burish, T.G. and Lyles, J.N. (1981). Effectiveness of relaxation training in reducing adverse reactions to cancer chemotherapy. *Journal of Behavioural Medicine*, **4**, 65–78.

28. Turner, J.A. and Chapman, C.P. (1981). Psychological intervention in chronic pain: A critical review. I. Relaxation and biofeedback. *Pain*, **12**, 1–21.

29. Benson, H., Rosner, B.A., Marzetts, B.A., and Klemchuk, H. (1974). Decreased blood pressure in pharmacologically treated hypertensive patients who regularly elicited the relaxation response. *Lancet*, **1**, 289–91. McGrady, A., Williams, S., Woerner, M., Bernal, G.A., and Higgins, J.T. (1986). Predictors of success in hypertensives

treated with biofeedback-assisted relaxation. *Biofeedback and Self-Regulation*, **11**, 95–103.

30. Patel, C. (1984). A holistic approach to cardiovascular disease. *British Journal of Holistic Medicine*, **1**, 30–41. Patel, C., Marmot, M.G., Terry, D.J., Carruthers, M., Hunt, B., and Patel, M. (1985). Trial of relaxation in reducing coronary risk. A 4-year follow-up. *British Medical Journal*, **290**, 1103–6.

31. Meares, A. (1981). Regression of recurrence of carcinoma of the breast at mastectomy site associated with intensive meditation. *Australian Family Physician*, **10**, 218–9. Meares, A. (1983). *Relief without drugs*. Fontana, London.

32. Fiore, N. (1974). Fighting cancer, one patient's perspective. *New England Journal of Medicine*, **300**, 284.

33. Simonton, O.C., Matthews-Simonton, S., and Creighton, J. (1978). *Getting well again*. Tarcher Books, Los Angeles. Achterberg, J. (1985). *Imagery in healing: shamanism and modern medicine*. Shambhala, Boston.

34. Kemmel, H.D. (1967). Instrumental conditioning of autonomically mediated behaviour. *Psychological Bulletin*, **67**, 337–45.

35. Miller, N.E. (1969). Learning of visceral and glandular responses. *Science*, **163**, 434–5.

36. Orne, M.T. (1979). The efficacy of biofeedback therapy. *Annual Review of Medicine*, **30**, 489–503.

37. Surwit, R.S., Pilon, R.N., and Fenton, C. (1977). Behavioural treatment of Raynaud's disease. *Annual meeting of the Assoc. for Advances in Behavioural Therapy*, Atlanta, Georgia.

38. Colgan, M. (1981). Medical uses of biofeedback: Principles and case studies. *New Zealand Medical Journal*, **93**, 49–51.

39. Patel, C., Marmet, M.G., and Terry, D.J. (1981). Controlled trial of biofeedback-aided behavioural methods in reducing mild hypertension. *British Medical Journal*, **282**, 2005–8.

40. Basmajian, J.V. (1978). Biofeedback in medical practice. *Canadian Medical Association Journal*, **119**, 10.

41. Cade, C.M. and Coxhead, N. (1987). *The awakened mind—Biofeedback and the development of higher States of Awareness*. Element, Shaftesbury, Dorset.

42. Luthe, W. (1976). *Creative mobilisation technique*, Grune and Stratton, New York.

43. Sargent, J.D., Green, E.E., and Walters, E.D. (1973). Preliminary report on the use of autogenic feedback training in the treatment of migraine and tension headaches. *Psychosomatic Medicine*, **35**, 129–35.

44. Huxley, A. (1974). *The art of seeing*, Montanu Books, Seattle.

18

Naturopathy and nutrition therapy

Background

Naturopathy, to quote the manifesto of the British Naturopathic and Osteopathic Association, is 'a system of treating human ailments which recognises that healing depends upon the vital curative force within the human organism'. This fundamental tenet underlies all natural therapies and certainly naturopathy. In practice it may range widely for, according to the American Naturopathic Association, it is 'a therapeutic system embracing a complete physianthropy employing nature's agencies, forces, processes, and products'.

It is customary for many systems of medical care to claim Hippocrates as their founder. Naturopathy can, perhaps, justify this claim more than most. When Hippocrates laid down guidelines for the maintenance of health in terms of the correct balance of rest and exercise, adequate nourishment and emotional stability, he was advocating those principles of bodily hygiene which are the foundations of naturopathy. These principles only came to be appreciated again in the past 150 years or so by a pioneering few. A revival in vitalism began in nineteenth-century Europe where individuals (not always those medically trained or involved in the fight against disease) discovered and developed the use of simple measures such as water applications, plain food, and herbs as ways of promoting the healing mechanisms of the body. The discoveries were generally empirical, rather than deliberately created under clinical conditions in the way that osteopathy or homeopathy were.

In the small village of Grafenberg, in the Silesian mountains, a farmer, Vincent Priessnitz, advocated fresh air, applications of cool water, and wholesome fare consisting of black bread, vegetables, and fresh milk from cows fed on the mountain pastures. Others learned from Priessnitz or discovered for themselves the value of nature's agents. Khune, a weaver, became famous for his dietary treatments, another farmer, Johannes Schroth, evolved a strict dietary regime combined with hydrotherapy for the treatment of rheumatic disorders which, in spite of its stringency, was, and still is, greatly esteemed by many sufferers from this complaint. However, it was to Father Sebastian Kneipp of Bad Worishösen in Bavaria that the tremendous popularity of hydrotherapy was due. Spas utilizing the methods he advocated were established throughout Europe.

Sometimes a chance observation led to the discovery of a system of treatment or diagnosis. Thus it was that a Prussian priest, Edmund von Peczely, founded the art of iris diagnosis, widely used by naturopaths to assess the vitality and the constitutional weaknesses of their patients. Von Peczely had a pet owl and, one day, when handling it, he accidentally broke its leg. He noticed that a blemish appeared in its eye which gradually changed in texture as the leg healed and this led him to pursue his observations; this became the foundation of modern iridology.

Fundamental concepts

As a system of health care which grew out of practical experience, naturopathy's philosophical concepts were not really laid down until an American doctor, Henry Lindlahr, wrote his *Philosophy of natural therapeutics* in the early part of this century. According to Lindlahr, 'health is the normal and harmonious vibration of the elements and forces composing the human entity on the physical, mental and moral planes of being in conformity with the constructive principle in nature'.[1] Disease is generally the result of the disobedience of nature's laws leading to an inharmonious vibration of those same elements and forces.

To the sceptic these definitions may seem to be gross oversimplifications; indeed they are, but they crystallize the thought that lies behind naturopathic practice. If the body possesses the capacity to heal cuts or mend broken bones then it must ultimately be capable of resolving other disorders. The concept of homeostasis, the self-regulating mechanism of the body, is generally accepted, and the immune process is under intense study in modern medicine. However, in concentrating attention on the minute biochemical details of disease, medicine has narrowed its view of the origin of disease and the requirements for recovery. Whereas the allopathic view might suggest that recovery is aided by removal of inflamed or degenerative tissue, destruction of bacteria, or intervention in a specific metabolic pathway, the naturopath would take steps to promote the body's ability to restore its own equilibrium.

Lindlahr wrote of the body's response to inimical forces by crisis which, if prolonged, would lead to exhaustion and devitalization of its resources. This is exemplified by the tendency for acute superficial disorders, if suppressed by drugs or unsatisfactorily resolved, to become chronic and lead to pathological change and degeneration. However, it was Professor Hans Selye, of Montreal, who first postulated in some detail the concept of a general adaptation syndrome. This is the adaptive process by which we have survived as a species.[2]

According to Selye, the body's response to any stress, be it emotional or physical, initiates a three-phase sequence. Initially in the *alarm stage* there is pain (due, for example, to injury), shock (from bad news), or inflammation (due to friction). Then, as the body adjusts to the crisis, there is a *stage of resistance* in which we adapt to, or withstand the 'invasion' (stiffen to protect a joint, or suppress the hurt feeling, etc.). If the traumas or emotional stresses are prolonged the body or the group of cells under siege can no longer adapt. It then enters a *stage of exhaustion* and collapse, or degeneration occurs.[3]

Naturopaths attach great importance to this adaptive capacity of the body and recognize that symptoms, such as inflammation or pain, are signs of the defences at work and not to be suppressed. Furthermore, the process of recovery from chronic ailments may necessitate a return to the stage of resistance—known in natural therapy as the *healing crisis*.

Therapeutic procedures are directed to the restoration of normality in all aspects of the human function but first it is necessary to determine at what level in the adaptive functions the breakdown has occurred.

Diagnosis

The patient who visits a naturopath for advice about a particular disorder may be surprised to be questioned about seemingly irrelevant aspects of his body function or lifestyle. Examination of the eyes or measurement of the blood pressure may not be expected by a person seeking advice about a gastric ulcer. For the naturopath, diagnosis is only partly the collection of data to arrive at a defined disorder. It is also an assessment of the total functional capacity of the individual. Naturopaths aim to diagnose the patient rather than the disease, although in practice they must do both.

Symptoms are only relevant as indicators of breakdown in adaptive mechanisms. Whilst palliative measures may be necessary it is the underlying disorder of bodily processes which must be corrected if the patient is to recover satisfactorily. Thus, when confronted with a skin rash, the naturopath is not particularly concerned with categorizing it among the host of medically defined dermatoses for he recognizes that it is most probably a manifestation of a deeper imbalance. That could be a disturbance in the metabolism of nutrients, or a blood dyscrasia (and the naturopath would check for these by the normal diagnostic procedure such as urine and blood analysis), but more often it may be a phase in the eliminative response to an underlying functional disturbance of organs such as the lungs or liver. It is this deeper cause of the rash which has to be sought.

Naturopathic assessment is also aimed at assessing the patient's vital reserve—his ability to respond to treatment. This information will be gleaned by standard methods of medical investigation which may, however, be interpreted cautiously. Levels of blood sugar or of certain vitamins or minerals which are considered within the 'normal range' may not always be acceptable to the naturopath, because under stress, these levels may be pushed way up or down. If this happens repeatedly, chronic, sometimes irreversible, changes take place. The most common example of this is what one naturo-path Martin L. Budd, has called the twentieth-century epidemic—hypoglycaemia.[4] This condition, otherwise known as low blood sugar, may occur in phases induced by repeated intake of refined carbohydrates (sugar, white flour), starchy snacks, and caffeine (in coffee, tea, or canned beverages). These are absorbed so rapidly that the pancreas becomes over-sensitive and produces too much insulin. The excess insulin brings down blood sugar below normal, which when repeated often, may eventually give rise to chronic disorders such as migraine, allergies, hyperactivity, depression, obesity, or alcholism. The hypoglycaemic pattern is fairly obvious from clinical signs and symptoms but it may be confirmed by a 6-hour glucose tolerance test, which measures changes in the blood sugar level at regular intervals after administration of 50 g of glucose by mouth. Treatment is the stabilization of blood sugar levels by diet.

The nutritional status as well as general vital reserve may be gauged by observation of skin tone, complexion, and the state of mucous membranes of the mouth and tongue. The nails can, for example, exhibit white spots, or leukonychia, which may suggest a deficiency of the trace element zinc. Some naturopaths use nair analysis as a means of assessing the levels of both the essential minerals and also the toxic metals such as aluminium, cadmium, and lead, which may cause insidious damage. Interpretation of hair analysis is still experimental; however it seems that the body's need for certain nutrients is not always reflected in the levels revealed by the more acceptable methods of assessment.

Iris diagnosis is among the most valuable diagnostic tools of the naturopath. It has not, thus far, been possible to establish definite anatomical evidence for a connection between the eye and other parts of the body but it seems highly probable that fine nervous connections do exist via the optic chiasma. The legacy of von Peczely's owl has become a sophisticated system of diagnosis which is now used the world over. The system was developed in Europe during the nineteenth century and there are now some German Heilpraktikers who rely almost exclusively on this method of diagnosis. Some practitioners take photographs of the iris as a permanent record whilst many others rely on direct observation with suitable illumination and magnification.[5]

Iris diagnosis is based on the principle that the general tone and level of inflammatory activity in various body tissues is reflected in the iris of the eye. Each system, such as stomach, intestines, autonomic nervous system, lymphatics, or skin, is represented in circular zones with radial divisions indicating the state of individual organs and mental faculties. Observation of the iris reveals the overall vital reserve of the patient and the areas of inherent weakness. Interpretation of the signs in the iris is made in functional terms, for example underactivity of skin, rather than a specific diagnosis such as eczema.

The treatment

The information accumulated by questioning, observation, and examination now has to be co-ordinated to form an overall impression of the patient and his requirements. The therapeutic regime will depend on a number of factors other than those immediately obvious from the examination, for example hereditary tendencies, constitution (both of which play a significant part in naturopathic assessment), past history, and previous treatments, especially use of drugs.[6]

From this information a decision can be reached as to whether therapy must be primarily anabolic (building up) or catabolic (breaking down). If the patient is devitalized, nutritionally deficient, and suffering from a chronic ailment he may need to be moved out of an over-stimulating catabolic phase requiring instead anabolic and tonic measures: a wholefood diet, rest and relaxation, and gentle manipulative procedures, with a constructive mental outlook. Nutritional measures will often be used to add the elements required by the patient, either by altering diet, or more usually by prescribing supplements of those substances to be taken orally or, in some instances (e.g. vitamin B_{12}), administered intramuscularly. For example, many micronutrients and trace elements have been shown to be important in treating conditions such as hypoglycaemia.[7]

In other cases, toxic accumulations must first be cleared by catabolic purificatory methods. Indeed, these eliminative methods in naturopathy used to rule supreme, especially in the early days of naturopathic hydros. Controlled catabolic activity is a necessary process in the management of chronic disorders to promote the functions of skin, lungs, or bowels. This may be done by dietary restriction or fasting, by hydrotherapy, both internal and external, and more stimulating exercise and manipulative procedures.

There are schools of naturopathy that still rely entirely on eliminative methods, with considerable success. The pure hygienic methods, pioneered by Shelton, will not admit of any external supplements or aids.[8] Spas and hydros offer a number of purificatory treatments, such as hot and cold spring and mineral baths, mud packs for skin conditions, bubbling aerated water, steam baths, and so on.[9]

It is sometimes necessary to promote a fever as a means of enabling the body to burn up toxic waste. This may be achieved by means of heat treatment and hydrotherapy, or the use of herbal substances. The stage at which these stimulating forms of treatment are introduced will depend upon the vitality of the patient—in those with sufficient vital reserve such treatments would be introduced at an early stage. These procedures may occasionally promote a crisis, and unless the naturopath can keep his patient under close observation, as, for example, in a residential clinic, he would be less inclined to impose prolonged eliminative procedures.

Fasting and other restricted diets

Under proper supervision the fast may be regarded as a most constructive, health-restoring procedure and should not be confused with starvation. The fact that it has been an important part of religious rituals in many parts of the world bears out its intellect-sharpening as well as physical benefits. Fasting constitutes a physiological rest which enables the body to divert its energy to the process of removing metabolic waste and restoring homeostasis.[10] Some authorities suggest that the element of metabolic shock in fasting induces an immune response. Fasting need not be total. A mono-diet is one in which a food or group of foods is eaten almost exclusively for a period of time. The most famous of these is the grape cure first advocated by Dr Johanna Budwig but graphically described by Basil Shackleton, who lived only on grapes (in South Africa where they are abundant) for almost 50 days and wrote '. . . after the twenty-third day an abscess came away from my one and only kidney and I was completely cured after all medical treatment had failed and made my condition worse'.[11]

The single most consistent factor in naturopathic practice has been the advocacy of a wholefood high fibre diet, preferably of foods which have been organically grown and are free from chemical additives.[12] For decades naturopaths have pointed out the harmful effects of chemicals and pesticide residues in food and, after encountering much opposition, are now finding more widespread acceptance and corroboration in medical research.[13]

The dynamics of structure

The need for an adequate transport system to and from each cellular unit is implicit in the requirement of good nutrition and adequate elimination. Freedom of circulation for the blood and lymph is, therefore, of paramount importance and the naturopath is very concerned with the removal of any obstacles to these in the form of joint restrictions and muscular spasm. Some naturopaths are also trained as osteopaths and can therefore bring to certain disorders, such as joint problems, the added dimension of the 'total lesion concept'. This means viewing restrictions of mobility and alignment not just from a mechanical standpoint but considering nutritional integrity, tissue tone, muscle balance, and even the influence of the emotions on the patient's postural habits.

The body-mind amalgam

The holistic view of health cannot ignore the powerful influence of thought, conscious or subconscious, on physical well-being. Naturopaths place varying degrees of emphasis on the role of the emotions in causing physical illness. A number of practitioners devote considerable time to counselling and other psychological approaches to physical illness. The fact that naturopaths give a great deal of time to their patients inevitably means that the social and psychological aspects of their ailments are considered in some depth. Some also teach relaxation methods. In general, where 'outrageous fortune' burdens the patient with stresses, such as marital disagreements or unreasonable work pressures, the naturopath will emphasize the need for sound nutrition to improve the person's ability to withstand the 'slings and arrows'.

The long-term effects of under-nutrition, or the constant abuse of digestive organs by over-refined or over-concentrated foods create a sensitivity to a wider and wider range of substances. It is now becoming fashionable in medical circles to attempt to identify these so-called allergens and in some cases such common foods as eggs or milk have been found to precipitate quite severe psychiatric disorders.[14] Exclusion of the offending foods achieves improvement although naturopathy attaches more importance to attaining the stability of the internal milieu.

Nutrition therapy

Nutrition therapy, or nutritional medicine, is a daughter specialization of naturopathy. It has grown so fast that the child is as big as, and in America towers over, its parent. It is the science of treating disease and promoting health by the use of specific nutritional factors, together with the elimination of toxic and allergenic materials from the diet.[15] It differs from naturopathy in several respects. First, it is more specialized: practitioners do not pay so much attention to hygienic, physical, or hydrotherapeutic aspects of traditional naturopathy. Secondly, it is more scientific. Practitioners draw their inspiration more from the 1000 nutritionally oriented scientific publications published in the world literature every year, than from the tenets of Hippocrates, Priessnitz, and Lindlahr. Thirdly it is more prescriptional: minerals, vitamins, essential fatty acids, amino acids, and other supplements are taken in therapeutic doses for a medicinal effect. Many naturopaths regard this as too interventionist for comfort, deviating from the basic naturopathic principles of self-cure.[16]

The basic principles of nutritional medicine are well defined in the summary issued by the British Society for Nutritional Medicine:

1. Man's diet, even in industrialised societies, may very often have only a borderline or indeed low content of certain essential nutrients. A 'normal' diet is not necessarily a healthy or optimum one.

2. Requirements for essential nutrients vary from individual to individual depending on genetic, physiological, lifestyle and other influences. What is adequate for one person may not be for another.

3. Illness is inevitably linked with an abnormal biochemistry and an alteration in the metabolism of nutrients and their by-products.

4. Specific nutrients such as vitamins, minerals, essential fatty acids and amino acids, as well as dietary manipulation in general, provide a potent means of influencing body biochemistry and thus disease processes.

5. By correcting fundamental biochemical abnormalities by nutritional means one can prevent certain diseases or alter the course of disease processes for the better.

In the last few years nutritional medicine has rapidly increased in popularity among both conventional and complementary health professionals. Doctors gain a set of options in addition to drugs to help manage some of the more intractable problems which reappear in their surgeries. For example, magnesium supplements, along with dietary changes, has been found useful as part of a combined treatment of high blood pressure and arrhythmias.[17] B vitamins and gamma linoleic acid are used for premenstrual, menopausal, and other conditions,[18] zinc and vitamin C for wound healing,[19] B vitamins in certain psychosomatic conditions,[20] and so on. Some clinical nutritionists who may or may not be medically qualified, use dietary factors as a health care system in its own right. Diagnosis would be essentially naturopathic, but would add hair mineral analysis, and a complete analysis of the diet and toxic constituents (including drugs) which the patient consumes. Treatment is given as a personally designed daily cocktail of vitamin, mineral, and other supplements.[21]

Nutritional therapists also pay attention to the possibility of food allergies, or more commonly, food sensitivities. Diseases such as infant gastrointestinal conditions, eczema, asthma, hyperactivity and sleep disturbance in children, migraine, colitis, obesity, malaise, headache and various so-called psychosomatic symptoms, *Candida* infections and autoimmune related conditions have all been associated with food allergies or sensitivities in a proportion of patients.[22] There is increasing medical research evidence to support this, for example studies at the Institute of Child Health have found that roughly two-thirds of children with hyperactivity and insomnia are cured by the removal of allergenic additives, particularly colourants and preservatives, from their diet.[23] Food allergies are diagnosed, conventionally, by a fast after which foods are restored one by one and the reactions carefully assessed. However, this method is difficult for patients to manage, and newer, less conventional methods are now employed, including testing of the reaction of the white blood cells of the patient, sublingual tests, applied kinesiology, and certain electrical equipment (see electroacupuncture page 129). These practices await solid clinical research backing, in particular it is not known to what extent patients treated by the elimination of additives and contaminants to the diet are responding because of elimination of allergic reactions, or the addition of necessary dietary factors along with the elimination of toxins and 'empty calories'.

Research

Because of its multidisciplinary approach, naturopathy as a complete therapy has not been subject to controlled research. Yet as some of its tenets, such as the harmful effects of animal fats on the circulation, have become obvious to conventional medical experts, these have been tested in academic establishments. This research has produced a considerable body of evidence to support much of naturopathic theory, referred to in references 6, 12, 15, 29, with some further examples below.

A stimulus towards acceptance of naturopathic tenets has been observation of the health and longevity of primitive tribal communities, or religious groups practising abstinence, particularly the Pennsylvania Amish.[24] At first this lent support to the view that the rich animal fat diet of the civilized world produced the degenerative disease load in its wake. However, subsequent analysis showed that some healthy tribes, such as the Masai and the Eskimos, eat a lot of meat. This drew attention to salt, milk and milk products, refined foods, a lack of certain polyunsaturated fatty acids and trace elements, combined with inadequate exercise and relaxation.[25]

Recently, more profound understanding of the primitive diet has emerged from a lengthy study of the nutritional status of early man.[26] Not only was his diet ten times richer in vitamin C than the recommended daily allowance today, but the ratio of polyunsaturated to saturated fats was three times that of today's diet. The meat of wild animals has eight times less fat than that of farm animals and contains the important protective fatty acid eicosapentanoic acid (EPA) which is in fish oil, but absent from today's meat. Together with a great deal of pharmacological and clinical work, the above evidence shifts the emphasis away from the question of dietary fat as such, towards consideration of content and quality.[27] EPA itself has been implicated in the prevention of cardiovascular, arthritic, and malignant conditions.[28]

There has been a tremendous amount of research on the effects of vitamins and micronutrients on health[7] and recovery from disease. The reader is referred to a number of books on the subject that review the evidence.[29] To cite one or two examples more or less at random, recent studies reported in the major medical journals include the finding of a proportional relation between the risk of cancer and unusually low levels of selenium and vitamins A and E in the blood,[30] and that vitamin E can have a remarkable effect on the prevention of scarring[31] and the treatment of peripheral vascular disease.[32] Orthomolecular medicine, the use of vitamins in large doses for curative purposes, is quite well researched, particularly the use of B vitamins in treating schizophrenia and hypoglycaemia, and vitamin C in treating a large number of infective conditions and cancer.[33] There is also classical research on the protection from cancer afforded by vitamin A. Other areas of dietary interactions with health that have been well researched include the toxic effects of small amounts of metals in the diet,[7] particularly lead,[34] the nature, absorption, and interconnections between dietary elements,[35] and the diseases associated with abnormal consumption of specific food items,[29] especially in relation to the common degenerative diseases.[36] On a positive side, the improvements in health available from a vegetarian or vegan diet have now been amply confirmed by researchers, including, for example, the recent finding that vegetarian women have a hormone pattern after the menopause that would tend to reduce the incidence of postmenopausal symptoms[37] and that vegetarians tend to have lower blood pressure[38] and reduced incidence of cancer.[39]

As far as non-dietary aspects of naturopathy are concerned, research is limited. The effectiveness of hydrotherapy is rarely explored outside Germany.[6,40] There is some work on the positive health benefits of negative ions in the atmosphere, which may account for some of the value of fresh air, especially by the sea or in the mountains.[41] Biorhythms and natural cycles have also been investigated to some extent.[42]

Uses and risks

Naturopathy is first and foremost a preventive system. The naturopath sees an important part of his work as that of education in the fundamentals of health—mechanical, biochemical, and emotional—and does not, therefore, attach great importance to the classification of disease. Nevertheless, there are certain categories of illness which naturopathy treats effectively.

Most respiratory disorders such as colds, coughs, tonsilitis, and sinusitis may be regarded as self-limiting but recovery is aided by naturopathic measures. Skin diseases are often closely related to lung disorders and are often successfully treated by naturopathy although inevitably there are cases in both categories which prove resistant to therapy. Sometimes this may be because the vital response of the patient has been considerably modified by previous therapy with drugs. Disorders of the gastrointestinal system can frequently be present without any evident cause in medical terms. These disorders may be associated with an inappropriate lifestyle and improve with a review of the patient's dietary habits—often simply the introduction of more fibre. Diseases of the heart and circulation may have a functional basis which responds well to naturopathic treatment aimed at restoring adaptability.

The normalizing procedures of naturopathy may be of benefit in treating functional disorders before they become degenerative. If they advance to irreversible degenerative pathology, for example such cases as osteoarthrosis or valvular heart disease, naturopathy can develop existing resources to aid the body's compensations for its physical shortcomings. The reduction of a catarrhal encumbrance in the patient with chronic bronchitis, or emphysema, coupled with breathing exercises and osteopathic mobilization of the chest and back will at least improve the patient's capacity and reduce the occurrence of infections. Naturopathy cannot claim to have any special answer to disorders such as cancer or severe neurological disorders but it has a definite contribution to make in terms of raising general resistance and improving nutrition and outlook.

Children are particularly amenable to naturopathic treatment. They have a much greater vital response and can, therefore, be subjected to more stimulating forms of treatment, such as hydrotherapy. Naturopaths commonly treat children with acute or chronic respiratory disorders, allergies, and urinary disturbances such as nocturnal frequency. The naturopath also has an important role to play in the care of the elderly by the application of constructive nutritional measures and the use of neuromuscular techniques for the alleviation of musculoskeletal disorders.

The naturopath aims to make his patient self-sufficient with regard to health but the attainment of that level of function may take weeks or months, and sometimes complete self-sufficiency may not be possible at all. The chronic arthritic, for example, may find periodic treatment necessary, perhaps every month or two for an indefinite period. There are no risks with properly qualified naturopathic practitioners, although in some cases fasts and purificatory procedures might make a patient feel temporarily worse and should be closely monitored.

References

1. Lindlahr, V.H. (1975). *Philosophy of natural therapeutics*. Maidstone

osteopathic clinic, Maidstone, Kent. Lindlahr, V.H. (1981). *Natural therapeutics* (2 Vols). C.W. Daniel, Saffron Walden.

2. Cannon, W.B. (1939). *The Wisdom of the body.* Norton, New York.
3. Selye, Hans (1976). *The stress of life.* McGraw-Hill, New York.
4. Cheraskin, E. and Ringsdorf, W. (1974). *Psychodietetics: Food as the key to emotional health.* Stein and Day, New York. Lesser, M. (1985). *Nutrition and vitamin therapy—the dietary treatment of mental and emotional ill-health*, Thorsons, Wellingborough.
5. Kriege, T. (1969). *The fundamental basis of iridiagnosis.* Fowler, London.
6. Kohnlechner, K. (1979). *Handbuch der Naturheilkunde* (2 Vols). Wilhelm Heyne Verlag, Munich.
7. Pfeiffer, C.C. (1975). *Mental and elemental nutrients: A physician's guide to nutrition and health care.* Keats Publishing, New Canaan, Connecticut. Holford, P. (1983). *The whole health guide to elemental health.* Thorsons, Wellingborough.
8. Shelton, H.M. (1969). *The hygienic system.* Health Research, Mokelumne Hill, California.
9. Roberts, P. (1981). Hydrotherapy: Its history, theory and practice. *Occupational Health*, **33**, 235–44.
10. Cott, A. *et al.* (1981). *Fasting: the ultimate diet.* Bantam, New York.
11. Brandt, J. (1971). *The grape cure.* Benedict Lust, Simi Valley, California.
12. The National Cancer Institute in the US at last acknowledges that the consumption of fruits and vegetables reduces the risk of certain cancer: Palmer, S. and Bakshi, K. (1983). Diet, nutrition and cancer, interim dietary guidelines. *Journal of the National Cancer Institute*, **70**, 1151–70. Null, G. (1984). *The complete guide to health and nutrition.* Arlington, London. Colditz, G., Branch, L.G.L., Lipnick, R.J., Willett, W.C., Rosner, B., Posner, B.M., and Hennekens, C.H. (1985). Increased green and yellow vegetable intake and lowered cancer deaths in an elderly population. *American Journal of Clinical Nutrition*, **41**, 32–6. Griggs, B. (1987). *The Food Factor.* Viking, London.
13. Hunter, B.T. (1972). *Consumer beware!* Simon and Schuster, New York. Body, R. (1987). *Report of House of Commons, Select Committee on Agriculture and Pesticides.* HMSO, London. Dohan, F.C. (1966). Cereals and schizophrenia: Data and hypothesis. *Acta Psychiatrica Scandinavia*, **42**, 125–52.
14. Cheraskin, E. and Ringsdorf, W. (1974). *Psychodietetics: Food as the key to emotional health.* Stein and Day, New York. Mackarness, R. (1985). *Not all in the mind.* Pan, London. Wurtman, R.J. (1983). Behavioural effects of nutrients. *Lancet*, **1**, 1145–8. Ferry, G. (1983). Eat your way to mental health. *New Scientist*, **100**, 46–7.

15. Davis, A. (1983). *Let's get well.* Unwin, London. Mindell, E. (1983). *The vitamin bible.* Arlington, London. Krause, M.V. and Hauscher, M.A. (1977). *Food, nutrition and diet therapy.* W.B. Saunders, Philadelphia. Garrison, R. and Somer, E. (1985). *Nutrition Desk Reference.* Keats Publishing, New Canaan, Connecticut. Mayes, A. (1985). A dictionary of nutritional health. Thorsons, Wellingborough.

16. Chaitow, L. (1984). Will the real naturopathy stand up? *Journal of Alternative Medicine*, **2(5)**, 20. Pizzorno, J. (1984). Family physicians the aim of American naturopathy college. *Journal of Alternative Medicine*, **2(6)**, 20. Cass, M. (1984). Alternative practitioners: the family physicians of the future. *Journal of Alternative Medicine*, **2(9)**, 10.

17. Seidl, A. (1987). Die bedentung von magnesium fur die therapie von herzerkrankungen. *Erfahrungsheilkunde*, **36**, 140–3. Editorial (1985). Magnesium, nature's calcium channel blocker. *Health Consciousness*, October issue, 1. Stamier, R., Stamier, J., Grimm, R., Gosch, F.C., Elmer, P., Dyer, A., Berman, R., Fishman, J., Van Neel, N., Civinelli, J., and MacDonald, A. (1987). Nutritional therapy for high blood pressure. Final report of a four-year randomized controlled trial. *Journal of the American Medical Association*, **257**, 1484–91.

18. Davis, A. (1965). *Let's get well.* Unwin, London. Horrobin, D. (ed.) (1982). *Clinical uses of essential fatty acids*, pp. 155–62. Eden Press, Montreal and London. Abraham, G.E. (1983). Nutritional factors in the etiology of premenstrual syndrome. *Journal of Reproductive Medicine*, **128**, 446–61.

19. Hamburger, B. (1962). Ascorbic acid and wound healing. *Military Medicine*, **127**, 723. Perger, F. (1987). Zinkmangel und storungen in immunreaktionen und bei diabetes. Erfahrungsheilkunde **36**, 285–90. Pasantes, M., Morales, H., Wright, C.E., Gaull, G.E. (1986). Protective effect of taurine, zinc and tocopherol on retinol-induced damage to human lymphoblastoid cells. *Journal of Nutrition*, **114**, 2256–61.

20. Cheraskin, E. and Ringsdorf, W. (1974). *Psychodietetics: Food as the key to emotional health.* Stein and Day, New York. Lesser, T. (1985). *Nutrition and vitamin therapy—the dietary treatment of mental and emotional ill-health.* Thorsons, Wellingborough. Crook, W.G. (1987). Nutrition, food allergies and environmental toxins. *Journal of Learning Disabilities*, **20**, 260–1. Schoenthaler, S. (1983). International Journal of Biosocial Research, **5**, 88–117. Ghadirian, A.M., Anath, J., and Engelsman, F. (1980). Folic acid deficiency and depression. *Psychosomatics*, **21**, 926–9.

21. Colgan, M. (1982). *Your personal vitamin profile.* Blond and Briggs,

London. Pizzorno, J. and Murray, M. (1985). *A textbook of natural medicine*. John Bastyr College Publications, Seattle.

22. Kenyon, J. (1985). Clinical ecology. In *Alternative therapies* (ed. G. Lewith). Heinemann, London.

23. Egger, J., Wilson, J., Carter, C.M., Turner, M.W., Soothill, J.F. (1983). Is migraine a food allergy? *Lancet*, **2**, 865-9. Egger, J., Graham, P.J., Carter, C.M., Gumley, D., and Soothill, J. (1985). Controlled trial of oligoantigenic treatment in the hyperkinetic syndrome. *Lancet*, **1**, 540-5.

24. Dubos, René (1968). *So human and animal*. Scribners, New York.

25. Krause, M.V. and Hauscher, M.A. (1977). *Food, nutrition and diet therapy*. W.B. Saunders, Philadelphia. Oski, F.A. (1985). Is bovine milk a health hazard? *Paediatrics*, **755**, 182-6. Medieros, D. and Borgman, R. (1985). Blood pressure in S. Carolina children; dietary aspects. *Journal of the Royal Society of Health*, **104**, 68-70. Clinical Science, **66**, 427-33 (1984). Mayes, A. (1985). *Dictionary of nutritional health*. Thorsons, Wellingborough.

26. Eaton, B. and Kooner, M. (1985). Paleolithic nutrition. *New England Journal of Medicine*, **312**, 283-9.

27. Woodcock, B.E., Smith, E., Lambert, W.H., James, W.M., Galloway, J.H., Greaves, M., Preston, F.E. (1984). Beneficial effect of fish oil on blood viscosity in peripheral vascular disease. *British Medical Journal*, **288**, 592-4. Simons, L., Hickie, J.B., Balasubramaniam (1985). On the effects of dietary n-3 fatty acids (MaxEPA) on plasma lipids and lipoproteins in patients with hyperlipidaemia. *Atherosclerosis*, **54**, 75-88. Garrison, R. and Somer, E. (1985). *Nutrition desk reference*. Keats Publishing, New Canaan, Connecticut.

28. Horrobin, D. (ed.) (1982). *Clinical uses of essential fatty acids*. Eden Press, Montreal and London. Sinclair, H. (1984). Essential fatty acids in perspective. *Human Nutrition Clinical Nutrition*, **38C**, 4, 245-60.

29. Null, G. (1984). *The complete guide to health and nutrition*. Arlington, London. Garrison, R. and Somer, E. (1985). *Nutrition desk reference*. Keats Publishing, New Canaan, Connecticut. Bland, J. (ed.) (1986). *Yearbook of nutritional medicine*. Keats Publishing, New Canaan, Connecticut.

30. Horvath, P. and Ip, C. (1983). Synergistic effect of vitamin E and selenium in chemoprevention of mammary carcinogenesis in rats. *Cancer Research*, **43**, 5335-41. Salonen, J., Salonen, R., Lapputeläinen, R., Mäenpää, P.H., Alfthan, G., Puska, P. (1985). Risk of cancer in relation to serum concentrations of selenium and vitamins A and E. *British Medical Journal*, **290**, 417-20.

31. Nockels, C.F. (1975). Protective effects of supplemental vitamin E

against infection. *Federation Proceedings*, **38**, 377-94. Hood, R.P. (1987). Nonspecific ulcerative colitis. Successful treatment with D-alpha tocopherol. *Townsend Letters*, **51**, 268-71.

32. Piesse J. (1984). Vitamin E and peripheral vascular disease. *International Journal of Clinical and Nutritional Reviews.*, **4**, 178-82.

33. Huemer, R.P. (ed.) (1986). *The Roots of molecular medicine: a tribute to Linus Pauling*. Freeman, New York. Pauling, L. (1974). Are recommended daily allowances for vitamin C adequate? *Proceedings of the National Academy of Sciences*, **71**, 4442-6. Pauling, L. (1986). *How to live longer and feel better*. W.H. Freeman, New York.

34. Bryce-Smith, D. *Chemistry in Britain*, **8**, 240 (1972). Barnes, J.E., Smith, P.E., and Drummond, C.M. (1972). *Archives Environmental Health*, **25**, 450.

35. Stevenson, N.R. (1974). Active transport of ascorbic acid in the human ileum. *Gastroenterology*, **67**, 952. Jensen, N.L. (1979). *Journal of Applied Nutrition*, **31**, 24-36. Garrison, R. and Somer, E. (1985). *Nutrition desk reference*. Keats Publishing, New Canaan, Connecticut.

36. National Advisory Committee on Nutritional Education (1983). *A discussion paper on proposals for nutritional guidelines for health education in Britain*. Health Education Council, London. Passwater, R. (1982). *Supernutrition for healthy hearts*. Thorsons, Wellingborough. Editorial (1983). *Journal of the American Medical Association*, **249**, 365-7.

37. Armstrong, B.K., Brown, J.B., Clarke, H.T., Crooke, D.K., Hähnel, R., Masarei, J.R., and Ratajczak, T. (1981). Diet and postreproductive hormones: A study of vegetarian and non-vegetarian postmenopausal women. *Journal of the National Cancer Institute*, **67**, 761-7.

38. Editorial (1984). *Lancet*, **1**, 671-3.

39. Colditz, G., Branch, L.G., Lipnick, R.J., Willett, W.C., Posner, B.M., Hennekens, C.H. (1985). Increased green and yellow vegetable intake and lowered cancer deaths in an elderly population. *American Journal of Clinical Nutrition*, **41**, 32-6.

40. Golland, A. (1981). Basic hydrotherapy. *Psysiotherapy*, **67**, 258-62. O'Hare, J., Heywood, A., Summerheyes, C., Lunn, G., Evans, J.M., Walters, G., Corrall, R.J.M., Dieppe, P.A. (1985). Observations on the effects of immersion in bath spa water. *British Medical Journal*, **291**, 1747.

41. Finnegan, M.J., Pickering, C.A., Gill, F.S., and Ashton, I. (1987). Effect of negative ion generators in a sick building. *British Medical Journal*, **294**, 1195-6.

42. O'Neil, B. and Phillips, R. (1975). *Biorhythms: How to live with your life cycles*. Signet, New York.

19

Osteopathy

Background and fundamental concepts

Andrew Taylor Still, although born in Virginia, spent most of his life in Missouri. His father was a Methodist minister who farmed and cared for the sick, as well as preached. This background influenced Still's devout behaviour and fierce opposition to alcohol. He was also an excellent mechanic. Shattered by the loss of three of his children in an epidemic of meningitis, Still was mystified by the impotence of the doctors, although he praised their attention and skill.[1] He turned his mind to the problem of health and disease, and developed an interesting but simplistic theory.

God, he reasoned, had created man in his own likeness and therefore the design of the human body was perfect. How then could man become ill? Because, as with the machines Still understood so well, man's structure got out of adjustment; if readjusted it would function normally. Still extended his loathing of alcohol to drugs. He could not believe the God he worshipped could have designed man without including in the package all necessary equipment and chemicals. He believed the body was its own medicine chest.

Still's theories were not based on observation but on personal and religious conviction, yet contemporary accounts of his successful treatment of many ailments show that he was soon putting them to the test. He announced his theory of osteopathy in 1874 when he was 46, and tried hard to gain acceptance by the medical profession of his methods of treating disease. The doctors would not listen and the local Methodist minister denounced him as being in league with the devil, forcing him to move to another town: Kirksville in Missouri. Here, in 1892, he founded the first school of osteopathy.

Within a few years John Martin Littlejohn enrolled as a student. Littlejohn held degrees in Law, Divinity and Arts at Glasgow University and had studied physiology for three years in Glasgow as part of a study of forensic medicine for which he was awarded the

William Hunter Gold Medal in 1892. It has been said that Littlejohn 'took A.T. Still's osteopathy and . . . dipped it well and truly in a bath of physiology and what is more, kept it there'.[2]

It was Littlejohn who first expressed the idea of osteopathy in what we would recognize as holistic terms. He called it the science of adjustment. Man as an organism lived in an environment which had physical, social, occupational, dietetic, and many other aspects. Health was present when man was in balance with these aspects although he had the adaptive capacity to adjust within a range. Ill health occurred when there was a breakdown in this adjustment and the task of the osteopath was to adjust the patient back to normal. This of course implies knowledge of psychology and dietetics as well as anatomy, physiology, and manipulative skills. Littlejohn returned to England in 1913 and set up the British School of Osteopathy in 1917.

Still's concept of pathology was naïve. He describes an early experience with a small child with severe diarrhoea. The child's spine was hot and its abdomen cold so he simply tried to move the heat to the cold parts. He was amazed at the child's rapid recovery. He ultimately came to the conclusion that minor strains, slips, dislocations, and subluxations caused pressure on arteries which impeded blood flow. Reduction in arterial blood flow was the key: 'Unobstructed blood will never form a tumor', he wrote. His method of treatment was to examine a patient for evidence of these factors and to devise a large number of manual techniques to resolve these problems to his satisfaction. However, Still's students had great difficulty in learning from him. They thought his diagnosis clairvoyant and he performed techniques so quickly that they could not follow him. Frequently he would use a technique only once. It was many years before satisfactory methods of teaching manual skills were devised.

There has been a gradual evolution in the interpretation of spinal diagnosis. Still was concerned only with variations from the normal position of the vertebrae. By the 1930s vertebral diagnosis was interpreted in terms of the range of motion of one bone on another. Also, by the 1930s many of the explanations advanced for successful treatment had dismissed the concept of arterial pressure in favour of that of disturbance of reflex activity.

The term *osteopathic lesion* was used early in the twentieth century to describe vertebral diagnostic observations. It is useful in terms of identifying a segment at which the examining fingers perceive something to be wrong but has led critics erroneously to deride osteopaths for having their own concept of pathology. The Americans dropped the term in favour of the less specific *somatic dysfunction* which was subsequently adopted by the World Health Organization. In the early 1970s the British School of Osteopathy dropped the term in favour of a diagnostic system which sought more specifically to identify the tissue that was responsible for the malfunction or pain and thus led to selection of more specific techniques.

Today, osteopathy largely treats back pain, cases of which have reached epidemic proportions, and spinal problems generally.[3] Many osteopaths, however, still see their role as being wider than this and will undertake to treat disturbances of function of the respiratory, gastrointestinal, genitourinary and cardiovascular systems, although they are selective in the conditions they undertake to treat. Those skilled in cranial techniques also tend to treat head symptoms, including some types of sinus problem and giddiness, and problems in infants and children which are related to birth injuries. Additionally, some osteopaths train in a combination of osteopathy and naturopathy and so view osteopathy from the standpoint of natural medicine; this colours the way in which they approach the patient and his treatment.

A suitable definition of an osteopath is therefore a practitioner who is an expert in the examination, treatment, and interpretation of abnormalities of function of the musculoskeletal system.

Diagnosis

The osteopath will first take the patient's history which will give him the patient's view of the onset, duration, characteristics, and so on of current and other problems. The patient is then observed standing still and performing active movements. He is then observed sitting. Areas which exhibit potential problems are examined more minutely using palpation and passive movements. The osteopath will also carry out various accepted clinical procedures employing percussion hammer, stethoscope, opthalmoscope, auriscope, etc. He may order or carry out X-rays and tests on blood and urine. At the end of this he is able to decide whether or not the patient needs further investigation, and whether or not he is likely to respond to osteopathic treatment.

The osteopath now has an overall and detailed assessment of the patient's musculoskeletal system. He may, for example, have detected the overall tension resulting from anxiety, or the solid, stiff feel of degenerative changes in the spine. He will certainly have a detailed picture of spinal function, segment by segment, which he must be able to relate to the symptoms. Symptoms are traced back into the patient's life habits. A pain in the lower back, for example, may be related to such features as an inequality of leg length, an area of stiffness in the thorax, altered gait caused by new footwear, loss of the long arch of one or both feet, or pressure at work or at home. Thus the treatment prescription will be individual and will seek to restore the individual to a harmonious relationship with his or her environment in its broadest sense as well as secure a better level of physical function.

Treatment

The techniques open to osteopaths have been classified in many ways. Perhaps one of the simplest is to divide them into direct and indirect techniques. The best known, especially in the United Kingdom, are the direct techniques.

Direct techniques

1. *Soft tissue techniques* suggest to the patient that he is being given a general massage but in fact only those tissues which need treatment are handled. Direction, amplitude, speed, and force are modified from moment to moment so that the practitioner almost appears to be enjoying a dialogue with the tissues under his hands. Soft tissue treatment may be a treatment in itself if the problem is confined to the muscles, or may be a preliminary to another technique which requires prior relaxation of the muscles. One special technique is called neuromuscular technique (NMT). The osteopath searches the soft tissue with a probing thumb, looking for stress bands, or tense, fibrosed, or contracted locations. The easing of the tensions can release physical knots, easing neighbouring joint problems. Tender 'trigger points' can also be massaged, which, like reflexology, can aid organ function of organs within the same reflex zone.[4] It has to be remembered that owing to the inter-relationship of all tissues the osteopath may well treat a disc problem merely by using soft tissue techniques. The change in the soft tissues not only

releases some pressure but creates a situation in which circulatory changes may occur, initiating healing.

2. *Articulatory techniques* involve the passive movement of joints. Techniques may be used to stretch or break down adhesions, stretch shortened ligaments, promote fluid movement, and exchange or treat muscles by stretching them. The osteopath is able to sense which tissue is restricting motion by the feel of the quality of the motion and the nature of its end-point. Again the essential feature is the impression of dialogue, one hand sensing the response in the tissues while the other provides the motive power and control. Springing is another form of articulation often used to provide shearing forces between joints which are not strictly speaking normal anatomical movements. It is often used on joints which normally have little active movement, for example sacro-iliac joints.

3. *High velocity thrust techniques* are sudden movements, often followed by a crack or pop, which startle the patient although in skilled hands they are painless. These techniques can be applied to the spine or peripheral joints. Ironically they owe more to the traditional bonesetter than to the founder of osteopathy who did not use and indeed disparaged them. Occasionally the technique can be very successful in causing dramatic relief from spinal pain. However, it is often used uncritically by many osteopaths because the patients believe in it and expect it. It is not clear what the technique achieves in scientific terms although clinically there is often a dramatic reduction of muscle tone.

4. *Muscle energy techniques* evolved in the US in the last 20 years. The patient supplies the motive power for these. The skill in this type of technique lies in the osteopath's sense of a barrier to motion. The joint is moved until a barrier is sensed. At this point the patient attempts to move the joint away from the barrier while the osteopath resists. The amount of power, the timing, and the patient's effort are all variables with therapeutic significance. The technique is fairly new to the UK but has been found valuable in certain acute cases, with nervous patients, or where thrust techniques may be contraindicated, for example, with elderly patients.

Indirect techniques

1. *Release techniques* also rely on a sense of barrier but here the

patient is passive. The osteopath moves a joint to the point of barrier and then applies a small extra force which is maintained. Frequently the osteopath becomes aware that the position is being maintained although the force has lessened, and relocates the boundary in its new position. On other occasions he becomes aware of the barrier slowly retreating to a new position. The technique is repeated until complete release has occurred or until it is judged that further release will not occur. This technique can also be used on soft tissue and organs, where accessible, in the abdominal and pelvic cavities.

2. *Functional techniques* were developed by Hoover, Bowles, and Johnston in the US over the last 40 years.[5] Here the joint is moved, with the patient's co-operation, through ranges of flexion, extension, sidebending, rotation, forward/backward, and sideways movements. The osteopath assesses where the joint prefers to be with reference to the ease of motion. Again the sense of ease and barrier to motion is paramount. A composite is found for all ranges where the joint is in its most favoured position. The patient's breath is held at the point of maximal ease. The tissues are felt to change and the joint is checked for improved function in motion. These are subtle techniques requiring a different range of skills and again are of great value in acute cases, although they can also be used effectively in chronic cases. Like all the indirect techniques they are difficult to explain. No force is involved but a subtle positioning. Inevitably not all osteopaths are attracted to these techniques.

3. *Cranial techniques.* Even more difficult to rationalize are the techniques which owe their origin to William Garner Sutherland.[6] Sutherland postulated that the sutures of the human skull permit a small but essential degree of motion. Manual encouragement of this motion assists the circulation of cerebro-spinal fluid. This could relieve local symptoms, and have more far-reaching effects, such as on pituitary function.[7] However, it is a controversial theory and excites considerable hostility among colleagues, partly because holding a patient's head without apparently performing any active function smacks of faith healing and is as far from thrust techniques as any manual skill can possibly be. However, research relating symptomatology of the newborn and learning disabilities in children with diagnosed disturbances of cranial function[8] lends considerable support to the protagonists of cranial techniques and it is likely that

although less than one in ten osteopaths are skilled in the technique at present, it is here to stay.

In an ideal situation all these techniques would be taught at under-graduate level. One school is attempting this at present but the more conservative schools rely on the longer-established direct tech-niques, leaving postgraduate departments to provide opportunities for extending skills in indirect techniques.

Research and development

Most research has been carried out in the US, beginning in the early part of this century. While it is inadequate by today's standards this early research yields some useful information: animal experiments suggested that vertebral lesions could affect the function of other tissues, including such factors as immunity.

More relevant research began at Kirksville in the 1950s when Denslow was able to demonstrate that where a skilled osteopath detected an osteopathic lesion there was an underlying alteration in neurological function: namely a facilitation of motor neurones.[9] Further research demonstrated that, with spinal defects, not only was motor function affected but the autonomic nervous system was also disturbed, leading to altered function in viscera and circula-tion.[10] For example, animal studies have shown that strains of the vertebra result in changes in the structure of organs on the same embryological segment.[11] Korr, one of the pioneers of this kind of research, has become quite well known in the scientific world for his discoveries that nerves act as channels, not only for electrical impulses, but also for substances needed by organs.[12] This has obvious implications for the osteopath, because mechanical inter-ference with nerves might affect the organs they supply (see also Chapter 9).

Clinical research has been hampered because diagnosis is coloured by the osteopath's individual model of spinal function.[13] Thus one osteopath sees his findings in terms of altered positional relation-ships, another in terms of mobility, another in terms of muscle tones, another in terms of involuntary function, and so on. When criteria are strictly laid down (e.g. is the vertebral joint more limited in flexion than extension, or in sidebending or rotation?) then there is a high level of correlation. Similarly, high levels of correlation have been found in respect of cranial findings where there has been agreement on criteria.[14]

Osteopathy is most commonly utilized in treating back pain yet research in this area is lacking. A central problem is, as ever, the requirements of the double-blind trial. It is not easy to imagine a dummy treatment in osteopathy against which actual treatments could be compared. However, different treatments can be compared with each other, for example conservative treatment versus osteopathy, and this work is beginning.[15] Another problem concerns the criteria. It is not possible to demonstrate instrumentally whether or not a person has back pain or whether or not he is better. There is no definitive X-ray or blood or urine test and osteopaths are forced to rely on subjective experience which scientists consider unreliable. In short, no-one knows what causes a back pain and it is not possible to separate what are probably many causes.

Uses and risks

A survey carried out by Burton[3] and work carried out for the Australian government (see Chapter 2, p. 33) shows that the patients select osteopaths in the belief that they have special skills which lend themselves to the treatment of musculoskeletal problems, particularly back pain which may spread to the limbs or head. Patients also sought treatment for other conditions including strains, sprains, migraines, headaches, cardiac, pulmonary, digestive, and neurological problems, although in smaller numbers. There is an obvious role for osteopaths in the treatment of sports injuries.[16]

It is unlikely that osteopathy can make much of a contribution where there is irreversible pathology. Even where such pathology affects muscles and joints, such as in rheumatoid arthritis, Paget's disease, the muscular dystrophies, and multiple sclerosis, osteopathy offers only marginal benefits. However, in the functional stages before such pathologies become established it may have some part to play by removing at least one important aetiological factor. Some osteopaths limit their practice by choice to musculoskeletal problems, some even to acute musculoskeletal problems only, while others would be prepared to treat tumours if they felt their treatment would help relieve pain and would not accelerate the process or cause injury or damage.

Osteopathic treatment in skilled hands is a remarkably safe

procedure. There is occasionally some discomfort after treatment for a day or two. More severe reactions occur only rarely. In such instances the patient should always return to the osteopath who treated him as severe reactions can usually be quickly modified.

Treatment almost invariably involves undressing down to underclothes. Gowns which tie up at the back allowing for complete exposure of the spine may be provided. For a first visit a patient may be required to attend for anything from 30 to 60 minutes while a subsequent treatment session may be 10 to 40 minutes, depending upon the osteopath and the type of problem.

Courses of treatment may be just one session or extend over many months. The trained osteopath will always discuss the prognosis and the likely length and cost of treatment.

References

1. Still, A.T. (1910). *Osteopathy—Research and practice*. Privately published, A.T. Still, Missouri.
2. Hall, T.E. and Wernham, J. (1978). *The contribution of John Martin Littlejohn to osteopathy*. Maidstone Osteopathic Clinic, Maidstone, Kent.
3. Burton, A.K. (1981). Back pain in osteopathic practice. *Rheumatology and Rehabilitation*, **20**, 239–46. Macdonald, R.S. and Peters, D. (1986). Osteopathy. *Practitioner*, **230**, 1073–6.
4. Chaitow, L. (1982). *Osteopathy: Head-to-toe health through manipulation*. Thorsons, Wellingborough. Lewis, K. and Simon, D. (1984). *Archives of Physical Medicine and Rehabilitation*, **65**, 452–6. McKechnie, A.A., Wilson, F., Watson, N., and Scott, D. (1983). Anxiety states: a preliminary report on the value of connective tissue massage. *Journal of Psychosomatic Research*, **27**, 125–9.
5. Johnston, W.L. (1966). Manipulative skills, *Journal of the American Osteopathic Association*, **66**, 389–407.
6. Sutherland, W.G. (1948). *The cranial bowl*. Sutherland Publishing, Mankato, Minnesota. Upledger, J. and Vredevoord, J. (1983). *Craniosacral therapy*. Eastland Press, Chicago.
7. White, W. (1985). The relation of the craniofacial bones to specific somatic dysfunction: A clinical study of the effects of manipulation. *Journal of the American Osteopathic Association*, **85**, 603–4.
8. Upledger, J.E. (1978). The relationship of craniosacral examination findings in grade school children with developmental problems. *Journal of the American Osteopathic Association*, **77**, 640–69.
9. Denslow, J.S., Korr, I.M., and Krems, A.D. (1947). Quantitative

studies of chronic facilitation in human motoneuron pools.' *American Journal of Physiology*, **150**, 229–38. Denslow, J.S. (1951). An approach to skeletal components in health and disease. *Journal of the American Osteopathic Association*, **50**, 399–403.

10. Korr, I.M., Wright, H.M., and Chace, J.A. (1964). Cutaneous patterns of sympathetic activity in clinical abnormalities of the musculoskeletal system. *Acta Neurovegetativa*, **25**, 589–606. Korr, I.M. (1978). *The neurobiologic mechanisms in manipulative therapy*. Plenum, New York.

11. Cole, W.V. and Sminers, M.H. (1953). Somatovisceral reflexes; effects of spinal fixation at thoracolumbar junction on certain visceral structures. *Journal of the American Osteopathic Association*, **52**, 309–17.

12. Korr, I.M., Wilkinson, P.N., and Chornok, F.W. (1967). Axonal delivery of neuroplasmic components of muscle cells. *Science*, **155**, 342–5. Mannino, R. (1979). The application of neurological reflexes to the treatment of hypertension. *Journal of the American Osteopathic Association*, **79**, 225–30.

13. Beal, *et al.* (1980). Classification of diagnostic tests used with osteopathic manipulation. *Journal of the American Osteopathic Association*, **79**, 451–5.

14. Upledger, J.E. (1977). The reproducibility of cranio-sacral examination findings. *Journal of the American Osteopathic Association*, **76**, 890–99.

15. Cummings, M. (1986). Evaluation of changes associated with osteopathic treatment of the lumbosacral region: a pilot study. *Complementary Medicine*, **3**, 10–12. Burton, A.K. (1986). Osteopathy in back trouble. *British Medical Journal*, **293**, 1482.

16. Moule, T.G. (1980). Sports injuries: How osteopathy can help. *Nursing*, **4**, 163–5.

20

Radionics and psionic medicine

Background

Radionics has been defined as a method of diagnosis and treatment at a distance, through the medium of an instrument, using what is known as the radiesthetic faculty, which is a form of extrasensory perception.

Radionics as a healing art emerged from the pioneering work and discoveries of the distinguished American physician Dr Albert Abrams, who was born in San Francisco in 1863. Something of a prodigy, Abrams completed his medical studies at such an early age that his degree could not be issued. He later became Professor of Pathology and Director of the Cooper Medical College of Stanford University, California. He wrote several successful medical textbooks and eventually won for himself a national reputation as a specialist in diseases of the nervous system.

At the beginning of this century Abrams made a strange discovery. In the course of a routine examination of a middle-aged male patient, who had a small cancerous growth on his lip, Abrams discovered that during the process of percussing the abdomen of the patient, the resonance of the note given off changed when the man faced west, and this in a very specific area above the navel. Abrams' curiosity was aroused and he went on to check a whole series of patients with cancer, all of whom without exception gave the same reaction. He then decided to check patients with other identifiable diseases, and found, for example, that those with tuberculosis exhibited the same repeatable phenomena, this time below the navel. Considering this to be an electromagnetic phenomenon, Abrams devised a box containing resistors, and by using this he found that he could measure the disease reactions in ohms, thus distinguishing one disease from another. He found that carcinoma reacted at 50 ohms, syphilis at 20, tuberculosis at 15 and so forth.

In Abrams' next experiment the patient was replaced by a healthy young male, who became known as the 'subject'. Abrams placed a dried spot of blood from a real patient in the box, and attached the electrode to the subject's forehead, while the subject stood on earthed metal plates. By setting the appropriate numbers (or rates as they were known) on the dials Abrams could, by percussing the abdomen of his subject, diagnose very accurately what was wrong with the patient who had donated the blood spot.

When Abrams announced this procedure and his theories about it, there was quite naturally a very hostile response from the orthodoxy of the day. It was only in 1924, the year of Abrams' death, that a concerted effort was made to test his methods. A medical committee under the chairmanship of Sir Thomas Horder ran a series of tests under controlled conditions. The results proved an overwhelming vindication of Abrams, to the astonishment of the distinguished medical men involved.[1] However, only a few perceptive physicians took his theories further. In the 1930s Ruth Drown, a chiropractor who practised in Hollywood, California, developed new approaches to radionics and new instrumentation. Her work was to attract many chiropractors and osteopaths into this field and was seen as a pioneering effort to establish a new form of medicine, one that employed subtle healing energies as opposed to drugs and surgical procedures.

Following the Second World War the engineer George de la Warr set up laboratories in Oxford, thus beginning a new phase of growth from which emerged new instruments based on the same principles as Drown's. There can be no doubt that the fertile minds of George de la Warr and his assistants fostered a whole new era of radionic development, the 1950s being one of the most intensive periods of organized research in the radionic field. The bulk, if not virtually all the work, was carried out at Oxford.

Fundamental concepts

Basic to radionic theory and practice is the concept that all life forms, including man, are submerged in and interpenetrated by a common field of energy. At the lowest level this field registers as the electromagnetic spectrum but there are many levels or planes of energy which cannot be measured by scientific instrumentation, and which lie beyond the electromagnetic field. All of these go into the make-up of man and any distortion in the life-field of an individual eventually registers as physical or psychological pathology.

Early radionic practitioners diagnosed and treated in medical and clinical terms, and saw the body basically in orthodox anatomical and physiological terms. Today most practitioners have adopted a model of the body directly drawn from theosophical and Eastern teachings, such concepts fitting in more easily with the idea of man as energy. They see man as being comprised of a totality of spirit, soul, and form, the latter being made up of the physical body, the etheric body (more recently referred to by some scientists as the bioplasmic body), the emotional body and the mental body. The four-fold form is that aspect of man wherein disease manifests itself, and it is to these bodies that the practitioner directs healing energies through specific instrumentation.[2]

This model of man lends itself readily to modern radionic practice, because practitioners since Drown have diagnosed and treated at a distance. Drown discovered that it was not necessary for a patient to be present for purposes of diagnosis or treatment, due to the fact that the human mind, through the energy field in which it was immersed, could connect with the patient no matter where he or she was. She posited that a beam of energy literally connected practitioner and patient, and that along this beam information could be derived relevant to the patient's health; similarly energy for treatment purposes could be 'broadcast' to the distant patient, the blood spot on the instrument acting as a link.

Ruth Drown created a whole series of rates or numbers representing the parts of the human body, and of man's known diseases. Each body-part rate and each disease rate is in effect the vibrational identification pattern of that particular object. While in practice the method worked, her theories can be seen to be a conglomeration of beliefs derived from radio waves and metaphysics. These beliefs have been promulgated over the years, and certainly none of them stand up to scientific examination. There is no evidence to support the concept that some form of physical radiation generated by the rates set up on the instrument goes out or is broadcast from the set to the patient at a distance. Despite the view of Abrams, it is likely that the instruments, although useful as a focus for the mind of the practitioner, do not in themselves have any intrinsic value beyond the fact that they can be used to objectify a process going on at mental levels. Thought connects the practitioner to the patient, and thought initiates the treatment process. Radionics is in fact a form of mental healing. When a practitioner tunes in to the patient, he literally brings that patient 'to mind' and on that plane of consciousness distance does not exist.

At this level the very act of making a diagnosis sets up a form of energy exchange which has a therapeutic impact upon the patient. This healing effect brought about by the diagnostic process has often been made clear to practitioners, by patients who telephone to exclaim how well they are feeling—and this before treatment in the accepted sense of the word has begun. Some would put it down to coincidence or imagination, but proper investigation of such cases would show that healing has taken place. Often in cases where pain had been intractable for weeks, it cleared at the time the diagnosis was made, and without the patient having any conscious knowledge of the work being done. Of course no practitioner should ever make a radionic analysis on an individual without his express permission; to do so is psychically to invade that patient, perhaps against his will. The only exceptions are in those cases of terminal illness where the patient cannot make his wishes known, and for children, where signed permission is given by the parents seeking help for their offspring.

Diagnostic and therapeutic practices

The primary aim of all radionic diagnosis and treatment at a distance is to identify fundamental causes of disease within an organism, and to set energies in motion which will eliminate these causes at their very root. In order to do this the practitioner employs a radionic diagnostic instrument in conjunction with a variety of procedures aimed at identifying the causes of a specific set of symptoms or disease patterns (see Fig. 20.1).

The instrument usually takes the form of a box covered by a panel. On the panel is a set of dials which are calibrated from 0 to 10 or possibly 0 to 44 depending upon which system is being used. There is normally a circular metal plate upon which the patient's 'witness' is placed (the 'witness' is either a blood spot or a small snippet of hair). This is said to provide the link between the practitioner, instrument, and the patient at a distance. One method of diagnosis takes a specific symptom, and subsequently places the rate or numerical

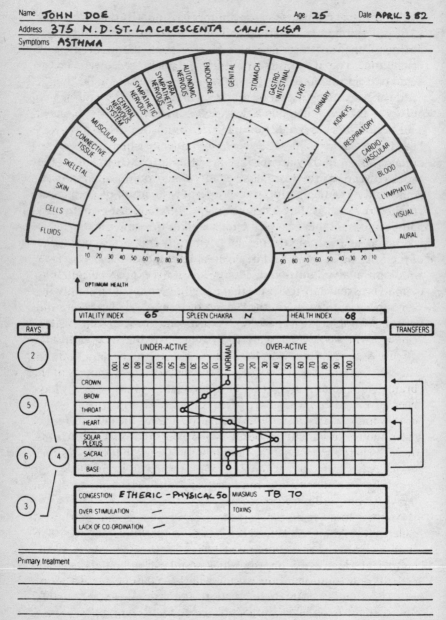

Name **JOHN DOE**   Age **25**   Date **APRIL 3 82**

Address **375 N.D.ST. LA CRESCENTA CALIF. USA**

Symptoms **ASTHMA**

VITALITY INDEX **65**   SPLEEN CHAKRA **N**   HEALTH INDEX **68**

RAYS

2

5

6   4

3

TRANSFERS

	UNDER-ACTIVE										NORMAL	OVER-ACTIVE									
	100	90	80	70	60	50	40	30	20	10		10	20	30	40	50	60	70	80	90	100
CROWN																					
BROW																					
THROAT																					
HEART																					
SOLAR PLEXUS																					
SACRAL																					
BASE																					

CONGESTION **ETHERIC – PHYSICAL 50**   MIASMUS **TB 70**

OVER-STIMULATION —   TOXINS

LACK OF CO-ORDINATION —

Primary treatment

Fig. 20.1: A radionic diagnostic chart.

value for that symptom on the appropriate dials of the instrument. The practitioner, having tuned his mind to the patient, asks a series of questions to determine which body systems are involved in the symptom. The responses to these mentally posed questions are externalized in two ways, depending upon which method the practitioner uses. If he uses a pendulum, for he is literally dowsing for disease, then the pendulum will swing, as a rule, from a simple oscillation to a clockwise movement to give a 'yes'. If a stick pad is built into the instrument, consisting of a rubber diaphragm over a rectangular metal plate, then the practitioner's fingers will literally stick to the pad instead of sliding easily across it as he mentally asks questions, giving a 'yes' in this way. These methods used to be termed radiesthesia. They are probably thousands of years old but nonetheless are very effective in the hands of a sensitive and properly trained operator.

Once a series of organ locations have been determined as being related to the symptom, then the rates representing each location are set on the dials in turn following the symptom rate, and the sublocations are determined relative to each organ involved. Having pinpointed the exact areas of the body, the practitioner then proceeds to find out precisely what the causative agent is that is creating the disease. For example, with headaches, a practitioner may find that there are residual toxins from measles located in the meninges of the brain. These toxins, similar to the homeopath's 'miasms', may have been left over from when the patient contracted the disease as a child or they may have come from a vaccination against the disease. In any event such toxins could not be identified by orthodox clinical means, and it is here especially that radionics in identifying these residual toxins, may have a role to play. Information is available to the properly trained sensitive mind that cannot be determined by, or derived from, ordinary procedures.

Another more comprehensive approach is to use an instrument called a Rae Analyser, named after its developer Malcolm Rae. This employs cards with geometric patterns on them in place of the numerical rates used on the older standard radionic sets. The procedure is to measure the mean deviation from perfect structure and function of each organ system. For this purpose an arbitrary scale of 0 as optimum health and 100 as maximum deviation from optimum health is used. The Analyser utilizes charts which readily provide the degrees of imbalance as the pendulum quite automatically seeks them out by swinging along the appropriate line.

Having now obtained an overall picture of the organ systems the practitioner, through a series of mentally posed questions, can seek out the causes of the imbalances he has detected. Once again a chart is used listing such causes as infection, toxins, allergies, emotional stress, congestion, miasms, and so forth. Some practitioners also analyse the states of the *chakras* to see if they are overactive, underactive, or normally active.

Chakras, according to Eastern philosophy, are a series of major force centres which lie along the cerebral spinal axis. They can be regarded as the points at which energy flows into the human system and maintains the integrity of the physical form by way of the etheric body. As such they provide a deep level at which treatment can occur. For example, the solar plexus *chakra* is the centre of emotional life. When it is overactive, the practitioner inevitably finds poor readings on the sympathetic nervous system and the skin, and of course the pancreas is working overtime too. This may relate to the onset of diabetes, which can often follow emotional shock. On the other hand a solar plexus *chakra* that gives an underactive reading will indicate a person who represses his deeper emotional feelings; cases of cancer often exhibit an underactive solar plexus *chakra*.

The analysis of the patient can be extended beyond the *chakras* to include the quality and characteristics of the energies of the transpersonal self, the mental, emotional, and etheric/physical bodies, and those of the personality as a whole. When all of the imbalances in the various bodies and their energy systems have been identified and measured for intensity, and the cause or causes similarly dealt with, then the practitioner is ready to determine what form of treatment is needed to remove the causes of disease within the patient.

Radionic treatment is determined by placing the patient witness on the detector plate of the instrument or, in the case of the Rae Analyser, upon the treatment chart, and asking a series of mentally posed questions. The main idea is to find the correct, and thus the most effective, form of treatment to remove those causes of disease which have been identified in the analysis. Some practitioners may then put a phial of an appropriate homeopathic remedy, such as *Morbillinum* or *Aconite*, on the plate next to the patient witness, with the intention of modifying the energy directed to the patient in such a way as to speed up his response and clear, for example, the measles virus, more quickly.[3]

Treatment with instruments employing geometric cards provides a more versatile approach. For example three cards may be used to set up a treatment. For the measles virus in the meninges, a card for *Morbillinum* is placed in the first slot, in the second a card for the crown *chakra*, and in the third a card representing the meninges. In this way a flow of energy is symbolized; the healing remedy is placed into and through the crown *chakra* which governs the brain and from there to the meninges. Many practitioners use colour as a therapeutic agent in their practices and this can be 'broadcast' in the same way that homeopathic remedies are. Often remedies such as the biochemic tissue salts, Bach flower remedies, homeopathic medicines, or vitamins and minerals where indicated, are recommended to the patient to be taken orally as an adjunct to his radionic treatment. If other forms of treatment, such as allopathic, manipulation, or acupuncture are indicated, then the practitioner advises the patient accordingly. Diet too is taken into account, particularly in those cases where allergies have been identified.[4]

Applications and contra-indications

Radionics can be employed in the treatment of any form of disease; there do not appear to be any contra-indications at all. By its very nature it can be used whilst other forms of therapy are being applied without in any way interfering with the healing processes they are designed to initiate. Like psychic healing, radionics has been found to be particularly effective in terminal illness, especially in reducing pain and engendering in the patient a realistic, calm, and relaxed attitude towards his illness and its subsequent outcome.

Like most therapies it enjoys an average rate of success. Having the advantage of being able to determine the presence of deeply hidden causes, it gets good long-term results with chronic cases that have not responded to other forms of therapy. Radionics has an application in dentistry[5] and is also employed in the field of agriculture, increasing crop yields and body weight of stock. Animals respond very well to radionic treatment and some practitioners treat animals only.

Research and development

Radionics by its very nature cannot provide scientific data through experimentation, so in the future we can only expect to see data emerging from practical work; where that data is of use it will be incorporated into radionics. An example of an emerging pattern that has been observed is that some children have exactly the same set of over- and underactive *chakras* as the mother, if during pregnancy the mother was highly tensed and subject to a great deal of stress. Radionics will obviously benefit from research demonstrating parapsychological phenomena in general, particularly in relation to healing and dowsing.[6] (See also Chapter 12.)

Obtaining treatment

As with any form of therapy it is always best to seek out a fully trained and qualified practitioner. The UK is the centre of radionics in the world today and information about practitioners is readily available from the relevant organizations. Having decided upon a practitioner the patient fills in a case history sheet giving his past medical history and present problem, and returns this to the practitioner together with signed permission for investigation and a small snippet of hair. When the analysis has been completed the practitioner sends a report of findings to the patient. At this point, if the practitioner and patient have not met or spoken to each other, it is not a bad idea to make such a contact. Often practitioners never see or speak to patients, especially those who live far away. In these cases the whole process of contact can be carried out through correspondence, which is satisfactory provided the channels of communication are kept alive by means of a monthly report from the patient and appropriate responses from the practitioner.

Psionic medicine

Psionic medicine is a composite diagnosis and treatment method involving basically similar concepts and practices to those of radionics. It was developed in the UK by a distinguished physician, George Laurence. He developed an energetic theory of the origin of disease that owes much to MacDonagh's unitary theory of disease, as well as to the teachings of Rudolf Steiner. He sees the source of many chronic diseases as miasms or vestiges of previous acute conditions, and treats homeopathically. Diagnosis and treatment are selected largely by pendulum. Psionic medicine is practised mostly by GPs, and therefore it is sometimes combined with conventional medicine. A good modern account of the subject has been published.[7]

References

1. Horder, T. (1925). The electronic reactions of Abrams. *British Medical Journal*, **1**, 179–185.
2. Wilcox, J. (1976). Radionics. *Nursing Times*, **72**, 568–70.
3. Silver, S. (1978). The radionic phenomenon, treatment at a distance. *Mims Magazine*, **2**, 377.
4. Westlake, T. (1973). *The pattern of health: A search for a greater understanding of the life force in health and disease*. Shambhala, Colorado.
5. Upton, C. (1980). Psionic medicine in dentistry. *Probe*, **22**, 9–11.
6. Williamson, T. (1977). Dowsing achieves new credence. *New Scientist*, **81**, 371–3.
7. Reyner, J.H., Laurence, G., and Upton, C. (1980). *Psionic medicine*. Routledge and Kegan Paul, London.

PART 3

Organizations and colleges

Acupuncture and Oriental medicine

COLLEGES AND TRAINING ESTABLISHMENTS

The British Academy of Western Acupuncture

Address: 12 Rodney Street, Liverpool L1 2TE; *Tel*:051 709 0479.

Date founded: 1975.

Major therapies taught: Acupuncture—formulae acupuncture incorporated into Western medical framework. Diagnosis based entirely on Western medicine.

Entry requirements: Medical practitioners, dental surgeons, nurses (min. qual. SRN) and physiotherapists (min. qual. SRN, SRP with 5 years' past experience).

Type and length of courses: Licentiate in Acupuncture (1 year part-time); Doctor of Acupuncture (3 years part-time, must be Lic.Ac.).

Subjects taught to trainees: Lic.Ac.: acupuncture technique, uses and practice; moxibustion; electro-acupuncture.

Average college attendance for trainees: 7 weekend training sessions plus home study.

Clinical experience (extent of supervised treatment of patients): 6 full clinical weekends.

Diplomas or certificates awarded: Lic.Ac.(AWA), D.Ac.(AWA).

Associated institutions: The Association of Western Acupuncture (professional association).

British College of Acupuncture

Address: Old Royal Free School of Medicine, 8 Hunter Street, London WC1N 1BN; *Tel*: 01 833 8164.

Date founded: 1964.

Major therapy taught: Acupuncture—combines traditional acupuncture with a Western medical approach.

Entry requirements: Qualified medical and paramedical practitioner or specified group of natural therapists or by interview and entrance exam.

Type and length of courses: Licentiate in Acupuncture (2 years part-time); Bachelor of Acupuncture (2 years part-time, must hold Lic.Ac.); Doctor of Acupuncture (1 year part-time, must hold B.Ac.).

Subjects taught to trainees: Acupuncture theory, technique, practice; moxibustion, clinical instruction; Electro-acupuncture.

Average college attendance for trainees: Lic.Ac.: First year: 8 weekends; second year: 7 weekends plus 28 days clinical experience; B.Ac.: First and second years: 6 weekends plus work in clinic.

Clinical experience: Lic.Ac.: 28 days in second year; min. 200 hours.

Number of students: At Summer Term, 1986: 150.

Diplomas or certificates awarded: Lic.Ac., B.Ac., D.Ac.

Associated institutions and societies: The British Acupuncture Association and Register (professional association).

Chung San Acupuncture School

Address: 15 Porchester Gardens, London W2 4DB; *Tel*: 01-727-6778.

Date founded: 1980.

Major therapy taught: 1. Foundation Course in Acupuncture; 2. Advanced Course in Acupuncture.

Entry requirements: 1.2 GCE A level science subjects; 2. degree qualification entry; 3. other professional qualifications (osteopathy, SRN, etc.).

Type and length of courses: Part-time (2–3 years).

Subjects taught to trainees: Basic scientific concepts; theory and practice of traditional Chinese channels and points; traditional diagnosis and technique.

Average college attendance for trainees: 1 full day every 2 weeks.

Clinical experience: 7 months.

Numbers of students: At Summer Term 1986: 30.

Diplomas or certificates awarded: Diploma in Acupuncture; Advanced Certificate in Acupuncture.

Associated institutions and societies: Chung San Acupuncture Society; Guangzhou College of Traditional Chinese Medicine.

College of Traditional Chinese Acupuncture

Address: Tao House, Queensway, Leamington Spa, Warwickshire CV31 3LZ; *Tel*: 0926 22121.

Date founded: 1963.

Major therapy taught: 5 element traditional Chinese acupuncture.

Entry requirements: 5 GCE O Levels and 2 GCE A Levels or equivalent of general education. Professional qualifications and work experience will be taken into account.

Type and length of courses: Licentiate in Acupuncture (3 years part-time); Bachelor of Acupuncture (2 years part-time, must be Lic.Ac.); Master of Acupuncture (2 years part-time, must be B.Ac.); Doctor of Acupuncture (3 years part-time, must be M.Ac.). Courses can also be taken full-time.

Subjects taught to trainees: Surface anatomy, physiology, biology of disease; acupuncture theory, technique and practice, traditional diagnosis, professional and ethical conduct, clinical training.

Average college attendance for trainees: For Lic.Ac. only: 15 × 2 days per year for 2 years; third year 1 day/week for 6 months plus 20 days then 1 day/month for 6 months; plus home study.

Clinical experience (extent of supervised treatment of patients): 10 days plus 1 day/week for 6 months then 1 day/month for 6 months.

Number of students: At Summer Term 1986: 388.

Diplomas or certificates awarded: Lic.Ac., B.Ac., M.Ac., D.Ac.

Associated institutions: Traditional Acupuncture Society (professional association); Council for Acupuncture; Acupuncture College Ltd (UK and Norway).

Institute of Bioenergetic Medicine

Address: 103 North Road, Parkstone, Poole, Dorset BH14 OLU; *Tel*: 0202 733762.

Date founded: 1982.

Major therapies taught: Vega test, neo-bioelectronic therapy (NBT), EAV, Mora therapy, Indumed therapy, all aspects of bio-regulatory medicine.

Entry requirements: Qualification in medicine or dentistry or recognized qualification in acupuncture or homeopathy.

Type and length of courses: Part-time (length varies according to course).

Subjects taught to trainees: Electronic diagnosis and therapy; homeopathy; acupuncture.

Numbers of students: No courses at present.

Certificate awarded: Certificate of attendance.

International College of Oriental Medicine UK Ltd

Address: Green Hedges House, Green Hedges Avenue, East Grinstead, Sussex RH19 1DZ; *Tel*: 0342 313106/7.

Date founded: 1972.

Major therapies taught: Acupuncture—classical acupuncture.

Entry requirements: At least 2 A Levels, one of which must be biology or human biology. Interview and references. Candidates for D.Ac. by invitation only and on completion of B.Ac. and at least 5 years clinical practice.

Type and length of courses: Bachelor of Acupuncture (3 years full-time); Master of Acupuncture (1 year part-time, must hold B.Ac.); Doctor of Acupuncture.

Subjects taught to trainees: Conventional physiology, anatomy, pathology; acupuncture theory, technique and practice; moxibustion; massage; medical discipline and ethics; clinic instruction; T'ai-chi; cupping.

Average college attendance for trainees: 3 years, each year comprising 3 terms of 11 weeks each. Each week usually consists of 3 days of lectures with a substantial amount of home study.

Clinical experience (extent of supervised treatment of patients): In second and third years, minimum of 100 hours training and fourth year clinical practice under supervision.

Number of students: At Summer Term 1986: 25.

Diplomas or certificates awarded: B.Ac., M.Ac., D.Ac.

Associated institutions: Council for Acupuncture.

London School of Acupuncture and Traditional Chinese Medicine

Address: 58 Gellatly Road, London SE14 5TT; *Tel*: 01-639 9313.

Date founded: 1984.

Major therapy taught: Traditional Chinese medicine.

Entry requirements: Minimum age 21 years. 5 O Levels; 2 A Levels. Applicants considered without the academic qualifications but with significant other experience.

Type of course: Part-time at weekends.

Subjects taught to trainees: Philosophy, pathology and practice of acupuncture, including diagnosis and point location; Western anatomy, physiology, pathology with some diagnosis and pharmacology.

Average college attendance for trainees: First year: 24 weekends plus 3 days; second year: 24 weekends, plus 3 days, plus 10 days; third year: 10 weekends, plus 6 days, plus 30 days.

Clinical experience: Minimum of 10 days observation; minimum of 30 days practice.

Numbers of students: At Summer Term 1986: 17.

Diplomas or certificates awarded: Diploma in Acupuncture and Moxibustion (Dip.Ac.).

Associated institutions and societies: Register of Traditional Chinese Medicine.

PROFESSIONAL ASSOCIATIONS AND SOCIETIES OF THERAPISTS

The Association of Western Acupuncture

Address: 12 Rodney Street, Liverpool L1 2TE; *Tel*: 051 709 0479.

Date founded: 1975.

Major therapy practised: Acupuncture—formulae acupuncture incorporated into Western medical framework. Diagnosis based entirely on Western medicine.

Types of membership: Full, Honorary, Associate.

Conditions and qualifications for entry: Full membership: graduates of the British Academy of Western Acupuncture.

Title of full members: MBAWA.

Number of members in association (inc. associate, honorary, foreign, and retired): 55.

Code of Practice: Yes.

Library: Yes.

Journal: *Academy Journal*.

Associated institutions and societies: Affiliated college: British Academy of Western Acupuncture; The Society of International Acupuncture.

Remarks: They are especially interested in new developments in the use of acupuncture in orthodox medicine.

British Acupuncture Association and Register

Address: 22 Hockley Road, Rayleigh, Essex SS6 8EB; *Tel*. 0268 742534.

Major therapy practised: Acupuncture.

Types of membership: Full, Overseas, Fellows, Life Members, Honorary Fellows.

Conditions and qualifications for entry: Full membership limited to graduates of the British College of Acupuncture or those passing Board of Governors examination; Associate membership limited to qualified practitioners lacking orthodox medical training.

Titles of full members: M.B.Ac.A., F.B.Ac.A., A.M.B.Ac.A.

Number of members in association (inc. associate, honorary, foreign, and retired): 411; Overseas 235.

Number of full members in practice in UK: 210.

Code of Practice: Yes.

Library: Yes.

Journal: *British Journal of Acupuncture*.

Associated institutions: The British College of Acupuncture (affiliated college); The Acupuncture Research Association; The International Organization of Acupuncture Associations; The Council for Acupuncture.

Remarks: Code of Practice produced in co-operation with the TAS and the Register of Oriental Medicine. The BAA holds conferences and public lectures.

British Medical Acupuncture Society

Address: 67–69 Chancery Lane, London WC2A 1AF.

Date founded: 1980.

Major therapy practised: Acupuncture—clinical acupuncture within an orthodox medical framework.

Types of membership: Full, Associate, Overseas, Honorary.

Conditions and qualifications for entry: Full—registered medical practitioners practising clinical acupuncture; Associate—registered medical practitioners interested in acupuncture.

Number of members in society (inc. associate, honorary, foreign, and retired): 600.

Number of full members in practice in UK: 300.

Code of Practice: BMA code of ethics.

Library: No.

Journal/newsletter: Yes.

Associated institutions and societies: International Council for Medical Acupuncture and Related Techniques (ICMART).

Remarks: The BMAS does not recognize any acupuncturists who do not have orthodox medical qualifications. It holds bi-annual national meetings and plans summer schools and p.g. meetings. Undertakes medical research into acupuncture, especially acupuncture anaesthesia. Runs training courses for qualified doctors.

The Register of Traditional Chinese Medicine

Address: 7A Thorndean Street, London SW18 4HE; *Tel*: 01-947 1879.

Date founded: 1975.

Major therapies practised: Acupuncture, traditional Chinese medicine.

Types of membership: Student, Fellow, Full.

Conditions and qualifications for entry: Graduates of the International College of Oriental Medicine and from the London School of Acupuncture and Traditional Chinese Medicine.

Title of full members: MRTCM.

Number of members in association (inc. associate, honorary, foreign, and retired): 78.

Number of full members in practice in UK: 76.

Code of practice: Yes.

Library: No.

Journal: No.

Associated institutions and societies: Council of Acupuncture.

Affiliated colleges: London School of Acupuncture and Traditional Chinese Medicine and International College of Oriental Medicine; recognized training colleges in Europe.

Remarks: They run occasional seminars on aspects of Oriental medicine.

Code of Ethics produced in co-operation with the TAS and the British Acupuncture Association and Register.

Society of Biological Medicine

Address: 398 Uxbridge Road, Hatch End, Middx. HAS 4HP; *Tel*: 01-428 4333.

Date founded: 1986.

Major therapies practised: Complex homeopathy, Vega system, Voll system, electro-acupuncture.

Types of membership: Full, Associate.

Conditions and qualifications for entry: Medical, paramedical, and complementary practitioners.

Title of full members: M.S. Bio.Med.

Number of members in society (inc. associate, honorary, foreign, and retired): 34.

Number of full members in practice in UK: 25.

Code of practice: Yes.

Library: No.

Journal: No.

Associated institutions and societies: Centre for Alternative Therapies.

The Traditional Acupuncture Society

Address: 1 The Ridgeway, Stratford upon Avon, Warwickshire CV37 9JL; *Tel*: 0789 298798.

Date founded: 1976.

Major therapy practised: Acupuncture—5 element traditional Chinese acupuncture.

Types of membership: Full, Associate, Fellowship, Friends.

Conditions and qualifications for entry: Graduates of the College of Traditional Chinese Acupuncture.

Titles of full members: M.T.Ac.S., F.T.Ac.S.

Number of members in society (inc. associate, honorary, foreign, and retired): 330.

Code of practice: Yes.

Library: No.

Newsletter: TAS Newsletter.

Associated institutions and societies: Affiliated college: The College of Traditional Chinese Acupuncture. Recognized training college in the US.

Remarks: They hold an annual weekend series of seminars. Code of Ethics and Register produced by the Council of Acupuncture.

Association of Irish Acupuncturists

Address: The Secretary, Association of Irish Acupuncturists, P.O.B. 124, Tralee, Ireland.

Activity: Professional body representing Irish acupuncturists awarding members an M.A.I.Ac.

SUPPORT ORGANIZATIONS

Acupuncture Society in the People's Republic of China and the Chung San Acupuncture School

Address: 15 Porchester Gardens, London W2 4DB; *Tel*: 01-229 0136.

Activity: Organizes groups of practitioners and students to China to study advanced courses in acupuncture at the Guangzhou (Canton) College of Traditional Chinese Medicine and the San Yatsen Medical University.

British Biomagnetic Association

Address: 179 Fore Street, Heavitree, Exeter, Devon; *Tel*: 0392 37366.

Activity: Supports using magnets in connection with acupuncture meridians.

Centre for the Study of Alternative Therapies

Address: 51 Bedford Place, Southampton, Hants SO1 2DG; *Tel*: 0703 334752.

Activity: The treatment of patients and education of medical practitioners in therapies, in particular acupuncture. Supplies electroacupuncture equipment and educates practitioners in their use.

The Pain Clinic

Address: Poole General Hospital, Poole, Dorset.

Activity: Acupuncture (NHS clinic).

The Society of Biophysical Medicine

Address: Salter Street, Stafford ST16 2JF; *Tel*: 0785 41671.

Activity: Supports all aspects of medical treatment using electromagnetic energy.

Alexander and Feldenkrais Techniques

COLLEGES AND TRAINING ESTABLISHMENTS

Alexander Technique Teachers' Training Course, North London

Address: 1 John's Avenue, London NW4; *Tel*: 01-203 2851.

Date founded: 1981.

Major therapy taught: Alexander Technique according to the principles set down by F.M. Alexander.

Entry requirements: Experience of the theory and practice of the Alexander Technique.

Type and length of course: Certificate Teacher Training Course (3 years full-time).

Subjects taught to trainees: Principles and practice of Alexander Technique; application of Alexander Technique; basic anatomy and physiology.

Average college attendance for trainees: 3 hours/day, 5 days/week, 3 terms/year of 12 weeks each.

Certificate awarded: Certificate, eligible for membership to STAT.

Associated institutions: Society of Teachers of the Alexander Technique (professional association).

Alexander Technique Training Centre

Address: King Edward VI College, Fore Street, Totnes, Devon TQ9 5RP; *Tel*: 0803 864218.

Date founded: 1980.

Major therapy taught: Alexander Technique based on the principles set out by F.M. Alexander.

Entry requirements: A basic practical and theoretical understanding of the Alexander Technique.

Type and length of course: Certificate Teacher Training Course (3 years full-time).

Subjects taught to trainees: Principles and practice of Alexander Technique; application of technique to daily life and to drama, music, sport, etc.; basic anatomy and physiology.

Average college attendance for trainees: 20 hours weekly class work plus home study; terms as for Dartington College of Arts.

Number of students: At Summer Term, 1986: 34.

Certificate awarded: Certificate and eligible to join STAT.

Associated institutions: Course run in association with Dartington College of Arts; Society of Teachers of the Alexander Technique (professional association).

The Constructive Teaching Centre Ltd

Address: 18 Lansdowne Road, Holland Park, London W11 3AG; *Tel*: 01-727 7222.

Date founded: 1973.

Major therapy taught: F.M. Alexander Technique.

Entry requirements: Some prior instruction in the Technique. Admitted for an initial probationary term.

Type and length of course: Certificate course in Alexander Technique (3 years full-time).

Subjects taught to trainees: Some anatomy and physiology; theory and practice of Alexander Technique according to F.M. Alexander; self-improvement of co-ordination; the control and/or change of behaviour to harmonize with demands of environment; learning a new skill; knowledge of the working of the self.

Average college attendance for trainees: Three years each of three 12-week terms.

Certificate awarded: Certificate giving entitlement to teach and eligibility for membership to STAT.

Associated institutions and societies: The School of Alexander Studies; The Society of Teachers of the Alexander Technique (professional body).

Macdonald's Training Course for the Alexander Technique

Address: 50a Belgrave Road, London SW1V 1RQ; *Tel*: 01-821 7916.

Major therapy taught: Alexander Technique.

Type and length of course: Teacher Training Course (3 years full-time).

Subjects taught to trainees: Principles and practice of the Alexander Technique.

Associated institutions: Associated with Society of Teachers of Alexander Technique.

PROFESSIONAL ASSOCIATIONS AND SOCIETIES OF THERAPISTS

Alexander Teaching Centre

Address: AT Centre, 188 Old Street, London EC1V 9BP; *Tel*: 01-250 3038.

Major therapy practised: Alexander Technique according to F.M. Alexander.

Type of membership: Qualified teachers only.

Conditions and qualifications for entry: Qualified Alexander teacher with a minimum of 3 years training.

Title of full members: Alexander teacher.

Number of members in association (inc. associate, honorary, foreign, and retired): 45.

Number of full members in practice in UK: 40.

Code of practice: No.

Library: Yes.

Journal/Newsletter: No.

Associated institutions: Affiliated with the Society of Teachers of the Alexander Technique.

Remarks: They run a variety of classes for people wishing to learn the Alexander Technique including evening, weekend, and summer courses.

The Society of Teachers of the Alexander Technique

Address: London House, 266 Fulham Road, London SW10 9EL; *Tel*: 01-351 0828.

Date founded: 1958.

Major Therapy practised: Alexander Technique according to the teaching of F.M. Alexander.

Types of membership: Full (qualified teachers), Student, Friends, Honorary.

Conditions and qualifications for entry: Full membership on completion of 3 year course at a registered training school.

Title of full members: Alexander teacher.

Number of members in society (inc. associate, honorary, foreign, and retired): 1100.

Number of full members in practice in UK: 285.

Code of Practice: Yes.

Library: No.

Journal: The Alexander Journal.

Associated institutions and societies: Mr. P.J. Macdonald's Training Course; The Alexander Institute; The New Alexander Teaching Centre; The Alexander Centre, Totnes, Devon; The North London Teachers' Training Course; The Constructive Teaching Centre Ltd; The Alexander Teachers' Training Centre, Oxford; The West Sussex Teacher Training course; (all recognized training centres in the UK).

Remarks: Society organizes lectures and seminars.

SUPPORT ORGANIZATIONS

The Feldenkrais Method

Address: 18 Kemplay Road, London NW3 1SY; *Tel*: 01-435 8145.

Activity: Runs courses on Feldenkrais technique for the public and professionals.

The Alexander Institute

Address: 16 Balderton Street, London W1Y 1TL; *Tel*: 01-722 1884.

Activity: A group of teachers associated with the Society of Teachers of the Alexander Technique who are developing the technique.

Anthroposophical medicine

COLLEGES AND TRAINING ESTABLISHMENTS

Artistic Therapy College

Address: Fox Elms House, Fox Elms Road, Tuffley, Gloucester GL4 0BH.

Date founded: 1973.

Major therapy taught: Artistic therapy, including the therapeutic use of painting, drawing, and modelling.

Entry requirements: Experience in social work, nursing or teaching, and artistic experience. Minimum age: 28 years.

Type and length of course: Artistic therapy course (Hauschka method), 2 years.

Subjects taught to trainees: Study of man as a being of body, soul, and spirit. Connection between illness tendencies and the healing possibilities in painting, drawing, and modelling, leading to basic principles of artistic therapy. Practice in therapeutically-orientated artistic work.

Clinical experience: Includes 6 months therapeutic experience.

Associated institutions and societies: The Anthroposophical Society.

Curative Eurythmy Training Course

Address: C/o London School of Eurythmy, Dunnings Road, East Grinstead, Sussex RH19 3NF.

Major therapy taught: Curative eurythmy within an anthroposophical framework.

Type and length of course: Diploma in Curative Eurythmy. 18-month postgraduate course following full four-year artistic eurythmy training.

Subjects taught to trainees: Curative eurythmy, anthroposophy, and anthroposophical medicine.

Clinical experience: Postgraduate training includes substantial periods of supervised clinical experience.

Diploma awarded: Diploma in Curative Eurythmy from the Medical Section of the School for Spiritual Science, Switzerland.

Associated institutions and societies: The Anthroposophical Society; Anthroposophical Medical Association; Medical Section of the School for Spiritual Science.

London School of Speech Formation

Address: Dunnings Road, East Grinstead, Sussex RH19 3NF; *Tel*: 0342 24384.

Date founded: 1971.

Major therapy taught: Speech therapy with an anthroposophical framework.

Entry requirements: (In general) equivalent of 5 O levels. Some knowledge of the work of Rudolf Steiner.

Type and length of course: Speech Diploma (4 years).

Subjects taught to trainees: Speech formation—a speech technique which seeks to release the forms, gestures, and movements of the sounds and rhythms of speech into the surrounding air on the freely-flowing breathstream. Subsidiary subjects: eurythmy, Greek gymnastics, painting, modelling, history of literature.

Average college attendance for trainees: 3 terms each year of 10–11 weeks each for four years.

Clinical experience: The course is an artistic training throughout, but during the third year a 'curative course' is included in the curriculum. This lasts for 1 year, with 1 class a week.

Number of students: At Summer Term 1986: 18.

Diploma awarded: Goetheanum Speech Formation Diploma.

Associated institutions and societies: The Anthroposophical Society. Liaises with The School of Speech Formation at Geotheanum and The London School of Eurythmy, East Grinstead.

Tobias School of Art

Address: Coombe Hill Road, East Grinstead, Sussex; *Tel*: 0342 31365.

Date founded: 1979.

Major therapy taught: Art therapy with an anthroposophical framework; painting (Hauschke method), modelling, drawing, sculpture.

Entry requirements: Prior knowledge of anthroposophy, i.e. Foundation Course at Emerson College (or equivalent).

Type and length of course: Diploma in Art Therapy. After 2 years an official certification may be obtained with 1 more year at St Albans, Goldsmiths', or equivalent.

Subjects taught to trainees: Artistic therapy, technique, theory and practice, therapeutic modelling, exercises, drawing, anthroposophical medicine, art history, introduction to approach and view of the human being.

Clinical experience: A 3-month placement is required in the second year, a 6-month placement requested at end of course.

Number of students: At Summer Term 1986: 6.

Diploma awarded: Diploma in Artistic Therapy.

Associated institutions and societies: The Anthroposophical Society; Emerson College.

PROFESSIONAL ASSOCIATIONS AND SOCIETIES OF THERAPISTS

Anthroposophical Medical Association

Address: Park Attwood Therapeutic Centre, Trimpley, Bewdley, Worcs. DY12 1RE; *Tel*: 02997 444.

Major therapy practised: Anthroposophically developed medicine.

Types of membership: Full, Associate, Student, Honorary.

Conditions and qualifications for entry: Open to qualified doctors and medical students who practise anthroposophical medicine.

Title of full members: AMA.

Number of members in association (inc. associate, honorary, foreign, and retired): 36.

Number of full members in practice in UK: 1986: 21.

Code of practice: Yes, as doctors, all are governed by GMC code.

Library: Yes.

Journal: No.

Associated institutions and societies: The Association of Eurythmy Therapists; The Medical Section of the School for Spiritual Science; The Goetheanum, Dornach, Switzerland; The Medical Group of the Anthroposophical Society; The Anthroposophical Society in Great Britain.

Remarks: The AMA holds 3 weekend conferences per year, arranges introductory seminars, and its members organize more advanced master classes and 'intensive lecture study' weeks. Practical clinical experience is given under individual practitioners and at Park Attwood Therapeutic Centre. More extensive training programmes are held in Switzerland, Holland, and Germany, and there are also a variety of research institutes.

Association of Eurythmy Therapists

Address: Rudolf Steiner House, 35 Park Road, London NW1 6XT; *Tel*: 01-723 4400.

Major therapy practised: Curative eurythmy.

Conditions and qualifications for entry: Holding a Diploma in Curative Eurythmy.

Title of full members: Curative Eurythmist.

Number of members in association (inc. associate, honorary, foreign, and retired): 42.

Number of full members in practice in UK: 42.

Journal: No.

Library: Yes.

Associated institutions and societies: As AMA above.

ASSOCIATED ORGANIZATIONS

Anthroposophical Society in Great Britain

Address: Rudolf Steiner House, 35 Park Road, London NW1 6XT; *Tel*: 01-723 4400.

Conditions and qualifications for entry: Open to any member of the public who recognizes the value of anthroposophical spiritual science.

Activities: Arranges national conferences and local group meetings in many parts of the country. Houses an extensive library of anthroposophical literature and a bookshop.

Publications: A journal—*Anthroposophy Today*.

Size: Approx. 2,500.

Associated institutions and societies: The Society is part of the General Anthroposophical Society with its centre in Dornach, Switzerland.

SUPPORT ORGANIZATIONS

The Medical Group of the Anthroposophical Society in Great Britain

Address: Garlon House, 4 Norton Road, Stourbridge, West Midlands OY8 2AE.

Activities: The furtherance of anthroposophical medicine. Holds weekend meetings at least twice a year.

Publications: *The Talander Journal* and Newsletter.

Remarks: Its secretariat provides an information service on anthroposophical medicine including a mailing service for various interests and professional groups.

Chiropractic

COLLEGES AND TRAINING ESTABLISHMENTS

Anglo-European College of Chiropractic

Address: 13–15 Parkwood Road, Boscombe, Bournemouth, Dorset BH5 2DE; *Tel*: 0202 431021.

Date founded: 1965.

Major therapy taught: Chiropractic—neurological and physical examinations supplemented with X-rays.

Entry requirements: 3 A level passes to include biology/zoology and chemistry; 5 O level passes to include english and physics.

Type and length of course: Diploma in Chiropractic (4 years full-time).

Subjects taught to trainees: Conventional and comprehensive instruction in basic medical sciences including radiology; chiropractic theory, examination procedures, techniques and application; clinical instruction.

Average college attendance for trainees: 1–3 years, 36 weeks/year; 4th year, 46 weeks including summer vacation clinicals, pre-clinical 1470 hours.

Clinical experience: Clinical—1926 hours; Clinic internship—820 hours.

Number of students: At Summer Term 1986: 90.

Diploma awarded: DC.

Associated institutions: British Chiropractors' Association (professional body); European Chiropractors' Union.

McTimoney Chiropractic School

Address: PO Box 127, Oxford OX1 1HH; *Tel*: 0865 246786.

Date founded: 1972.

Major therapy taught: The John McTimoney development of traditional chiropractic. Developed for animal application as well as human.

Entry requirements: O and A standards of education are desirable but not essential. An entrance examination may be required.

Type and length of course: Certificate in Chiropractic (4 years part-time).

Subjects taught to trainees: Conventional anatomy; chiropractic philosophy, art and science of chiropractic palpation, analysis, and manipulative techniques and application; clinical instruction; additional fourth/fifth year studying animal chiropractic.

Average college attendance for trainees: Monthly tutorials supplemented by weekly home-study notes.

Clinical experience: 2 years clinical practice.

Number of students: At Summer Term 1986: 26.

Certificate awarded: Practitioner's certificate, leading to MIPC.

Associated institutions: Institute of Pure Chiropractic.

PROFESSIONAL ASSOCIATIONS AND SOCIETIES OF THERAPISTS

British Chiropractors' Association

Address: 5 First Avenue, Chelmsford, Essex CM1 1RX; *Tel*: 0245 353078. *Executive Sec.*: Ground Floor, 1 Arthington Avenue, Harrogate, North Yorkshire HG1 5NB; *Tel*: 0423 525863.

Date founded: 1925.

Major therapy practised: Chiropractic—neurological and physical examinations supplemented with X-rays.

Types of membership: All members qualified chiropractors.

Conditions and qualifications for entry: Membership limited to graduates of recognized chiropractic colleges.

Title of full members: None.

Number of members in association (inc. associate, honorary, foreign, and retired): 250.

Number of full members in practice in UK: 1985: 220.

Code of practice: Yes.

Library: Yes.

Journal: Contact.

Recognized colleges: Anglo-European College of Chiropractic; The European Chiropractors' Union; The Chiropractic Advancement Association (lay support group).

Remarks: Publish a series of booklets for the public on spinal dysfunctions and chiropractic. Hold annual symposium.

SUPPORT ORGANIZATIONS

The Chiropractic Advancement Association

Address: 38a Upper Richmond Road West, East Sheen, London SW14 8DD; *Tel*: 01-878 3989.

Activity: Chiropractic Support Group for British Chiropractic Association. Organizes local groups, lectures, discussions etc. Encourages chiropractic as a career.

Size: Over 600 members.

Scottish Chiropractic Association

Address: 12 Walker Street, Edinburgh EH3 7LP; *Tel*: 031 225 7743.

Activity: Professional body representing Scottish Chiropractors' Register.

Size: 15 members.

Creative and sensory therapies

COLLEGES AND TRAINING ESTABLISHMENTS

Nordoff-Robbins Music Therapy

Address: 3 Leighton Place, London NW5 2QL; *Tel*: 01-267 6296.

Major therapy taught: Music therapy with the emphasis on practical work based on the creative use of music to equip students to work with handicapped children.

Entry requirements: Professional musical qualification, experience of working with handicapped children desirable.

Type and length of course: Diploma course in music therapy (1 year full-time).

Subjects taught to trainees: Musical studies; introduction to child psychiatry, pathologies etc.; provisions made for handicapped children (includes visits to centres, etc.); practical instruction.

Average college attendance for trainees: Not known. Course run in co-operation with the City University, London.

Clinical experience: Duration not known.

Diploma awarded: Diploma in Music Therapy.

Associated society: British Society of Music Therapy.

PROFESSIONAL ASSOCIATIONS AND SOCIETIES OF THERAPISTS

Association of Professional Music Therapists in Great Britain

Address: The Meadows, 68 Pierce Lane, Fulborne, Cambridge CB1 5BL; *Tel*: 0223 880377.

Date founded: 1971.

Major therapy practised: Music therapy.

Types of membership: Full, Student.

Conditions and qualifications for entry: Diploma in Music Therapy from recognized training course.

Title of full members: Member.

Number of members in association (inc. associate, honorary, foreign and retired): 120.

Number of full members in practice in UK: 1986: 100.

Code of Practice: Yes.

Library: No.

Journal: Yes.

Associated institutions and societies: The British Society for Music Therapy.

British Association of Art Therapists

Address: 13c Northwood Road, London N6 5TL (enquiries by letter with s.a.e. only).

Date founded: 1964.

Major therapy practised: Art therapy.

Types of membership: Registered Art Therapist (qualified), Associate Members (general public), International Members and Corporate Members (institutions).

Conditions and qualifications for entry (full members): Registered members *must* hold a postgraduate Diploma in Art Therapy.

Title of full members: Registered Art Therapist (R.A.Th.).

Number of members in association (inc. associate, honorary, foreign, and retired): 550.

Number of full members in practice in UK: 250.

Code of Practice: Yes.

Library: No.

Journal: *Inscape* (bi-annual).

Associated institutions: Close affiliations with 3 colleges (see below).

Remarks: Recognized Diploma courses run by Goldsmiths' College, Hertfordshire College of Art, and Sheffield University. The BAAT also organizes regional group seminars, workshops, and support groups.

British Association for Dramatherapists

Address: PO Box 98, Kirkbymoorside, York. YO6 6EX.

Date founded: 1977.

Major therapy practised: Dramatherapy, including remedial drama, psychodrama, role play, etc.

Types of membership: Full, Associate, Student.

Conditions and qualifications for entry (full members): Practising dramatherapists who have satisfied conditions of entry (usually through the satisfactory completion of a recognized dramatherapy qualifying course).

Title of full members: R.D.Th.

Number of members in association (inc. associate, honorary, foreign, and retired): 300.

Number of full members in practice in UK: 85.

Code of Practice: In preparation.

Library: No.

Journal/Newsletter: *Journal of Dramatherapy*; *Dramatherapy Newsletter*.

Remarks: Meetings, workshops, research, national conference, regional conferences, workshops and training committee.

ASSOCIATED ORGANIZATIONS

British Society for Music Therapy

Address: 69 Avondale Avenue, East Barnet, Herts. EN4 8NB; *Tel*: 01-368 8879.

Date founded: 1958.

Major therapy practised: Music therapy.

Types of membership: Ordinary, Student.

Conditions and qualifications for entry: Open to all interested in promoting use and development of music therapy.

Title of full members: None.

Number of members in society retired: 500.

Journal: *Journal of Music Therapy*.

Associated institutions: The Association of Professional Music Therapists in Great Britain.

Remarks: They hold regional branch meetings and an annual conference. The society organizes weekend and day courses at the request of local medical and educational authorities.

International Association of Colour Therapists

Address: Brook House, Avening, Tetbury GL8 8NS; *Tel*: 045 383 2150.

Date founded: 1969.

Major therapies practised: Colour and sound therapy.

Type of membership: Associate, Full.

Title of full members: Colour therapist, MIACT.

Number of members in association (inc. associate, honorary, foreign, and retired): 55.

Number of full members in practice in UK: 1986: 10.

Code of Practice: Yes.

Library: Yes.

Journal: *The Colour Circle*.

Remarks: Manufacturers and retailers of colour-sound therapy equipment. Conduct research in colour, sound, and light and their effects on biological structures. Conduct therapy and healing courses over 5 weekends. Hold 'advanced' summer schools in UK, US, West Germany, Holland.

SUPPORT ORGANIZATIONS

International Association of Colour Healers

Address: 33 St Leonards Ct, East Sheen, London SW14 7NG.

Activity: Colour therapy support group, education.

Education: Diploma postal courses—short 30-hour courses.

Universal Colour Healers

Address: 70 Iveagh Close, Northwood, Middlesex HA6 2TF; *Tel*: 09274 20132.

Activity: Colour therapy support group.

Ethnic medicine

PROFESSIONAL ASSOCIATIONS AND SOCIETIES OF THERAPISTS

ASH-SHIFA—The School of Oriental Herbal Medicine—TIBB

Address: 446 East Park Road, Leicester LE5 5HH; *Tel*: 0533 734633.

Major therapies taught: Herbal medicine; gem therapy.

Type and length of course: Professional—part-time (3 years).

Subjects taught to trainees: The philosophy and practice of Tibbi and Unani medicine.

Clinical experience: Minimum of 200 hours.

Associated institutions and societies: Society of Hakims.

Association of Ayurvedic Practitioners in the UK

Address: 12 Agar Street, Leicester LE4 6ND; *Tel*: 0533 666746.

Date founded: 1982.

Major therapies practised: Ayurvedic and Unani medicine.

Type of membership: Limited to qualified practitioners.

Conditions and qualifications for entry: Fully qualified Ayurvedic practitioners holding the official Indian Bachelor of Ayurvedic Medicine and Surgery degree.

Title of full members: MAAP.

Numbers of full members in practice in UK: 1986: 10.

Code of Practice: Yes.

Newsletter: Yes.

SUPPORT ORGANIZATIONS

Chinese Cultural Arts Association

Address: 377 Edgware Road, London W2 1BT.

Activity: Chinese medicine, philosophy, culture and religion; education centre.

Education: Various courses and classes.

Publication: Pamphlets.

Size: 20 to 100 members.

Society for Ayurveda

Address: 139 Cleveland Road, London W13 0EN; *Tel*: 01-997 2303.

Date founded: 1984.

Major therapies supported: Membership for any person interested in the philosophy and practice of Ayurveda.

Activities: Newsletter.

Study Group for Tibetan Medicine

Address: The Secretary, Hawthorne Cottage, Hampstead Lane, Yalding, Maidstone, Kent ME18 6HG; *Tel*: 0622 812607.

Major therapy supported: Tibetan medicine.

Activities: Acts principally as a central point of information in the West. In the UK it works in close collaboration with The Dharma Therapy Trust (Bristol) and Rigpa Meditation Centre (London).

Education: Study groups, meetings, courses.

Publication: Bi-annual journal: *Myrobalan*.

Size: Under 20 members.

Healing

COLLEGES AND TRAINING ESTABLISHMENTS

Claregate College

Address: Great North Road, Potters Bar, Herts. EN6 1JL; *Tel*: 01-774 2341.

Date founded: 1977.

Major therapies taught: Esoteric healing; the ancient wisdom; metaphysics.

Entry requirements: Anyone with interest.

Type and length of courses: Correspondence; Degree of Bachelor of Metaphysics (2 years; individuals can take as long a time as they wish).

Subjects taught to trainees: Origin of man; esoteric healing; astrology.

Numbers of students: Enrolled: 250; qualified: 200.

Diplomas or certificates awarded: Degree in Metaphysics: B.Mph.

College of Healing

Address: Runnings Park, Croft Bank, West Malvern, Worcs. WR14 4BP; *Tel*: 06845 65253.

Date founded: 1963.

Major therapies taught: Healing and colour therapy.

Entry requirements: None.

Type and length of course: 3-part course in the art, science, philosophy, and practice of healing (3 × 6 days).

Subjects taught to trainees: Wide curriculum covering many esoteric subjects, anatomy and physiology, self-healing, counselling, and nutrition.

Numbers of students: At Summer Term 1986: 16.

Diploma awarded: Diploma of the College of Healing.

Associated institutions and societies: Confederation of Healing Organizations (affiliated).

Maitreya School of Healing

Address: 7 Penland Road, Bexhill-on-Sea, East Sussex TN40 2JG; *Tel*: 0424 211450.

Date founded: 1974.

Major therapy taught: Mental colour therapy (healing by the laying on of hands with mental colour projection).

Entry requirements: Interest in healing as a service to humanity.

Type and length of courses: Colour healing and absent healing (13 weeks). Follow-up course including use of astrology, numerology, and hypnotherapy in healing (6 weeks).

Subjects taught to trainees: Basic anatomy; subtle anatomy (the etheric body, chakras, etc.); principles and practice of colour and absent healing; clinic instruction.

Average college attendance for trainees: 14 weeks of approximately 2 hours each in London, Bexhill, Brighton, Birmingham, and Crawley.

Clinical experience: Gained under supervision after course completion.

Number of students: At Summer Term 1986: 100.

Diplomas or certificates awarded: Certificate for 14-week course; Diploma for 20-week course.

Associated institutions and societies: Founder Member, Confederation of Healing Organizations.

Westbank Natural Health Centre

Address: Westbank—Strathmiglo, Fife, Scotland KY14 7QP; *Tel*: 03376 233.

Date founded: 1959.

Major therapies taught: Predominantly healing (absent and laying on of hands), also massage, reflexology, yoga, dowsing, meditation, Bach Flower, and vegetarianism.

Entry requirements: Possession of healing potential.

Type and length of courses: 1-, 2-, and 5-day courses in Britain and abroad. Longer periods including clinical experience up to 2 years by individual arrangement.

Subjects taught to trainees: As above plus the formation, organization, and administration of groups and centres.

Average college attendance for trainees: Train practitioners either as full-time residential students or through specific courses lasting 1 week. Mostly for self-help. Few become practitioners.

Clinical experience: Varying periods up to 2 years.

Associated institutions and societies: Natural Health Network; British Society of Dowsers; National Federation of Spiritual Healers.

PROFESSIONAL ASSOCIATIONS AND SOCIETIES OF THERAPISTS

Aetherius Society

Address: 757 Fulham Road, London SW6 5UU; *Tel*: 01-736 4187 or 01-731 1094.

Date founded: 1956.

Major therapies practised: Metaphysical society which also practises contact healing, absent healing, and colour healing.

Types of membership: Full, Associate.

Conditions and qualifications for entry: No restriction on members. Membership of the Aetherius Society Absent Healing Band is open to all Full and Associate Members. Membership of the Aetherius Society Spiritual Healing Team is open to all Full and Associate Members who have completed their course on spiritual healing.

Title of full members: Aetherius Society Spiritual Healer.

Number of members in society (inc. associate, honorary, foreign, and retired): Unspecified.

Number of full members in practice in UK: 1981: 263.

Code of Practice: Yes, but not written code.

Library: No.

Journal/Newsletter: *The Aetherius Society Healing Bulletin*; *Cosmic Voice*.

Associated societies: The Aetherius Society also has branches and groups in America, Australia, New Zealand, and Africa.

Remarks: The society holds twice-weekly healing sessions in London and has various spiritual healing sanctuaries where members do contact and absent healing. They run a series of training courses at the Aetherius Society College of Spiritual Sciences.

British Alliance of Healing Associations

Address: 23 Nutcroft Grove, Fetcham, Leatherhead, Surrey KT22 9LD; *Tel*: 0372 373241.

Date founded: 1977.

Major therapy practised: Spiritual healing.

Types of membership: Non- (inter-) denominational. Members of member organizations deemed to be members through their parent association.

Conditions and qualifications for entry: Practising healer from one of the member organizations.

Title of full members: Full healer member.

Numbers of members in association (inc. associate, honorary, foreign, and retired): 3500.

Numbers of full members in practice in UK: 2500.

Code of Practice: Yes.

Library: No.

Journal: *The Alliance Review*.

Member associations: Bristol District and Somerset Association of Spiritual Healers; Devon and Cornwall Healers' Association; Dorset Hants and Wilts Spiritual Healers' Association; Essex Healers' Association; Home Counties Association of Spiritual Healers; Jewish Association of Spiritual Healers; Kent Healers' Association; Lancs and District Healing Association; Lincoln and District Healing Association; Moreton and Plymouth Healing Fellowships; Norfolk Healers' Association; Scottish Association of Spiritual Healers; Suffolk Healers' Association; Surrey Spiritual Healers' Association; Sussex Spiritual Healers' Association; The Aquarian Truth and Healing Foundation; The Body Harmonies Association; The Edna Ashby Foundation; The Christian Spiritualist Society Healers' Association; The Warwickshire Spiritual Healers' Foundation; The Yorkshire Healers' Association; The Greater World Spiritual Healing Fellowship; The Invictu Healers' Association; The Pegasus Spiritual Healers' Association; The Spiritualist Association of Great Britain; The Seekers' Trust; The Research and Enlightenment Centre; The Spiritual Venturers' Association.

Remarks: The Alliance was formed to allow representatives of member organizations to discuss matters concerning healing, standards of conduct of members, the exchange of views, etc. Addresses of member associations can be obtained from the Alliance.

Friends' Fellowship of Healing

Address: Secretary: Lilian Palmer, 5 Old Manor Close, Ifield, Crawley RH11 0HQ; *Tel*: 0293 21267.

Date founded: 1935.

Major therapy practised: Spiritual healing—absent healing and prayer.

Types of membership: Individual, prayer group, postal group.

Conditions and qualifications for entry: None.

Numbers of members in association (inc. associate, honorary, foreign, and retired): 800.

Code of Practice: No.

Library: No.

Remarks: The Fellowship runs 2 centres: Claridge House, Dormansland, Lindfield, Surrey RH7 6QH (*Tel*: 0342 832150) and Lattendales, Berrier Road, Greystoke, Penrith, Cumbria CA11 0UE (*Tel*: 08533 229). Available for individual guests and for conferences and study.

Greater World Christian Spiritualist Association

Address: 3 Lansdowne Road, Holland Park, London W11 3AL; *Tel*: 01-727 7264 and 9795.

Date founded: 1961.

Major therapy practised: Spiritual healing by laying on of hands and absent prayer healing.

Type of membership: Full member.

Conditions and qualifications for entry: Probationary healers become healers on presentation of evidence of patient's testimony supported by healing leader's recommendation at the church where healing takes place.

Title of full members: Member of the Greater World Spiritual Healing Fellowship.

Number of members in association (inc. associate, honorary, foreign, and retired): 300.

Numbers of full members in practice in UK: 1986: 200.

Code of Practice: Yes.

Library: Yes.

Journal: *The Greater World*.

Associated institutions and societies: Branches throughout the world.

SNU Guild of Spiritualist Healers

Address: 36 Newmarket, Otley, W. Yorks LS21 3AE.

Date founded: 1964.

Major therapies practised: Contact and absent healing.

Types of membership: Trainee, Approved, Associate, Honorary.

Conditions and qualifications for entry: Class B member of the SNU or a member of an SNU church healing group.

Title of full members: Approved Practising Healer.

Number of members in Guild (inc. associate, honorary, foreign, and retired): 1985: 2371.

Number of full members in practice in UK: 1985: 2291.

Code of practice: Yes.

Library: No.

Newsletter: Yes.

Associated institutions and societies: The Guild is a branch of the Spiritualists' National Union Ltd.

Remarks: There are 2 healing training courses available from the SNU, all newly qualified Approved Guild Healers have had 12 months as a trainee healer and studied and passed one of these courses. The Guild is made up of 14 District Guilds throughout the UK. The National and District Guilds arrange seminars, lectures, and demonstrations throughout the UK. There is a referral system for putting patients in touch with available healers.

The Harry Edwards Spiritual Healing Sanctuary

Address: Burrows Lea, Shere, Guildford, Surrey GU5 9QG; *Tel*: 048 641 2054.

Date founded: 1946.

Major therapy practised: Spiritual healing—contact and absent healing.

Conditions and qualifications for entry: No formal requirements.

Code of Practice: No.

Library: No.

Journal: *The Spiritual Healer*

Associated institutions and societies: The National Federation of Spiritual Healers; The British Alliance of Healing Associations.

Remarks: Publishes a selection of books, cassettes, and records—primarily a private healing sanctuary.

National Federation of Spiritual Healers

Address: Old Manor Farm Studio, Church Street, Sunbury-on-Thames, Middlesex TW16 6RG; *Tel*: 0932 783164.

Date founded: 1955.

Major therapy practised: Spiritual healing by prayer or meditation, and by laying-on of hands.

Types of membership: Healer, Probationer Healer, Associate (for medically and paramedically qualified), Member of the International Fellowship of Healing (for friends of the NFSH).

Conditions and qualifications for entry: Healer—sponsorship and authenticated evidence of spiritual healing acceptable to a panel of NFSH executives.

Title of full members: Healer Member of the NFSH.

Numbers of members in society/association (inc. associate, honorary, foreign, and retired): 4200.

Numbers of full members in practice in UK: 1986: 2078.

Code of Practice: Yes.

Library: No.

Journal: *Healing Review*.

Associated institutions and societies: Founder Member of Confederation of Healing Organizations.

Remarks: There is an NFSH national scheme of development groups for probationer healers. Educational and training courses within a structured syllabus are held in London and the provinces. The NFSH organizes a major national conference annually and seminars (residential and non-residential). A national and international referral service puts patients in touch with healers and is operated from NFSH HQ office.

Spiritualists' National Union

Address: General Secretary, Britten House, Stansted Hall, Stansted Mountfitchet, Essex CM24 80D; *Tel*: 0279 812705.

Date founded: 1901.

Major therapy practised: Spiritual healing.

Types of membership: Full members and trainees.

Conditions and qualifications for entry: Open to SNU-trained healers.

Title of full members: Either DSNU (diploma holder), CSNU (Certificate of Recognition for Speakers or Administrators), MSNU (Minister), FSNU (Fellow-academic), LSSNU (Long Service over 25 years).

Number of members in association (inc. associate, honorary, foreign, and retired): 2100.

Number of full members in practice in UK: 2100.

Code of Practice: Yes.

Library: Yes.

Journal: Yes.

Associated institutions and societies: The Guild of Spiritualist Healers is a branch of the SNU.

Remarks: The SNU runs diploma courses open to all full SNU members either by postal tuition or in study groups working under the direction of a leader, in spiritualism, administration, healing (basic and advanced), and mediumship.

The White Eagle Lodge

Address: New Lands, Rake, Brewells Lane, Hampshire GU33 7HY; *Tel*: 0730 893300.

Date founded: 1936.

Major therapy practised: Christian healing—contact and absent.

Type of membership: Full members of organization only. (*Note*: This does not imply healer training which is separate.)

Conditions and qualifications for entry: No formal requirements.

Title of full members: None.

Numbers of members in association (inc. associate, honorary, foreign, and retired): 5000.

Numbers of full members in practice in UK: 1986: 750.

Code of Practice: Yes.

Library: Yes.

Journal: *Stella Polaris*.

Associated institutions and societies: 8 lodges in the UK.

Remarks: The above information covers all 8 lodges.

World Federation of Healing

Address: 134 Darnley Road, Gravesend, Kent DA11 0SN; *Tel*: 0474 62304. Or 133 Gatley Road, Gatley, Cheadle, Cheshire; *Tel*: 061 428 4980.

Major therapy practised: Healing.

Types of membership: Practitioner (medical); Healer (minister of religion/spiritual healer); Practitioner (complementary therapist, paramedical); Friend.

Conditions and qualifications for entry: Full membership open to qualified practitioners of any healing discipline, registered medical practitioners, and ministers of recognized religious bodies who personally practise the ministry of healing.

Journal: *WFH Journal*.

Associated institutions and societies: Branches worldwide.

Remarks: Organizes annual conferences. Involved in work to foster understanding between orthodox and complementary medicine, maintain standards, etc.

SUPPORT ORGANIZATIONS

Burrswood

Address: Groombridge, near Tunbridge Wells, Kent TN3 9PY; *Tel*: 089276 353.

Activity: Prayer and contact healing—residential and healing centre.

Education: Short courses.

Assoc. with: International Fellowship.

Size: 30 beds.

Carthage Trust

Address: Bay Tree House, The Street, Wallerton, Arundel, W. Sussex; *Tel*: 02435 52265.

Activity: Healing and natural therapies centre.

Education: Occasional conferences.

Size: Under 20 members.

Christian Fellowship of Healing (Scotland)

Address: c/o Holy Corner Church Centre, 15 Morningside Road, Edinburgh EH10 5DP; *Tel*: 031 447 9383.

Activity: Prayer and sacramental healing.

Size: 60 members.

The Churches' Council for Health and Healing

Address: St Marylebone Parish Church, Marylebone Road, London NW1 5LT; *Tel*: 01-486 9644.

Date founded: 1944.

Activities: Encouraging and co-ordinating the Healing Ministry in all the churches; acting as a resource centre for the Healing Ministry and publishing literature, audio and video tapes; teaching and training in Christian Healing Ministry.

Size: Over 50 member bodies: all the major church denominations and Royal Colleges of Medicine and allied disciplines, together with hospital chaplaincy associations and healing groups and associations.

College of Psychic Studies

Address: 16 Queensbury Place, London SW7 2EB; *Tel*: 01-589 3292/3.

Activity: Absent healing; parapsychology; information service.

Education: Workshops and short courses on healing and relaxation. Extensive teaching in parapsychology.

Publications: Journal. ('*Light*')

Confederation of Healing Organizations (CHO)

Address: 113 Hampstead Way, London NW11 7JN; *Tel*: 01-455 2638.

Major therapy supported: Healing through the hands or at a distance, whether spiritual healing or not.

Activities: Umbrella organization working towards provision of healing to all and its adoption by the medical profession: controlled trials conducted by independent medical scientists are under way.

Size: 16 healing organizations, comprising over 7500 healers.

Crystal Research Foundation

Address: 37 Bromley Road, St. Annes-on-Sea, Lancashire FY8 1PQ; *Tel*: 0253 723735.

Activities: The promotion of crystals in healing and the supply of information on their use.

Divine Healing Fellowship (Scotland)

Address: Linn Horen, Avonbridge, Falkirk FK1 2NN.

Activity: Healing—support group.

Size: Under 100 members.

Guild of Health

Address: Edward Wilson House, 26 Queen Anne Street, London W1M 9LB; *Tel*: 01-580 2492.

Activity: Religious organization—healing through prayer and counselling. Nationwide: 150 groups involved in prayer, meditation, and other healing acts for the benefit of local communities and group members. Residential and day conferences. Large number of publications and library. Quarterly magazine.

Education: Training courses in Christian counselling; meetings; lectures in prayer and meditation.

Publications: Magazine, books.

Associated with: Churches' Council of Healing.

Size: 800 full members of the guild.

Guild of St Raphael

Address: St. Marylebone Church, Marylebone Road, London NW1 5LT; *Tel*: 01-935 6328.

Date founded: 1915.

Activity: Healing; support group; lectures.

Size: 2000 members.

Methodist Church: Division of Social Responsibility: Family, Healing and Personal Concerns Committee

Address: Methodist Church, 1 Central Buildings, Matthew Parker Street, Westminster, London SW1H 9NH; *Tel*: 01-222 8010.

Activity: Religious organization; healing; health education and promotion.

Size: Under 100 members.

The Presbyterian Church of Wales Healing Committee

Address: Madryu, Meadow Gardens, Llandudno, Gwynedd L30 1UW; *Tel*: 0286 2951.

Activity: Healing—specific therapy support group.

Size: Under 20 members.

The Seekers' Trust

Address: Centre for Prayer and Spiritual Healing, The Close, Addington Park, near Maidstone, Kent ME19 5BL; *Tel*: 0732 843589.

Activity: Religious group, residential and healing centre.

Education: Healing course of 10 1–2 hour sessions plus home study; monthly lectures.

Publication: Journal; information literature.

Associated with: Worldwide network.

Size: Under 100 members.

The Spiritualists' Association of Great Britain

Address: 33 Belgrave Square, London SW1X 8QB; *Tel*: 01-235 3351.

Activity: Healing—support group.

Associated with: 23 Commonwealth Spiritualist Churches in the UK.

The United Reformed Church Committee on Health and Healing

Address: 86 Tavistock Place, London WC1H 9RT; *Tel*: 01-837 7661.

Activity: Promoting the work of health and healing throughout the denomination.

Unity Teaching and Healing Trust

Address: The Priory, Thornsbury, Holsworthy, Devon EX22 7DA; *Tel*: 040 926273.

Activity: Healing; meditation; acupressure; homeopathy and spiritual massage.

Publications: Bi-annual journal.

Remarks: The Trust has a country house which is available for lectures, etc. and which also includes a sanctuary and accommodation for courses.

Herbalism

COLLEGES AND TRAINING ESTABLISHMENTS

The School of Herbal Medicine (Phytotherapy)

Address: 148 Forest Road, Tunbridge Wells, Kent TN2 5EY; *Tel*: 0892 30400.

Date founded: 1864 (renamed 1978).

Major therapies taught: Herbalism, Phytotherapy.

Entry requirements: Full time—2 A levels in natural sciences; Tutorial—O levels; Certificate in Herbal Studies—open to any interested lay person.

Type and length of courses: Diploma in Phytotherapy (3½ years full-time); Special Course for Qualified Doctors (1 year part-time); Tutorial Course—Membership of Nat. Instit. of M. Herb. (4 years part-time); Certificate in Herbal Studies (1 year part-time).

Subjects taught to trainees: Basic medical sciences including pharmacology; *materia medica*; physiomedical philosophy; posology; herbalism theory and practice; clinical instruction; medical discipline and ethics.

Average college attendance for trainees: Full time—3 days per week plus home study; Tutorial—weekly seminar once each year approx. 40 hours per year plus 20–30 hours home-study per week.

Clinical experience (extent of supervised treatment of patients): Minimum 300 hours over 4 years.

Number of students: Full-time approx. 60; part-time approx. 250; doctors approx. 6; laymen approx. 380.

Diploma or certificate awarded: Diploma in Phytotherapy; Certificate in Herbal Studies; Membership of National Institute of Medical Herbalists.

Associated institutions: The National Institute of Medical Herbalists.

PROFESSIONAL ASSOCIATIONS AND SOCIETIES OF THERAPISTS

The General Council and Register of Consultant Herbalists Ltd

Address: Marlborough House, Swanpool, Falmouth, Cornwall TR11 4HW; *Tel*: Falmouth 317231.

Major therapy practised: Herbal medicine.

Types of membership: Full members and Fellows.

Conditions and qualifications for entry: Correspondence course training with practical clinical-experience at selected clinics situated in different areas of the UK.

Title of full members: Registered Medical Herbalist (MRH).

Number of members in association (inc. full, fellows, honorary, foreign and retired): 300.

Number of full members in practice in UK: 250.

Code of practice: Yes.

Library: Yes.

Journal: No.

Associated institutions and societies: The British Herbalists' Union Ltd; The Osteopathic and Naturopathic Guild Ltd.

National Institute of Medical Herbalists Ltd

Address: General Secretary, 41 Hatherley Road, Winchester SO22 6RR; *Tel*: 0962 68776.

Date founded: 1864.

Major therapies practised: Herbalism ('physiomedical system'); Phyto-therapy.

Types of membership: Full member, Fellow.

Conditions and qualifications for entry: Graduate of the School of Herbal Medicine.

Title of full members: MNIMH.

Number of members in society/association (inc. associate, honorary, foreign, and retired): 171.

Number of full members in practice in UK: 1986: 127.

Code of Practice: Yes.

Library: Yes.

Journal: *New Herbal Practitioner*.

Associated institutions and societies: The School of Herbal Medicine.

Remarks: Has its own research department.

Register of Chinese Herbal Medicine

Address: C/o Wendy Owen, 138 Prestbury Road, Cheltenham GLS2 2DP.

Date founded: 1985.

Major therapies practised: Chinese herbal medicine; acupuncture.

Types of membership: Full, Foreign.

Conditions and qualifications for entry: 1. Successful completion of course in Chinese herbalism taught by Ted Kaptchuk (or equivalent); 2. Membership of one of the acupuncture societies (RTCM, BAAR, TAS, BROM).

Title of full members: Member of the Register of Chinese Herbal Medicine (MRCHM).

Number of members in association (inc. associate, honorary, foreign, and retired): 41.

Number of full members in practice in UK: 30.

Code of practice: Yes.

Library: No.

Journal: No.

Remarks: The Register was born out of the need to establish a body to regulate and set educational standards, share information on supplies etc., and organize further seminars/courses etc.

SUPPORT ORGANIZATIONS

Aromatherapy Training Centre

Address: 4 Eltham Road, London SE12 8TF; *Tel*: 01-852 7591.

Activity: Aromatherapy; educational institution.

Education: 3-day intensive courses.

Size: 150 therapists in the UK in 1980.

British Herbal Medicine Association

Address: PO Box 304, Bournemouth, Dorset BH7 6JT *Tel*: 0202 433691.

Activity: Herbalism; support group for herbal use, manufacture and legislation.

Education: Meetings and seminars.

Publications: *British Herbal Pharmacopoeia*; newsletter.

Associated with: National Institute of Medical Herbalists; herbal manufacturers and suppliers.

Size: Under 100 members.

The Herb Society

Address: 77 Great Peter Street, London SW1P 2EZ; *Tel*: 01-222 3634.

Activity: Herbalism; support group; information service; lectures.

Publications: Quarterly magazine *The Herbal Review*.

Associated with: National Institute of Medical Herbalists.

Remarks: Founded in 1927. Library. The society's structure includes a scientific and publications committee involved in the collection and assessment of historical and contemporary data and the publication of previously unpublished materials. The society is also involved in the establishment of a National Herb Collection.

Size: Over 2000 members.

International Association of Aromatherapists

Address: 46 Dalkeith Road, London SE21 8LS.

Activities: Support for aromatherapy practitioners.

London School of Aromatherapy

Address: PO Box 780, London NW6 5EQ.

Activities: Postal courses, with weekend tuition, leading to aromatherapy diploma. Affiliated with London and Counties Society of Physiologists.

Natural Medicines Group

Address: Natural Medicines Society, Regency House, 97–107 Hagley Road, Edgbaston, Birmingham B16 8LA; *Tel*: 021-454 9390.

Activities: Organizations of herbal manufacturers (NMG) and the concerned public (NMS) to press for protection of the right to make, supply, and sell herbal, homeopathic, and anthroposophical remedies. Information, seminars, and political action in support of natural remedies.

Homeopathy

COLLEGES AND TRAINING ESTABLISHMENTS

British School of Homeopathy

Address: PO Box 8, Liphook, Hants GU30 7JD.

Date founded: 1986.

Major therapy taught: Homeopathy.

Entry requirements: Postgraduates preferred but undergraduates considered according to age, education, and work experience.

Type and length of course: Extension—by checksheet and tutorial (approx. 1 year).

Subjects taught to trainees: Homeopathic principles and philosophy, *materia medica*, repertory, cases, clinical work.

Clinical experience: About 200 hours.

Number of students: Enrolled: 5.

Diploma awarded: Postgraduate Diploma in Homeopathy.

Associated institutions and societies: London School of Osteopathy; International Academy of Nutrition (UK).

The College of Homeopathy

Address: 26 Clarendon Rise, London SE13 5EY.

Date founded: 1978.

Major therapy taught: Hahnemannian homeopathy.

Entry requirements: Education to A level standard preferred. Minimum age 21.

Type and length of courses: 4-year part-time professional course of which the first year is a foundation year; 3-year full-time professional course.

Subjects taught to trainees: Principles and philosophy of homeopathy; *materia medica*; medical sciences; clinical instruction and practice.

Average college attendance for trainees: 1. Part-time course: 11 weekends per year plus clinical training in third and fourth year; 2. Full-time course: 24 hours per week plus clinical training in second and third year.

Clinical experience: 100 hours observation and participation plus assessed case taking.

Number of students: July 1986: 400.

Diplomas or certificates awarded: Licentiate of the College of Homeopathy; Membership of the College of Homeopathy.

Associated institutions and societies: The Society of Homeopaths (professional body).

The Hahneman College of Homeopathy

Address: 243 The Broadway, Southall, Middx. UB1 1NF; *Tel*: 01-574 4281.

Date founded: 1978.

Major therapy taught: Homeopathy.

Entry requirements: Paramedics or members of the public by interview.

Type and length of courses: Part-time (3 years and 2 years). Also postgraduate course for medical practitioners.

Subjects taught to trainees: All aspects of homeopathy.

Clinical experience: 3 months supervised clinical experience required after examination.

Number of students: Enrolled: 28.

Diplomas or certificates awarded: Diploma. D.Hom.(Med.), MHMA or FHMA after membership of professional body.

Associated institutions and societies: Register and Council of Homeopathy; UK Homeopathic Medical Association (professional association); The Society of Holistic Medicines Practitioners.

Northern College of Homeopathy

Address: 21 Leazes Park Road, Newcastle-upon-Tyne NE1 2PF; *Tel*: 0434 605401.

Date founded: 1981.

Major therapy taught: Homeopathy.

Type and length of course: Licentiate of College of Homeopathy (3 years part-time).

Conditions and qualifications for entry: Practising chiropodists with recognized qualifications and state registration. Associate on joining and after homeopathic training becomes full member.

Title of full members: MIPAHM; FIPAHM.

Number of members in association (inc. associate, honorary, foreign, and retired): Associate—210; Full—75; Fellow—25.

Number of full members in practice in UK: 310.

Code of Practice: Under preparation.

Library: Yes—Homeopathy and Chiropody, 97 Highfield Avenue, London NW11.

Journal: *Homeo-Chiropody*.

Associated institutions and societies: International Homeopathic Medical League (Pakistan, India, Sri Lanka, Bangladesh); Hahnemann Society for Promotion of Homeopathy in UK; British Homeopathic Association; Institute of Chiropodists; English Chiropodists, Association; the Association of Homeopathic Chiropodists UK.

Subjects taught to trainees: Basic medical sciences; Homeopathy – basic principles, practices, *materia medica*; Clinic instruction.

Diploma awarded: Licentiate of College of Homeopathy.

Associated societies: Society of Homeopaths.

The North West College of Homeopathy

Address: 23 Wilbraham Road, Fallowfield, Manchester M14 6FB; *Tel*: 061-224 6809.

Date founded: 1984.

Major therapy taught: Homeopathy.

Entry requirements: A Level GCE or similar or practical experience.

Type and length of course: Part-time (4 years).

Subjects taught to trainees: Homeopathic principles and philosophy; homeopathic *materia medica*; repertory use and case analysis; anatomy, physiology, pathology, clinical examination.

Average college attendance for trainees: 10 weekends of lectures. 12 hours each weekend each year for 4 years.

Clinical experience: With qualified and registered practitioners in the college and elsewhere by arrangement during the third and fourth years. Minimum of 75 hours.

Numbers of students: Enrolled: 75.

Diplomas or certificates awarded: Licentiate of the college.

Associated institutions and societies: The Society of Homeopaths.

PROFESSIONAL ASSOCIATIONS AND SOCIETIES OF THERAPISTS

The Faculty of Homeopathy

Address: The Royal London Homeopathc Hospital, Great Ormond Street, London WC1N 3HR; *Tel*: 01-837 3091 ext 72.

Date founded: 1844.

Major therapy practised: Homeopathic medicine.

Types of membership: Associate, Full, Fellows, Student.

Conditions and qualifications for entry: Full member only open to doctors with an orthodox medical degree after written and clinical entrance exam, Associate membership open to veterinary surgeons pharmacists, dental surgeons and SRNs.

Title of full members: M.F. Hom.

Numbers of members in society/association (inc. associate, honorary, foreign and retired): 411.

Numbers of full members in practice in UK: 350.

Code of Practice: GMC code.

Library: Yes.

Journal: British Homeopathic Journal.

Associated institutions and societies: The Homeopathic Trust for Research and Education.

Remarks: The Faculty runs pot-graduate courses: (a) 2 year part-time course, comprising several 2- and 3-day mini-courses; (b) 6 months full-time course – introductory, intermediate and advanced (for doctors and veterinary surgeons only).

International Podiatric Association of Homeopathic Medicine

Address: 134 Montrose Avenue, Edgware, Middlesex; *Tel*: 01-959 5421.

Date founded: 1978.

Major therapies practised: Homeopathy, chiropody.

Types of membership: Associate and Full Membership; Fellow Member and Honorary Fellowship.

The Society of Homeopaths Ltd

Address: 47 Canada Grove, Bognor Regis, West Sussex PO21 1OW; *Tel*: 0243 860678.

Date founded: 1978.

Major therapy practised: Hahnemannian homeopathy.

Types of membership: Associate, Full, Graduate.

Conditions and qualifications for entry: Associate membership open to anyone. Full membership and entry in the Register of Homeopaths on submission of evidence of competence to practise and approval by an examination committee.

Title of full members: R.S.Hom. (registered with Soc. of Hom.).

Number of members in society (inc. associate, honorary, foreign, and retired): 600.

Number of full members in practice in UK: 53.

Code of Practice: Yes.

Library: No.

Journal: *The Homeopath* (quarterly journal).

SUPPORT ORGANIZATIONS

Blackie Foundation Trust

Address: C/o 101 Harley Street, London W1N 1DF.

Activity: Homeopathy—research and educational support group (awards grants).

British Association of Homeopathic Pharmacists

Address: 19a Cavendish Square, London W1M 9AD; *Tel*: 01-629 3205.

Activity: Represents pharmacists who dispense homeopathic remedies.

British Association of Homeopathic Veterinary Surgeons

Address: Chinham House, Stanford-in-the-Vale near Faringdon, Oxon SN7 8NQ.

Activities: Support, training, research, information for veterinary surgeons in homeopathy.

Size: 113 members.

The British Homeopathic Association

Address: 27a Devonshire Street, London W1N 1RJ; *Tel*: 01-935 2163.

Date founded: 1902.

Major therapy supported: Homeopathy support group.

Journal: *Homeopathy* (bi-monthly).

Activities: Holds regular annual seminars in various parts of the UK, and a series of Homeopathic First Aid lectures. Library for the use of members only. Training courses held for pharmacists, and when possible, symposiums for veterinary surgeons. On enquiry, provides geographical lists of medical doctors, pharmacists, and veterinary surgeons who are also fully qualified in homeopathic medicine.

Size: 5000 members.

British Homeopathy Research Group

Address: C/o 101 Harley Street, London W1N 1DF: *Tel*: 01-580 5489, 01-730 4235 (messages).

The Dr Edward Bach Centre

Address: Mount Vernon, Sotwell, Wallingford, Oxfordshire OX10 0PZ; *Tel*: 0491 39489.

Activity: Preparation and supply of Bach flower remedies; help and advice given freely.

Publications: Newsletter; books and information leaflets.

Size: Under 20 members.

The Hahnemann Society for the Promotion of Homeopathy

Address: Avenue Lodge, Bounds Green Road, London N22 4EU; *Tel*: 01-889 1595.

Activity: Homeopathy—support group.

Publications: Magazine, *Homeopathy Today*.

Remarks: Holds occasional seminars and meetings.

Size: 3000 members 1981.

Homeopathic Development Foundation

Address: Harcourt House, 19a Cavendish Square, London W1M 9AD; *Tel*: 01-629 3205.

Activity: Homeopathy—research/information service.

Homeopathic Hospitals (providing in- and out-patient facilities within the NHS)

The Royal London Homeopathic Hospital, Great Ormond Street, London WC1N 3HR; *Tel*: 01-837 3091, outpatients 01-837 7821.

The Glasgow Homeopathic Hospital, 1000 Great Western Road, Glasgow G12 ORN; *Tel*: 041-339 0382.

Outpatients Department, 5 Lynedoch Road, Glasgow C3; *Tel*: 041-332 4490.

Outpatients Clinic, Baillieston Health Institute, Buchanan Street, Baillieston, Glasgow; *Tel*: 041-771 7396/7.

Liverpool Clinic, The Mossley Hill Hospital, Park Avenue, Liverpool L18 8BU; *Tel*: 051-724 2355.

The Bristol Homeopathic Hospital, Cotham Road, Cotham, Bristol BS6 6JU; *Tel*: 0272 731231, outpatients 0272 32007.

Tunbridge Wells Homeopathic Hospital, Church Road, Tunbridge Wells, Kent; *Tel*: 0892 42977.

Homeopathic Manufacturers

A. Nelson and Co. Ltd, Manufacturing Laboratories, 5 Endeavour Way, Wimbledon, London SW19 9UH; *Tel*: 01-946 8527.

Weleda (UK) Ltd, Heanor Road, Ilkeston, Derbyshire DE7 8DR; *Tel*: 0602 303151.

The Homeopathic Trust for Research and Education

Address: Hahnemann House, 2 Powis Place, Great Ormond Street, London WC1N 3HT; *Tel*: 01-837 9469.

Activity: Homeopathy—research and educational group.

Size: Under 20 members.

Activity: Homeopathy discussion group—advice on research.

Publications: Newsletter, *Communications*.

Size: 30 members.

Hypnotherapy

COLLEGES AND TRAINING ESTABLISHMENTS

School of Hypnosis and Advanced Psychotherapy

Address: Registrar, 28 Finsbury Park Road, London N4 2JX; *Tel*: 01-359 6991.

Date founded: 1981.

Major therapies taught: Hypnotherapy and psychotherapeutic techniques—emphasis on the methods of the hypnotist Milton H. Erickson, includes methods of visualization, dream therapy, age-regression and self-hypnosis, neuro-linguistic programming and advanced psychotherapeutic techniques.

Entry requirements: Entry to Part I is flexible. Entry to Part II is dependent on the successful completion of Part I. Lower age limit of 25 years.

Type and length of course: 3-part course: Part I (complete in itself for the layman or foundation course for trainees): 60 hours; Part II leads to examination for SHAP Intermediate certification: over 60 hours; Part III (for graduates of the Intermediate Certificate).

Subjects taught to trainees: Part I—Psychotherapeutic and hypnotherapeutic principles and methods, self-hypnosis, neuro-linguistic programming; Part II—NLP, principles and methods and practice, behaviour modification, super-learning, schools of psychological thought; Part III—Extension of the Part II work, and preparation for setting up in practice.

Average college attendance for trainees: Part I—60 hours approx. (part-time, weekends); Part II—57 hours approx.; Part III—60 hours approx.

Clinical experience: 6 months post-Diploma period of clinical supervision.

Number of students: 1986: 39.

Diplomas or certificates awarded: SHAP Intermediate Certificate. SHAP Diploma in Therapeutic Hypnosis and Psychotherapy (Diploma).

Associated institutions and societies: The Society of Advanced Psychotherapy Practitioners (professional association).

UK Training College of Hypnotherapy and Counselling

Address: 10 Alexander Street, London W2 5NT; *Tel*: 01-221 1796.

Date founded: 1984.

Major therapies taught: Hypnotherapy (especially Ericksonian); counselling; TA; Gestalt.

Entry requirements: Equivalent of 2 A levels and an interview.

Type of courses: Foundation; Diploma.

Subjects taught to trainees: Basic hypnotic skills, basic counselling skills, areas of concern such as depression, anxiety, unwanted habits (e.g. smoking), performance anxiety, reframing procedures, psychodynamics, relationship work, use of metaphor, etc.

Average college attendance for trainees: Foundation course—9 weekends plus exam weekend; Diploma course—18 weekends plus exam weekend.

Clinical experience: 1 year supervised experience post-Diploma, at least one client per week during Diploma.

Number of students: Summer 1985: 64.

Diplomas or certificates awarded: Joint Skills Testing Certificate/Diploma with City and Guilds of London Institute.

Associated institutions and societies:Association for Professional Therapists; Association for Applied Hypnosis.

Stephen Brooks Associates

Address: 23 Godwin Close, Cambridge CB1 4QS; *Tel*: 244125.

Date founded: 1986.

Major therapies taught: Professional training in Ericksonian hypnosis and psychotherapy.

Entry requirements: Preferably degree level although each applicant is considered on personal merit.

Type and length of course: Intense training in the techniques of Milton H. Erickson with emphasis on experiential learning (3 years).

Subjects taught to trainees: Indirect suggestion, induction techniques, problem solving, deep trance phenomena, post-hypnotic suggestions, stategic therapy, NLP, metaphorical communication, developing creativity and flexibility, utilization approaches, research skills, practice management.

Average college attendance for trainees: 9 weekends plus 15 evenings per year.

Clinical experience: Most trainers are medically qualified specialists in their field. All training takes place at London teaching hospitals.

Number of students: 1986: 25.

Diplomas awarded: The Practitioner Diploma (first year); Advanced Practitioner Diploma (second year); Master Practitioner Diploma (third year).

Associated institutions and societies: The British Hypnosis Research Association.

PROFESSIONAL ASSOCIATIONS AND SOCIETIES OF THERAPISTS

The Association for Applied Hypnosis

Address: 33 Abbey Park Road, Grimsby, South Humberside DN32 0H2; *Tel*: 0472 47702.

Date founded: 1980.

Major therapy practised: Hypnotherapy, including psychotherapy and stress reduction.

Types of membership: Student, Associate, Fellow.

Conditions and qualifications for entry: Membership is granted only after successful completion of training and is dependent also on examination results.

Title of full members: Member of Association for Applied Hypnosis.

Code of Practice: Yes.

Library: No.

Journal/Newsletter: Yes.

Associated institutions and societies: UK Training College of Hypnotherapy and counselling.

Remarks: The Association runs a 2-year training course involving home study, 6-week training sessions, and supervised practice.

Association of Qualified Curative Hypnotherapists

Address: 10 Balaclava Road, Kings Heath, Birmingham B14 7SG; *Tel*: 021 444 5435.

Date founded: 1985.

Major therapy practised: Curative hypnotherapy.

Types of membership: Full, Licentiate, Associate, Overseas.

Conditions and qualifications for entry: Written exam and interview.

Title of full members: MAQCH.

Number of members in association (inc. associate, honorary, foreign, and retired): 45.

Number of full members in practice in UK: 43.

Code of practice: Yes.

Library: No.

Journal: Yes.

The British Association of Therapeutical Hypnotists (UK)

Address: Secretary, 95 Prospect Road, Woodford Green, Essex 1G8 7ND; *Tel*: 01-505 8720.

Date founded: 1951.

Major therapies practised: Hypnotherapy, clinical hypnosis, psychology, statistics, relaxation therapy, regression therapy, counselling, hypno-analysis, deep sleep therapy, dream analysis, hypnopictography.

Types of membership, and conditions and qualifications for entry: Licentiate (1 year initial training course); Associateship (full training course with B.A.T.H. or by set thesis); Member B.A.T.H. (after set period and dissertation); Fellow.

Title of full members: MBATH.

Number of members in association (inc. associate, honorary, foreign, and retired): 85.

Number of full members in practice in UK: 40.

Code of practice: Yes.

Library: Yes.

Journal: Newsletter.

Associated institutions and societies: Institute of Curative Hypnotherapists (UK); World Federation of Hypnotherapists; American Association of Professional Hypnotherapists; International Institute of Hypnotists.

British Society of Medical and Dental Hypnosis

Address: Secretary (Metropolitan Branch), 42 Links Road, Ashtead, Surrey KT21 2HJ; *Tel*: 27 73522.

Major therapies practised: Hypnotherapy used within an orthodox medical framework.

Conditions and qualifications for entry: Membership open to qualified doctors and dentists only.

Title of full members: MBSMDH.

Number of members in society (inc. associate, honorary, foreign, and retired): 1000.

Code of Practice: GMC code.

Library: No.

Journal: Proceedings of the BSMDH.

Remarks: They run a programme of lectures and seminars throughout the autumn and winter including a 2-day course on the theory, technique, practice, and application of hypnosis in dentistry and medicine for doctors and dentists only. Branch groups operate throughout the UK.

British Hypnotherapy Association

Address: 67 Upper Berkeley Street, London W1; *Tel*: 01-723 4443.

Major therapy practised: Hypnotherapy within a psychiatric/psychoanalytic framework.

Types of membership: Fellows, Members, Associates.

Conditions and qualifications for entry: Minimum 4 years of relevant postgraduate training. The prospective practitioner should have adequate therapy himself.

Title of full members: MBHA.

Code of Practice: Yes.

Library: Yes.

Journal/Newsletter: No.

Institute of Curative Hypnotherapists

Address: Equity House 49-51 London Road, Waterlooville, Hampshire PO7 7EX; *Tel*: 07014 65880.

Major therapy practised: Hypnotherapy—specializing in the treatment of addiction, phobias and compulsive behaviour.

Types of membership: Licentiate, Full.

Conditions and qualifications for entry: Licentiate must practise for 3 years to qualify for full membership. Membership also open to qualified hypnotherapists from other associations.

Title of full members: MICH.

Number of members in association (inc. associate, honorary, foreign, and retired): 100.

Code of Practice: Yes.

Library: No.

Journal/Newsletter: Yes.

National Association of Hypnotists and Psychotherapists

Address: Marine Villa, Ferry Road, Earlsferry, Elie Fife KY9 1AJ; *Tel*: 0333 330364.

Date founded: 1977.

Major therapies practised: Hypnotherapy, psychotherapy, counselling.

Types of membership: Full, Associate, Subscribing.

Conditions and qualifications for entry: 1. Associations own training and examinations followed by supervisory period (1 year); 2. In exceptional circumstances, other qualified/experienced therapists.

Title of full members: MNAHP.

Number of members in association (inc. associate, honorary, foreign, and retired): 196.

Number of full members in practice in UK: 172.

Code of practice: Yes.

Library: No.

Journal/Newsletter: Yes.

Associated institutions and societies: Institute of Neurophysiological Psychology.

National Council of Psychotherapists and Hypnotherapy Register

Address: Secretary, Stream Cottage, Wish Hill, Willingdon, E. Sussex BN20 9HQ; *Tel*: Eastbourne 501540.

Date founded: 1971.

Major therapies practised: All forms of hypnotherapy and psychotherapy.

Types of membership: Licentiate, Full.

Conditions and qualifications for entry: Open to all professional psychotherapists and hypnotherapists. Entry at Licentiate level by open exam. Progression to full membership after 1 year on evidence of competence to practise and thesis, if entered as Licentiate.

Title of full members: MNCPHR.

Number of members in society/association (inc. associate, honorary, foreign, and retired): 137.

Code of Practice: Yes.

Library: No.

Journal: The Journal.

Remarks: As a multidisciplinary council it is open to all therapists who can offer proof of competence, or by written or oral examination. No official training course but training can be arranged. Holds seminars and annual 3-day residential conference.

The Professional Hypno-Therapists Centre

Address: 136 Harley Street, London W1. Or Lodbury House, 74 Amhurst Park, London N16 5AP; *Tel*: 01-800 4045.

Major therapies practised: Psychotherapy, hypnotherapy, hypno-analysis, and practical philosophy.

Types of membership: Full UK and foreign members.

Number of members in society/association (inc. associate, honorary, foreign, and retired): 40.

Library: No.

Journal/Newsletter: No.

Remarks: No formal training courses but private tuition in hypnotherapy given to suitable candidates. Also give lectures.

The Society of Advanced Psychotherapists and Parapsychologists

Address: C/o SHAP, 28 Finsbury Park Road, London N4 2JX; *Tel*: 01-226 6963.

Date founded: 1981.

Major therapies practised: Hypnotherapy, psychotherapy and Ericksonian psychotherapy.

Types of membership: Full, Associate, Student, Fellowship.

Conditions and qualifications for entry: Successful graduation from the SHAP three-part course; acceptance by the Council of the Society (SAPP).

Title of full members: MSAPP.

Numbers of members in society (inc. associate, honorary, foreign, and retired): 113.

Numbers of full members in practice in UK: 1986: 93.

Code of Practice: Yes.

Library: No.

Journal/Newsletter: Yes.

Associated institutions and societies: School of Hypnosis and Advanced Psychotherapy (affiliated college).

SUPPORT ORGANIZATIONS

British College of Hypnotherapy

Address: 117 Granville Road, London SW18 5SF.

Activity: Runs 6-month courses in hypnotherapy and two 6-month courses in psychotherapy.

Size: 20 members.

British Hypnosis Research Association

Address: 118–120 Springfield Road, Chelmsford, Essex CM2 6LF; *Tel*: 0277 221063.

Activity: Co-ordinating research.

Institute of Applied Psychology and Hypnosis

Address: 1 Walmsley Gardens, High Raincliffe, Scarborough YO12 5DE; *Tel*: 0723 64162.

Activity: Professional group of hypnotherapists derived from various colleges.

The Proudfoot School of Hypnosis and Psychotherapy

Address: 9 Belvedere Place, Scarborough, N. Yorks. YO11 2QX; *Tel*: 0723 363638.

Activities: Runs courses in hypnosis, hypnotherapy, neuro-linguistic programming, self-hypnosis, and advanced hypnotherapy.

Manual therapies

COLLEGES AND TRAINING ESTABLISHMENTS

The Bayly School of Reflexology

Address: Monks Orchard, Whitbourne, Worcester WR6 5RB; *Tel*: 0886 21207.

Date founded: 1968.

Major therapy taught: Reflexology—imbalances in body corrected by massage to reflexes in the feet.

Entry requirements: None.

Type and length of courses: Introductory and Advanced courses.

Subjects taught to trainees: Theory and principles of reflexology and interrelationship with the nerves, glands, and circulation. Practical instruction.

Average college attendance for trainees: 4 days intensive over 2 weekends and examination.

Clinical experience: None, apart from 14 hours of supervised practical instruction.

Number of students: Enrolled: approx. 1500; qualified: approx. 350.

Certificate awarded: Certificate in reflexology.

Associated institutions and societies: British Reflexology Association.

The British School for Reflex Zone Therapy of the Feet

Address: 87 Oakington Avenue, Wembley Park, Middlesex HA9 8HY; *Tel*: 01-908 2201.

Date founded: 1982.

Major therapies taught: Reflex zone therapy of the feet; relaxation.

Entry requirements: Previous training as physiotherapist, nurse, doctor, or recognized training in other therapies.

Type and length of courses: Introductory (3 8-hour days); Advanced (3 8-hour days after treating at least 50 patients).

Subjects taught to trainees: Treatment procedure; indications and contra-indications; relationship of organs and structures in the body to reflex zones in the feet, back, and hands; acupuncture points relating to this treatment; relaxation procedures and bi-manual techniques.

Average college attendance for trainees: 6 days college attendance occupy 48 working hours of theory and practice. Observation in the care of the sick is a pre-requisite.

Clinical experience: This is gained in the students' own time.

Numbers of students in UK: Summer 1986: 280.

Certificate awarded: A certificate is awarded from the International School.

Associated institutions and societies: International School—Reflex Zone Therapy, D-7744 Königsfeld-Burgberg, W. Germany.

British School of Shiatsu

Address: Admin. office: 14 Brooklyn Road, Larkhall, Bath BA1 6TE; *Tel*: 0225 331357. Teaching venue: East–West Centre, 188 Old Street, London EC1V 9BP.

Date founded: 1983.

Major therapy taught: Shiatsu therapy. Course includes studies in Oriental medicine and philosophy, anatomy and physiology, diet and health, corrective exercises, meditation, counselling, shiatsu theory and practice.

Entry requirements: Open to anyone.

Type and length of course: Part-time (16 weeks or 1 year).

Subjects taught to trainees: Shiatsu: Oriental medicine and philosophy; Sotai corrective exercises; anatomy and physiology; Do-In self-massage for injury and stress control; principles of diet and your health; meditation and yoga techniques; counselling technique.

Average college attendance for trainees: Either 2 evenings weekly plus 1 weekend per month, or 1 weekend per month.

Clinical experience: Recorded treatments are part of assessment programme. Supervised practical sessions.

Numbers of students: Summer 1986: 150.

Certificate awarded: BSS Practitioner Certificate; ITEC Certification also.

Associated institutions and societies: Bristol School of Shiatsu; East Anglia School of Shiatsu; Pennsylvania Shiatsu Association, USA.

Fylde School of Natural Therapies

Address: 21 St Albans Road, Lytham St. Annes, Lancashire FY8 1TG.

Date founded: 1979.

Major therapies taught: Remedial massage, osteopathic manipulations, acupuncture, reflexology, aromatherapy, sports injuries.

Entry requirements: At least 3 O levels inc. English.

Type and length of courses: Full-time and part-time (up to 4 years for osteopathic course; 1 year for basic course in remedial massage).

Subjects taught to trainees: Anatomy, physiology, practice management, massage techniques, osteopathic and chiropractic techniques.

Clinical experience: Experience given to all students at school's own clinic: St Annes Remedial Clinic.

Number of students: Summer 1986: 55.

Diplomas awarded: Diploma in: Remedial Therapies, Osteopathic Techniques, Reflexology, Acupuncture; ITEC Diploma in Anatomy, Physiology, and Massage.

Associated institutions and societies: Faculty of Osteopathy.

International Institute of Reflexology

Address: POBox 34, Harlow, Essex CM17 0LT.

Major therapy taught: Reflexology.

Entry requirements: None, but a knowledge of anatomy and physiology is an advantage.

Type and length of courses: 2 basic; 2 advanced (about 1 year).

Subjects taught to trainees: Anatomy and physiology, reflexology.

Number of students: Summer 1986: 172.

Diplomas or certificates awarded: Diploma.

Associated institutions and societies: International Institute of Reflexology, POBox 12642, St Petersburg, Florida 33733, USA.

Midland School of Reflexotherapy

Address: 5 Church Street, Warwick CV35 8EN; *Tel*: 0926 491071.

Date founded: 1976.

Major therapies taught: Reflex therapy, nutrition, counselling.

Entry requirements: Background knowledge of anatomy and physiology.

Type and length of course: Part-time (1 year).

Subjects taught to trainees: Anatomy, physiology, nutrition, reflex therapy, the holistic approach.

Average college attendance for trainees: 7 weekends/year.

Clinical experience: Continual practical assessment.

Number of students: Summer 1986: 28.

Diplomas or certificates awarded: Certificate.

Northern Institute of Massage/Northern College of Physical Therapies

Address: 100 Waterloo Road, Blackpool FY4 1AW; *Tel*: 0253 403548.

Date founded: 1924.

Major therapies taught: Therapeutic massage, manipulative therapy, electrotherapy, and allied therapies including osteopathic and chiropractic procedures.

Entry requirements: Must have completed Remedial Massage Diploma course to qualify for the Advanced Massage and Manipulative Therapy course and must have completed this to qualify for classes in osteopathy/manipulation.

Type and length of courses: Body Massage and Physical Culture—occupational course. Professional courses: Diplomas in: Remedial Massage; Advanced Remedial Massage; Manipulative Therapy (Ord.); Manipulative Therapy (Hons.).

Subjects taught to trainees: Basic medical sciences: general body massage and fitness studies; therapeutic application of remedial massage at basic and advanced levels; electrotherapy; hypnotherapy; manipulative therapy and osteopathic/chiropratic procedures at basic and advanced levels.

Average college attendance for trainees: Body massage and Physical Culture: 60 hours; Remedial Massage: 105 hours; Advanced Remedial Massage: 205 hours; Manipulative Therapy (Ord.): 225 hours; Manipulative Therapy (Hons.): 135 hours.

Clinical experience: Remedial Massage: 150 hours; Advanced Remedial Massage: 800 hours; Manipulative Therapy (Ord.): 800 hours; Manipulative therapy (Hons.): 800 hours.

Numbers of students: Summer 1986: 900.

Diplomas awarded: As above.

Associated institutions and societies: London and Counties Society of Physiologists (professional association).

'Touch for Health' Foundation

Address: 39 Browns Road, Surbiton, Surrey KE5 8ST.

Date founded: 1972.

Major therapies taught: Applied kinesiology (muscle testing and activation, energy balancing, etc.)—emphasis on basic principles of self-help preventive health care rather than training of practitioners.

Entry requirements: None.

Type and length of course: Training programme in self-help health care (3 weekends part-time).

Subjects taught to trainees: emotional stress release; basic applied kinesiology (muscle testing); food sensitivity testing; energy balancing.

Average college attendance for trainees: 3 weekends; continuous practice session; instructors' training workshop (8 days residential course).

Certificates awarded: Certificate awarded on completion of each section. Instructor's certificate awarded on completion of all courses.

Associated institutions and societies: Touch for Health Foundation, California, USA; British Touch for Health Association.

PROFESSIONAL ASSOCIATIONS AND SOCIETIES OF THERAPISTS

British Association of Manipulative Medicine Ltd

Address: 16 Wimpole St, London W1M 7AB; *Tel*: 01-636 9871.

Date founded: 1962.

Major therapies practised: Manipulation; injection; TNS.

Types of membership: Associate membership open to all medical practitioners. Full membership restricted to those in substantially full-time manipulative practice.

Conditions and qualifications for entry: Registrable medical degree (UK).

Title of full members: None.

Numbers of members in association (inc. associate, honorary, foreign, and retired): 230.

Numbers of full members in practice in UK: 1986: 85.

Code of Practice: No, but members abide by GMC/BMA codes.

Library: No.

Journal: Yes.

Associated institutions and societies: Affiliated as British Member of Fédération Internationale de Medecine Manuelle.

Remarks: BAMM teaches manipulative medicine in weekend courses.

Chiltern Institute of Reflexology

Address: 193 Tring Road, Aylesbury, Bucks. HP20 1JH; *Tel*: 0296 24854.

Date founded: 1982.

Major therapy practised: Reflexology.

Types of membership: Student, Associate.

Conditions and qualifications for entry: Associate: Holds the Institute's Certificate after attending the Institute's basic and advanced courses and passing the Institute's examinations.

Title of full members: Associate of the Chiltern Institute of Reflexology.

Number of members in institute (inc. associate, honorary, foreign, and retired): 55.

Numbers of full members in practice in UK: 37.

Code of practice: Yes.

Library: No.

Journal: No.

Associated institutions and societies: Association of Reflexologists.

Independent Professional Therapists International

Address: Storcroft House, London Road, Retford, Nottingham DN22 7EB; *Tel*: 0777 707371.

Major therapies practised: Primarily beauty therapy and massage.

Types of membership: Fellow, Full (UK and Foreign), Student.

Conditions and qualifications for entry: Diplomas and qualifications from any school of any complementary therapy, especially that of the International Therapists' Examining Council.

Title of full members: MIPTT.

Number of members in society/association (inc. associate, honorary, foreign, and retired): 350.

Code of Practice: No.

Library: No.

Journal: Yes.

Associated institutions and societies: The Churchill Centre; International Therapists' Examining Council.

Independent Register of Manipulative Therapists Ltd

Address: 32 Lodge Drive, London N13 5JZ; *Tel*: 01-886 3120.

Date founded: 1963.

Major therapies practised: Manipulative medicine, massage.

Numbers of members in society/association (inc. associate, honorary, foreign, and retired): 122.

The London and Counties Society of Physiologists

Address: Sec., 100 Waterloo Road, Blackpool FY4 1AW; *Tel*: 0253 403548.

Date founded: 1919.

Major therapies practised: Massage and allied skills including osteopathy, chiropractic, manipulative therapy, remedial massage, beauty therapy, and chiropody.

Types of membership: Full, Fellows, Honorary, Student, Associate.

Conditions and qualifications for entry: Full membership (a) those qualified in massage and allied therapies and/or chiropody from a recognized training establishment (b) graduates of the Northern Institute of Massage. Diploma courses after 2 years practice in both cases.

Title of full members: LCSP (Phys.) or LCSP (B.Th.) or LCSP (Chir.).

Number of members in society (inc. associate, honorary, foreign, and retired): 1477.

Number of full members in practice in UK: 1005.

Code of Practice: Yes.

Library: Yes.

Journal/Newsletter: *Skill Bulletin*.

Associated institutions and societies: The Northern Institute of Massage (recognized training college).

Remarks: The LCSP is probably both the oldest and largest of this type of independent professional organisation in the UK. It co-operates in postgraduate Advanced Study Groups arranged through the Northern Institute of Massage and is involved in continuing research into all areas of physical therapy.

The Metamorphic Association

Address: 67 Ritherdon Road, London SW17 8QE; *Tel*: 01-672 5951.

Date founded: 1979.

Major therapy practised: The Metamorphic Technique — also known as prenatal therapy, works on the spinal reflexes of the feet, hands, and head in order to free energy 'blocked' during gestation.

Types of membership: Full, 'Friends'.

Conditions and qualifications for entry: Open to all practitioners of this technique with the necessary training and experience.

Title of full members: Member of the Metamorphic Association.

Numbers of members in association (inc. associate, honorary, foreign, and retired): 200.

Numbers of full members in practice in UK: 1986: 115.

Code of practice: Yes.

Library: No.

Newsletter: *Metamorphic* Association Newsletter.

Remarks: Holds 12 hour training sessions for would-be practitioners, and weekend seminars and practical workshops.

The Shiatsu Society

Address: 19 Langside Park, Kilbarchan, Renfrewshire PA10 2EP; *Tel*: 05057 4657.

Date founded: 1981.

Major therapy practised: Shiatsu.

Types of membership: Ordinary membership: open to everybody. Registered Student. Registered Practitioner.

Conditions and qualifications and entry: Registered Practitioners have studied for a minimum 2 year period, with over 200 tuition hours, and must pass an assessment panel.

Title of full members: Shiatsu Society Registered Practitioner.

Number of members in society (inc. associate, honorary, foreign, and retired): 300.

Numbers of full members in practice in UK: 50.

Code of practice: No.

Library: Yes.

Journal: Quarterly newsletter.

Associated institutions and societies: Informally linked with the American Shiatsu Association.

SUPPORT ORGANIZATIONS

British Reflexology Association

Address: 12 Pond Road, London SE3 9JL; *Tel*: 01-852 6062.

Activities: Holds seminars and courses, publishes a newsletter. Associated with the Bayly School of Reflexology.

British Touch for Health Association

Address: C/o Charles Benham, 2a Bushey Close, High Wycombe, Bucks. HP12 3HL; *Tel*: 0494 37409.

Activity: Applied kinesiology—support group.

Size: 170 members.

Compton House

Address: 87 High Street, Hampton, Middlesex; *Tel*: 01-979 3119.

Activity: Reflexology and massage—residential education centre.

Size: Under 20 members.

Edinburgh School of Natural Therapy

Address: 2 London Street, Edinburgh EH3 6NA; *Tel*: 031-557 3901.

Activities: Courses in massage, beauty therapy, reflexology, aromatherapy.

Eve Taylor Institute for Clinical Aromatherapy

Address: 22 Bromley Road, London SE6 2TP; *Tel*: 01-690 2149.

Activity: Aromatherapy teaching and support.

Independent Therapists Examining Council (ITEC)

Address: James House, Oakelbrook Mill, Newent, Glos. GL18 1HD.

Activity: Beauty therapy, massage and physical therapy (inc. sports therapy).

Remarks: A major independent examining body in the UK, providing professional examination system for all English speaking countries.

International Institute of Reflexology

Address: 32 Coppetts Road, Muswell Hill, London N10 1JY; *Tel*: 01-444 6354.

Activity: Courses in reflexology, register of reflexologists.

London School of Manipulative Therapies

Address: 13 Copleigh Close, Redhill, Surrey RH1 5BJ.

Activity: Courses in therapeutic massage and manipulation. Affiliated with Health Practitioners Association.

Moorlands Natural Medicine Teaching Centre

Address: 'Moorlands', 24 South Road, Newton Abbot, Devon TQ12 1HQ; *Tel*: 0626 65493.

Activity: Runs mostly weekend courses to registered and qualified medical personnel only, teaching acupuncture, acupressure, reflextherapy, applied kinesiology, homeopathy, physiopathy and osteopathy. Specializes in the naturopathic approach to sports injuries and Chinese osteopathy.

Polarity Therapy Association of the UK

Address: 48 Devonshire Buildings, Bath BA2 4SU.

Activity: Register of practitioners in the UK. Weekend workshops run through the Polarity Therapy Educational Trust.

The Reflexology Centre

Address: 8 Russell Court, London Lane, Bromley, Kent BR1 4EX; *Tel*: 01-464 9401.

Activity: The Centre concentrates on teaching reflexology.

The Rolfing Network

Address: 6 Powis Gardens, London W11 1JG; *Tel*: 01-727 4903.

Activity: Massage as taught by Ida Rolf—'Rolfing' (structural integration).

West London School of Therapeutic Massage and Reflexology

Address: 41 St Luke's Road, London W11 1DD; *Tel*: 01-229 4672/7411.

Activity: Short professional qualifying courses in therapeutic massage, anatomy, and physiology. Four months Holiday Study Programme for Overseas Visitors. Professionally qualifying reflexology courses.

Mind–Body therapies

COLLEGES AND TRAINING ESTABLISHMENTS

Centre for Autogenic Training

Address: 101 Harley Street, London W1Y DF; *Tel*: 01-935 1811.

Date founded: 1978.

Major therapy taught: Autogenics.

Entry requirements: Medical degree, degree in clinical psychology, SRN nurses with psychiatric nursing experience, or psychotherapists with suitable qualifications and experience.

Type and length of courses: Basic courses for trainees (also run autogenic therapy sessions)—2 months; Certificate courses for trainers—Basic course and 1 week intensive.

Subjects taught to trainees: 6 standard autogenic exercises and basic training positions; medical and non-medical applications and contra-indications; practical instruction.

Average college attendance for trainees: 8 weekly 1½ hour group or individual sessions.

Clinical experience: Trainees: None. Trainers: 2 years.

Number of students: At Summer Term 1981: 21; Qualified 1981: 21.

Certificates awarded: Basic and Advanced ICAT Certificates for trainers.

Associated institutions and societies: The International Committee for the Co-ordination of Clinical Application and Teaching of Autogenic Therapy (ICAT); British Association for Autogenic Training and Therapy (BAFATT).

Institute for Psychobiological Research

Address: 26–28 Wendell Road, London W12 9RT; *Tel*: 01-743 1518.

Major therapy taught: Biofeedback.

Entry requirements: None.

Type and length of courses: Workshops (1 day); Courses in evenings and summer courses.

Subjects taught to trainees: Biofeedback (psychocybernetics and psychotechnics, meditation). Use of biofeedback instruments.

Associated institutions and societies: Audio Ltd.

Relaxation for Living

Address: 29 Burwood Park Road, Walton-on-Thames, Surrey KT12 5LH; *Tel*: 0932 227826.

Date founded: 1972.

Major therapies taught: Physical relaxation techniques.

Entry requirements: For teacher training: basic knowledge of anatomy and physiology. Must have attended at least 1 series of sessions as a pupil. Plus continuing study.

Type and length of courses: Teacher training course (2 weekends full-time); study days open to the public (3 per year); classes and correspondence courses for public.

Subjects taught to trainees: Teacher training course—relaxation therapy, thorough knowledge of the physiology of stress and neuro-muscular systems, constructive self-awareness, simple loosening and breathing movement, deep relaxation skills, teaching practice.

Certificate awarded: Relaxation for Living Teacher. Letter of Credential for those teachers not wishing to join Relaxation for Living.

School of T'ai-chi Ch'uan (Centre for Healing)

Address: 5 Tavistock Place, London WC1H 9SN; *Tel*: 01-459 0764.

Date founded: 1973.

Major therapy taught: T'ai-chi Ch'uan.

Entry requirements: Open to all.

Type and length of courses: Wide variety of courses for guidance, healing, and self-help. T'ai-chi teaching (4 years) and intuitive foot massage.

Subjects taught to trainees: T'ai-chi Ch'uan (long Yang form); consulting the I Ching; basic Chinese and holistic philosophy; basic spiritual science including subtle anatomy; philosophy and practice of natural breathing; posture and body alignment; basic nutrition; applied meditation and symbolism.

Diplomas or certificates awarded: T'ai-chi teaching; Intuitive Foot Massage Certificate.

Associated institutions and societies: Centre for Healing and Spiritual Understanding.

SUPPORT ORGANIZATIONS

Centre for Yoga Studies

Address: 48 Devonshire Buildings, Bath BA2 4SU; *Tel*: 0225 26327.

Activity: Individual yoga therapy. Practitioner therapy/teacher training. Register of qualified yoga therapists.

Institute for Neuro-physiological Psychology

Address: Warwick House, 4 Stanley Place, Chester; *Tel*: 0244 311414.

Activity: The Institute was established to research into the effect central nervous system dysfunctions have on children with learning difficulties and adults suffering from neuroses, and to develop appropriate CNS remedial and rehabilitation programmes. It treats children and adults and trains therapists.

International Stress and Tension Control Society (UK Branch)

Address: The Priory Hospital, Priory Lane, Roehampton, London SW15 5JJ; *Tel*: 01-876 8261.

Activity: Practical, scientific self-help methods for stress and tension control. Information service; details of members active in stress and tension control. Organizes conferences, workshops, etc., sale of books and tapes.

The Relaxation Society

Address: St Mary Woolnoth Church, Lombard Street, London EC3V 9AN; *Tel*: 01-626 9701.

Activity: Psychophysical development group; general health promotion group.

Size: Under 100 members.

Salisbury Centre

Address: 2 Salisbury Road, Edinburgh EH16 5AB; *Tel*: 031-667 5438.

Activity: Natural therapies—educational and residential centre.

Education: Continuous classes and weekend workshops in healing, yoga, meditation, massage, and T'ai-chi Ch'uan.

Size: Under 100 members.

Naturopathy and nutrition therapy

COLLEGES AND TRAINING ESTABLISHMENTS

Brantridge Forest School

Address: Highfield, Dane Hill, Haywards Heath, Sussex RH17 7EX; *Tel*: 0825 790214.

Date founded: 1961.

Major therapies taught: Natural healing sciences—see below.

Type and length of courses: Correspondence only.

Subjects taught to trainees: Homeopathy, botanic medicine, naturopathy, drugless healing, massage, colour healing and psychology, diet and nature, Schuessler's biochemistry, psychology, psychotherapy, super-science, philosophy, radiesthesia and radionics.

Average college attendance for trainees: All postal home study courses.

Clinical experience (extent of supervised treatment of patients): None, but if students require practical work they are referred to a suitable practitioner.

British College of Naturopathy and Osteopathy

Address: 6 Netherhall Gardens, London NW3 5RR; *Tel*: 01-435 7830.

Date founded: 1949.

Major therapies taught: Naturopathy and osteopathy.

Entry requirements: 2 A levels minimum, preferably chemistry, biology, zoology, physics.

Type and length of courses: Diploma in Naturopathy (4 years full-time); Diploma in Osteopathy (4 years full-time).

Subjects taught to trainees: Basic medical sciences including psychology and dietetics; principles, philosophy, and techniques of naturopathy; principles, philosophy, and techniques of osteopathy; clinic instruction in naturopathy and osteopathy.

Average college attendance for trainees: 3 12-week terms per year. Minimum 80 per cent attendance.

Clinical experience (extent of supervised treatment of patients): 5 supervised clinics per week to third and fourth year students.

Diplomas or certificates awarded:DO, ND. Eligible to join the British Naturopathic and Osteopathic Association.

Associated institutions and societies: The British Naturopathic and Osteopathic Association (professional association).

School of Natural Medicine

Address: Bright Haven, Robin's Lane, Lolworth, Cambridge CB3 8HH; *Tel*: 0954 81074.

Date founded: 1986.

Major therapies taught: Iridology, herbal medicine, naturopathy, natural medicine.

Entry requirements: Several O levels.

Type and length of courses: Iridology Diploma: 1 year (prerequisite for Herbal Medicine and Naturopathy); Herbal Medicine: 2 years; Naturopathy: 1 year after Iridology; Natural Medicine: 4 years minimum study and Diplomas in Iridology, Herbal Medicine, Naturopathy, and thesis.

Subjects taught to trainees: Iridology, herbal medicine, naturopathy, Bach Flower remedies, anatomy and physiology, nutrition, constitutional medicine, subtle healing, fasting, water cure, tongue diagnosis, botany, pharmacy, practical herbal treatments.

Average college attendance for trainees: 5 weekends, 4-day summer school, tutorials, apprenticeship.

Clinical experience: Completely dependent on the students' individual needs.

Number of students: Summer 1986: 200.

Diplomas or certificates awarded: Diplomas awarded.

College of Dietary Therapy

Address: Hillsborough House, Ashley, Tiverton, Devon EX16 5PA; *Tel*: 0884 255879.

Major therapies taught: Dietary therapy; iridology (supplementary).

Entry requirements: None.

Type and length of courses: Diploma course in dietary therapeutics: 1 year;

Correspondence course in nutrition; Advanced Diploma course: 1 extra year; Iridology course.

Subjects taught to trainees: Principles and practice of nutrition and dietary therapy.

Average college attendance for trainees: Diploma course: 11 weekends.

Clinical experience: Supervised clinical work during Advanced Diploma course.

Numbers of students: 1986: 120.

Diploma awarded: Dietary Therapy Diploma.

PROFESSIONAL ASSOCIATIONS AND SOCIETIES OF THERAPISTS

British Dental Society for Clinical Nutrition

Address: Flat 5, 30 Harley Street, London W1N 1AB; *Tel*: 01-580 6284.

Date founded: 1984.

Major therapies practised: Nutrition and factors which interfere with nutrition.

Types of membership: Full, Associate, Student.

Conditions and qualifications for entry: Full: Dental degree or licence; Associate: at discretion of committee.

Title of full members: Member.

Number of members in society (inc. associate, honorary, foreign, and retired): 90.

Number of full members in practice in UK: 82.

Code of practice: As dentists.

Library: No.

Journal: Newsletter.

The British Naturopathic and Osteopathic Association

Address: Frazer House, 6 Netherhall Gardens, London NW3 5RR; *Tel*: 01-435 8728.

Date founded: 1946.

Major therapies practised: Naturopathy and osteopathy.

Types of membership: Qualified practitioners only.

Conditions and qualifications for entry: Mainly graduates of the British College of Naturopathy and Osteopathy. Otherwise must have a diploma in naturopathy, osteopathy, or chiropractic and pass entrance exam.

Title of full members: MBNOA Registered Naturopath and Osteopath.

Number of members in association (inc. associate, honorary, foreign, and retired): 260.

Number of full members in practice in UK: 230 naturopaths.

Code of Practice: Yes.

Library: No.

Journal: Yes.

Associated institutions and societies: The British College of Naturopathy and Osteopathy.

Remarks: Hold bi-annual conferences.

British Society for Nutritional Medicine

Address: 4 Museum Street, York YO1 2ES; *Tel*: 0904 52378.

Date founded: 1984.

Major therapy practised: Promotion of use of nutrition in clinical medicine.

Types of membership: Full: medically qualified practitioners only; Associate: qualified members of related professions (e.g. nurses, dieticians, bio chemists, etc.) and bone fide academic researchers in related fields; Student: medical students only.

Conditions and qualifications for entry: As above.

Number of members in society (inc. associate, honorary, foreign, and retired): 330.

Number of full members in practice in UK: Approx. 150.

Incorporated Society of Registered Naturopaths/British Register of Naturopaths

Address: Registrar BRN: 1 Albemarle Road, The Mount, York YO2 1EN; *Tel*: 0904 23693; Hon. Sec. ISRN: 328 Harrogate Road, Leeds LS17 6PE; *Tel*: 0532 685992.

Date founded: 1934.

Major therapies practised: Straight nature cure—'hygienic' system, including fasting, massage, and manipulative therapy.

Types of membership: Full members.

Conditions and qualifications for entry: To the ISRN: qualified naturopaths trained by the Edinburgh School of Natural Therapeutics or at least a minimum of 4 years tuition at a school or college of natural therapeutics, whose standards are acceptable to the council. To the BRN: registration is open to anyone whose standards of training, practice, and professional conduct are satisfactory to the council.

Title of full members: No titles given.

Number of members in society/association (inc. associate, honorary, foreign, and retired): Small (undisclosed) membership.

Number of full members in practice in UK: 1980: 27; 1981: 20.

Code of practice: Yes.

Library: No.

Journal/Newsletter: No.

Associated institutions and societies: Edinburgh School of Natural Therapies.

National Council and Register of Iridologists

Address: 80 Portland Road, Bournemouth BH9 1NQ, Dorset; *Tel*: 0202 529793.

Date founded: 1983.

Major therapies practised: Iridology, iris diagnosis.

Conditions and qualifications for entry: Completion of 18-month course and acceptance by the National Council.

Associated institutions and societies: Society of Iridologists, support group at same address.

The Nutrition Association

Address: 36 Wycombe Road, Marlow, Buckinghamshire SL7 3HX; *Tel*: 06284 4383.

Major therapies practised: Nutrition and diet therapy.

Types of membership: Members, listed in the TNA Directory; Associates.

Conditions and qualifications for entry: Members: 1. Practitioners of complementary or conventional medicine who have trained 4 years in their discipline. 2. Nutritional consultants: 3 years experience in clinical nutrition after training. 3. Nutrition advisors: knowledge of clinical nutrition and 12 months in full-time practice.

Code of practice: No.

Library: No.

Journal: Newsletter.

SUPPORT ORGANIZATIONS

Bath Spa Trust

Address: Old Royal Baths, Hot Bath Street, Bath BA1 1ST.

Activity: Balneology—support group for Bath Spa.

Publications: Information booklet.

Size: Under 20 members.

British Associated Professions Specialist Courses—Clinical Nutrition

Address: PO Box 8, Liphook, Hants GU30 7JD.

Activity: Correspondence courses and seminars for postgraduates and undergraduates. Graduates are enrolled on a Register of Clinical Nutritionists.

The British Natural Hygiene Society

Address: 'Shalimar', First Avenue, Frinton-on-Sea, Essex CO13 9E7; *Tel*: 025 562823.

Activity: Pure nature cure—support group.

Publication: Magazine.

Associated with: International Federation of Hygienists; the American Natural Hygienic Society; Organizations in Greece, Australia, and India.

Size: 200–400 members 1981.

Green Farm Nutrition Centre

Address: Burwash Common, East Sussex TN19 7LX; *Tel*: 0435 882180.

Activity: Teaching of 3-month courses in nutrition and self-care; seminars and the marketing of supplements.

The Institute for Optimum Nutrition

Address: 5 Jerdan Place, London SW6 1 BE; *Tel*: 01-385 7984.

Activity: Run self-help nutritional therapy programmes. Also 2-year nutrition consultants' diploma course, a 6-month course for health professionals, a 13-week home study course, as well as day plus weekend courses. Individuals can become members. They receive mailings plus quarterly magazine.

International College of Natural Health Sciences

Address: 100 Wigmore Street, London W1H 0AE; *Tel*: 01-486 0431.

Activity: Correspondence courses in nutrition and homeopathy.

Iridology Research

Address: 36/37 Featherstone Street, London EC1Y 8RN; *Tel*: 01-251 4429.

Major therapies supported: Iridology and all holistic therapies and treatment systems with main-stream medicine.

Activity: Iris photography service for practitioners; iris analysis service for practitioners with difficult or non-responding patients; education in iridology for practitioners of all therapies; short and long-term research projects.

Kushi Institute

Address: 188 Old Street, London EC1V 9BP; *Tel*: 01-251 4076.

Activity: Macrobiotics—Oriental medicine (diagnosis, acupressure, acupuncture).

Education: Weekend and short courses.

Publications: Books.

Associated with: East West Centre, Community Health Foundation.

Size: 600 graduates.

The McCarrison Society

Address: 24 Paddington Street, London W1M 4DR.

Activity: Nutrition—health education and preventive medicine.

Education: Conferences.

Publication: Journal, conferences proceedings.

Size: Over 600 members.

Nutrition Science Research Institute

Address: Mulberry Tree Hall, Brookthorpe, Glos. GL4 0UU; *Tel*: 0452 813471.

Activity: Dietary and vitamins, information and research centre, laboratory service.

Publication: Books and pamphlets.

Osteopathy

COLLEGES AND TRAINING ESTABLISHMENTS

Andrew Still College of Osteopathy and Natural Therapeutics

Address: Registrar: 7 Sidewood Road, London SE9 2EZ.

Date founded: 1980.

Major therapy taught: Osteopathy.

Entry requirements: 5 passes at GCSE, including 2 at advanced level. Mature students may be admitted at the discretion of the principal.

Type and length of course: Diploma in Osteopathy (DO) (5 years part-time).

Subjects taught to trainees: Anatomy, physiology, biochemistry, pathology, radiology, naturopathy, osteopathic principles and techniques, clinical instruction.

Average college attendance for trainees: 3 full days per month.

Clinical experience: 500 hours.

Number of students: At Summer Term 1986: 20.

Diploma awarded: Diploma in Osteopathy.

Associated institutions and societies: British and European Osteopathic Association.

The British School of Osteopathy

Address: 1–4 Suffolk Street, London SW1Y 4HG; *Tel*: 01-930 9254.

Date founded: 1917.

Major therapy taught: Medically orientated osteopathy—training includes conventional medical diagnostic techniques and practices.

Entry requirements: 5 GCE passes including 2 A levels. English language necessary plus A levels, preferably in the natural sciences. Special arrangements for mature students.

Type and length of courses: Diploma in Osteopathy (4 years full-time); Course for registered medical practitioners only (18 months full-time);

Course for physiotherapists (3½ years); Course for registered medical practitioners only (2½ years part-time).

Subjects taught to trainees: Basic sciences; conventional medical sciences (anatomy and physiology to second MB standard); osteopathic principles, theory, and practice; nutrition; clinic instruction.

Average college attendance for trainees: 3 10-week terms per year plus vacation work in second, third, and fourth years.

Clinical experience: Approximately 2000 hours supervised work in the School's clinics.

Number of students: At Summer Term 1986: 400.

Diploma awarded: DO.

Associated institutions and societies: The General Council and Register of Osteopaths; The Osteopathic Association of Great Britain (professional bodies).

European School of Osteopathy

Address: 104 Tonbridge Road, Maidstone, Kent ME16 8SL; *Tel*: 0622 671558.

Date founded:1965 (in GB).

Major therapy taught: Osteopathic medicine (non-allopathic) including use of conventional diagnostic techniques, X-rays, and laboratory tests.

Entry requirements: 4-year course: 2 A levels in sciences; 6 years post-graduate course: open only to French-speaking state-registered physio-therapists.

Type and length of course: Diploma in Osteopathy (4 years full-time); Postgraduate course (in French) (6 years full-time).

Subjects taught to trainees: Basic sciences; general medicine; psychological medicine; osteopathic theory, practices, and technique; clinical osteopathic practice; applied nutrition; medical jurisprudence; ethics.

Average college attendance for trainees: 4-year course: 3 terms/year of 12 weeks each; 6-year course is run on a seminar basis.

Clinical experience: Full-time course—a teaching clinic is attached to the school. Students are required to complete a minimum of 1000 hours.

Diploma awarded: DO.

Associated institutions and societies: The Society of Osteopaths, SBO and RTM (Belgium), AFDO (France) (professional bodies). Osteopathic

Education and Research Limited (Registered in England) (controlling body).

The London College of Osteopathic Medicine

Address: 8–10 Boston Place, London NW1 6ER; *Tel*: 01-262 5250.

Date founded: 1946.

Major therapy taught: Osteopathy—combining osteopathic and medical techniques of treatment and diagnosis.

Entry requirements: Medically qualified practitioners registered with the GMC.

Type and length of course: Postgraduate training (1 year full-time).

Subjects taught to trainees: Applied medical sciences; osteopathic principles, technique, and practice; clinic instruction.

Average college attendance for trainees: Minimum 3 days/week. Minimum of 800 hours theoretical and clinical supervised work.

Clinical experience: Approximately 400 hours in the Osteopathic Association Clinic.

Diploma awarded: Diploma MLCOM.

Associated institutions and societies: Postgraduate teaching unit of: Osteopathic Association Clinic, Association of Osteopathic Trusts Ltd, British Osteopathic Association, The Osteopathic Medical Association.

PROFESSIONAL ASSOCIATIONS AND SOCIETIES OF THERAPISTS

British and European Osteopathic Association

Address: 70 Galahad Road, Bromley, Kent BR1 5DT; *Tel*: 01-850 1785.

Date founded: 1976.

Major therapy practised: Osteopathy.

Types of membership: Practising Full Members or Fellows only.

Conditions and qualifications for entry: 4 years full-time training or equivalent at a recognized college or completed formal college course and been in practice for at least 5 years.

Title of full members: MBEOA.

Numbers of full members in practice in UK: 68.

Code of practice: Yes.

Library: Yes.

Journal/Newsletter: *BEOA Osteopathic Journal; BEOA Members'
Newsletter*.

Associated institutions and societies: Andrew Still College of Osteopathy
and Natural Therapeutics.

Remarks: Publishes information booklet on back care. Runs weekend postgraduate training seminars (2 per year). Some members also members of
other professional associations.

The British Osteopathic Association

Address: 8–10 Boston Place, London NW1; *Tel*: 01-262 5250.

Date founded: 1911.

Major therapy practised: Osteopathy according to Andrew Still's principles—all practitioners must be qualified physicians.

Types of membership: Full, Fellow.

Conditions and qualifications for entry: Physicians only who are: (a)
medical graduates of the London College of Osteopathic Medicine or (b)
graduates of any recognized school of osteopathic medicine eligible for
membership of the American Osteopathic Association.

Title of full members: MLCO (Member of the London College of Osteopathic Medicine) or FLCO.

Numbers of full members in practice in UK: 80.

Code of practice: Yes, GMC Code.

Library: Yes.

Journal: Yes.

Associated institutions and societies: Professional body for The London
College of Osteopathic Medicine, Osteopathic Association Clinic,
American Osteopathic Association.

Remarks: Holds postgraduate meetings twice yearly.

The College of Osteopaths

Address: Administrative Services, 110 Thorkhill Road, Thames Ditton,
Surrey KT7 0UW; *Tel*: 01-398 3308.

Date founded: 1946.

Major therapy practised: Classical osteopathy—naturopathy.

Types of membership: Full, Fellows, Honorary Fellows, and Members.

Conditions and qualifications for entry: Graduates of the College of Osteopaths' Educational Trust (or similar standard); entrance examination equivalent to College of Osteopaths' Educational Trust Final Examination.

Title of full members: MCO, FCO.

Number of members in society/association (inc. associate, honorary, foreign, and retired): 106.

Number of full members in practice in UK: 1986: 86.

Code of practice: Yes.

Library: Yes.

Remarks: Holds annual seminar at AGM, a mid-year seminar, plus periodic lectures for members. Membership includes some chiropractors.

Cranial Osteopathic Association

Address: 478 Baker Street, Enfield, Middlesex EN1 3QS; *Tel*: 01-367 5561.

Major therapy practised: Cranial osteopathy.

Type of membership: Full members.

Conditions and qualifications for entry: Qualified osteopaths only.

Title of full members: M.Cr.OA.

Numbers of members in association (inc. associate, honorary, foreign, and retired): 20–25.

Associated institutions and societies: College of Osteopathy.

Remarks: The Association runs postgraduate courses in cranial osteopathy (over 1 week, several weekends, or 1 day/week for 9 months) in association with the College of Osteopathy.

The General Council and Register of Osteopaths Ltd

Address: Reg. and admin. office: 1–4 Suffolk Street, London SW1Y 4HG; *Tel*: 01-839 2060.

Date founded: 1936.

Major therapy practised: Osteopathy.

Types of membership: Full, not practising, overseas.

Conditions and qualifications for entry: Qualified osteopaths from schools or colleges recognized by the General Council and Register.

Title of full members: Registered Osteopath, DO, MRO.

Number of members in society/association (inc. associate, honorary, foreign, and retired): 850.

Number of full members in practice in UK: 1986: 800.

Code of Practice: Yes.

Library: Yes.

Journal: Yes.

Associated institutions and societies: the British School of Osteopathy; the Osteopathic Association of Great Britain; London College of Osteopathic Medicine; British Osteopathic Association; European School of Osteopathy; Society of Osteopaths.

The Natural Therapeutic and Osteopathic Society and Register

Address: 11 Roseberry Close, Cranham, Upminster, Essex RN14 1NL; *Tel*: 04022 28716.

Date founded: 1948.

Major therapies practised: Osteopathy and natural therapy, particularly combined with physiotherapy.

Types of membership: Associate, Full or Professional, Fellowship, Honorary.

Conditions and qualifications for entry: Professional membership open to any properly qualified practitioner of osteopathy or branch of natural therapeutics, subject to examination by examining committee of the London School of Osteopathy. Graduates of LSO and other schools recognized by NTOS.

Title of full members: MNTOS.

Number of members in society (inc. associate, honorary, foreign, and retired): 63.

Number of full members in practice in UK: 1986: 46.

Code of practice: Yes.

Library: Yes.

Journal: Yes.

Associated institutions and societies: Association of Osteopathic Practitioners.

Remarks: The NTOS is the governing body of the London School of Osteopathy (LSO) and graduates can automatically become members and be included on the register of the NTOS. The London School runs a 5-year integrated curriculum in osteopathic principles and practice. The society has a programme of ongoing post graduate education.

The Osteopathic Association of Great Britain

Address: 206 Chesterton Road, Cambridge, Cambs. CB4 1NE.

Date founded: 1925.

Major therapy practised: Osteopathy.

Types of membership: Full.

Conditions and qualifications for entry: Practitioners eligible for membership to the General Council and Register of Osteopaths Ltd. Mostly graduates of the British School of Osteopathy.

Title of Full Members: Registered Osteopath, DO MRO.

Number of members in association (inc. associate, honorary, foreign, and retired): 465.

Number of full members in practice in UK: 1986: 450.

Code of practice: Yes.

Library: Yes.

Journal: *British Osteopathic Journal*.

Associated institutions and societies: The British School of Osteopathy; The General Council and Register of Osteopaths.

Remarks: Organizes academic conventions and postgraduate studies. Distributes technical literature. Furthers research projects.

The Osteopathic Medical Association

Address: 6 Dorset Street, London W1H 3FE; *Tel*: 01-580 6147.

Date founded: 1961.

Major therapy practised: Medical osteopathy—diagnosis and treatment combines osteopathic and conventional medicine.

Type of membership: Ordinary.

Conditions and qualifications for entry: Any medical practitioner practising full-time osteopathy satisfying training and technical requirements.

Title of full members: None.

Code of Practice: No (apart from BMA Code of Ethics).

Library: No.

Newsletter: Yes.

Remarks: Postgraduate evening and weekend refresher courses and lectures. Lectures to GPs on osteopathy. Meetings with other groups from America, France, and New Zealand.

Society of Osteopaths Ltd

Address: Secretary, 12 College Road, Eastbourne, Sussex BN21 4HZ; *Tel*: 0323 638606.

Date founded: 1971.

Major therapy practised: Medically orientated osteopathy.

Types of membership: Full, Associate, Student.

Conditions and qualifications for entry: Graduates of the European School of Osteopathy; practising osteopaths able to pass the qualifying exams of the ESO.

Title of full members: DO, MSO.

Code of Practice: Yes.

Library: Yes.

Journal: *Journal of the Society of Osteopaths*.

Associated institutions and societies: Officially recognized colleges: The European School of Osteopathy.

Remarks: Organizes occasional postgraduate courses.

SUPPORT ORGANIZATIONS

Maidstone College of Osteopathy

Address: 30 Tonbridge Road, Maidstone, Kent ME16 8RT; *Tel*: 0622 52375.

Activity: New full-time course in osteopathy, affiliated with Institute of Applied Osteopathy. Also recognized by the College of Osteopaths.

Association of Osteopathic Physicians

Address: see the Institute for Complementary Medicine (p. 364).

Activity: An informal federation of several osteopathic organizations for the purpose of mutually improving standards.

Radionics and psionic medicine

PROFESSIONAL ASSOCIATIONS AND SOCIETIES OF THERAPISTS

The Psionic Medical Society and Institute of Psionic Medicine

Address: Garden Cottage, Beacon Hill Park, Hindhead, Surrey; *Tel*: 042 873 5752.

Date founded: 1968.

Major therapies practised: The study, diagnosis, and homeopathic treatment of constitutional causes of disease and their prevention.

Types of membership: Full and Associate (non-practising supporters of the aims of the Society and Institute).

Conditions and qualifications for entry: Must have conventional medical or dental qualifications for full membership.

Title of full members: Members (in case of doctors or dentists qualified in the techniques, Fellow or Member of the Institute of Psionic Medicine).

Number of members in society (inc. associate, honorary, foreign, and retired): 300 approx.

Number of full members in practice in UK: 1986: 20.

Code of Practice: No (apart from BMA Code of Ethics).

Library: No.

Journal/Newsletter: *Psionic Medicine*, journal of the Society. *Newsletter of the Institute of Psionic Medicine*.

Remarks: The Institute provides psionic medical training for medical and dental practitioners and promotes research.

The Radionic Association Ltd

Address: 16A North Bar, Banbury, Oxon. OX16 OTF; *Tel*: 0295 3183.

Date founded: 1943.

Major therapy practised: Radionics—a method of distant healing with the aid of an instrument and the radiesthetic (dowsing) faculty.

Types of membership: Fellow, Member, Licentiate, Associate.

Conditions and qualifications for entry: Students of the training schools approved by the Association may apply for Licentiateship. After a further period of supervision they are eligible to apply for full Membership.

Title of full members: M.Rad.A., F.Rad.A.

Number of members in association (inc. associate, honorary, foreign, and retired): 573.

Number of full members in practice in UK: 1986: 69.

Code of Practice: Yes.

Library: Yes.

Journal: Radionic Quarterly.

Associated institutions and societies: The School of Radionics (affiliated college); The British Society of Dowsers; The Confederation of Healing Organizations and The Holistic Contact group.

Remarks: Association supplies books on radionics and pendulums.

SUPPORT ORGANIZATIONS

De la Warr Laboratories Ltd

Address: Radleigh Park Road, Oxford OX2 9BB; *Tel*: 0865 244388 or 248572.

Activity: Radionic diagnosis and therapy; development and manufacture of radionic instruments; information service.

Publications: Newsletter, instruction manuals.

International College of Radionics

Address: Highfield, Dane Hill, Haywards Heath, Sussex RH17 7EX; *Tel*: 0825 790 214.

Activity: Correspondence courses in radionics.

Miscellaneous and general

Association for New Approaches to Cancer

Address: 231 Kensal Road, London W10 5DB; *Tel*: 01-969 1684.

Activity: Cancer support group: natural therapies.

Education: Lectures; conferences.

Associated with: Health for the New Age; Bristol Cancer Help Centre.

Size: Under 20 members.

Bretforton Trust

Address: Bretforton Hall Clinic, Vale of Evesham, Worcestershire WR11 5JH; *Tel*: 0386 830537.

Activity: Naturopathic research; medical application of cymatic sound; classes, lectures, seminars; cymatic medical training classes.

British Association for Holistic Health

Address: 179 Gloucester Place, London NW1 6DX; *Tel*: 01-262 5299.

Activity: A holistic medicine association for all holistically oriented practitioners to promote holistic medicine, to act as a forum for holistic medicine, and educate the public and authorities. Has regional groups.

Publications: Newsletter; *British Journal of Holistic Medicine*.

Size: 300 practitioner members.

British Holistic Medical Association

Address: 179 Gloucester Place, London NW1 6LX; *Tel*: 01-262 5299.

Activity: The BHMA is the central holistic medical organization for the medically qualified. Associate membership is available for the general public. BHMA has a network of regional groups throughout the country; runs regular workshops, lectures, and conferences.

Publications: Newsletter and the quarterly journal *Holistic Medicine*.

Size: approx. 1500 members.

Associated with: British Association for Holistic Health.

Bristol Cancer Help Centre

Address: Grove House, Cornwallis Grove, Clifton, Bristol BS8 4PG; *Tel*: 0272 743216.

Activity: Day and residential courses for patients to include doctor's consultation, psychotherapy, dietary advice, relaxation, meditation, and healing. Day and residential seminars.

The Centre for the Study of Alternative Therapies

Address: 51 Bedford Place, Southampton, Hants SO1 2DG; *Tel*: Southampton 334752.

Activity: Teaching, both medical students and at postgraduate level, in acupuncture, clinical ecology, and homeopathy. Research into many different aspects of complementary therapy, both from the point of view of basic research and clinical trials, into homeopathy, spinal manipulation, clinical ecology, and acupuncture. Postgraduate degree at the University of Southampton also supervised here.

College of Health

Address: 18 Victoria Park Square, London E2 9PF; *Tel*: 01-980 6263.

Activity: A variety of activities such as seminars, publications, and political and consumer-oriented action intended to help people make the most effective use of the NHS, and find alternative sources of help.

Publications: Quarterly journal *Self-Health*, range of publications.

Size: 10,000 members.

College of Holistic Medicine

Address: Old Hall, East Bergholt, Colchester CO7 6TG; *Tel*: 0206 298294.

Activity: Education centre: teaches 1 year part-time. Professional training courses in therapeutic massage and courses in preventative medicine for practitioners. Plans several other courses in aspects of holistic medicine. Courses are run in London and Glasgow.

Community Health Foundation

Address: 188–194 Old Street, London EC1V 9BP; *Tel*: 01-251 4076.

Activity: Macrobiotics; holistic health; health promotion; educational centre. Classes and courses evenings and weekends in macrobiotic cookery & philosophy, Shiatsu massage, iridology, reflexology, yoga, Tai-chi Chuan. Therapists also available for treatments.

Size: Over 1000 members.

Council for Complementary and Alternative Medicine (CCAM)

Address: Suite 1, 19a Cavendish Square, London W1M 9AD; *Tel*: 01-409 1440.

Activity: A central council representing the major complementary professions. Represents the interests of complementary medicine nationally, acts as a political body and a forum for communication and development of professional bodies in complementary medicine.

Exeter University's Centre for Complementary Health Studies

Address: Streatham Court, Rennes Drive, Exeter EX4 4PU; *Tel*: 0392 33828.

Activities: runs seminars for medical professionals and lectures for non-medical students, research into complementary medicine, and a resource or information centre.

FORDEAH (Foundation Offering Relief of Disability through Education, Arts and Healing)

Address: PO Box 484, London NW3 4HW; *Tel*: 01-794 9432.

Activity: To develop holistic health care facilities and develop holistic approaches to aid the disabled.

Foresight

Address: The Old Vicarage, Church Lane, Witley, Godalming, Surrey GU8 5PN; *Tel*: 0428 794500.

Activity: Preconceptual care. Mainly parents who have had previous birth tragedies or problems, stillbirth, anomalies, miscarriage. Help for infertile couples. Dietary advice, advice on allergies and mineral metabolism. Provides information to professionals and parents.

Education: Symposia, seminars.

Publications: Reports; booklets for patients.

Size: 2,600 members.

Geddes Positive Health Associates

Address: 'Sanda', 89 Woodfield Road, Thames Ditton, Surrey KT17 0DS; *Tel*: 01-398 4556.

Activity: Healing; massage; reflexology; relaxation techniques; natural therapies centre and support group.

Size: Under 20 members.

Hawkwood Adult College and Conference Centre

Address: Painswick Old Road, Stroud, Glos. GL6 7QW; *Tel*: 0536 4607.

Activity: Natural therapies—educational and residential centre.

Education: Wide variety of short and weekend courses, some on natural therapies.

The Holistic Council for Cancer

Address: Runnings Park, Croft Bank, West Malvern, Worcester WR14 4BP; *Tel*: 06845 65286.

Activity: To aid cancer-help clinics, develop standards, and promote holistic therapies.

Holistic Pharmacists' Association

Address: 50 St Gabriels Road, London NW2 4SA; *Tel*: 01-452 0371.

Activity: To promote the use of a holistic approach in pharmacy and holistic patient care. To advise patients, pharmacists, and pharmaceutical organizations on holistic medicine.

Human Potential Resources

Address: 35 Station Road, Hendon, London NW4; *Tel*: 01-202 4941.

Activity: Psychotherapeutic information centre.

Education: Occasional short courses.

Publications: Handbook/resource guide.

Information and Study Centre for Alternative Medicine

Address: 64 Bower Mount Road, Maidstone, Kent ME16 8AT; *Tel*: 0622 54858.

Activity: Natural therapies—information centre.

Publication: Booklets.

Institute for Complementary Medicine
Association for Complementary Medicine

Address: 21 Portland Place, London W1N 3AF; *Tel*: 01-636 9543.

Activity: Independent charity, information and research centre; data bank on natural healthcare.

Education: Public lectures, conferences, short courses, classes.

Associated with: The Healing Research Trust.

Publications: Journal ('Complementary Medicine').

Remarks: Maintains a public information and documentation centre covering many aspects of complementary medicine relevant to practitioners, patients, and researchers. For details of service phone 01-636 9543. Administers a national network of Provincial Information Points (PIPs) to provide local information about complementary medicine.

Size: Over 100 members.

Institute of Symbiotic Studies

Address: 5 Fairlight Place, Brighton, Sussex BN2 3AH; *Tel*: 0273 695880.

Activity: Trains practitioners of complementary and conventional medicine in symbiotic therapy, which is a natural method of re-establishing the body's beneficial micro-organisms, to promote health and treat certain diseases.

International Guild of Natural Medicine Practitioners

Address: 9 Lancaster Road, Southall, Middlesex; *Tel*: 01-574 8746.

Activity: Establishing a register of all practitioners and publishes quarterly magazine (*Focus*).

Journal of Alternative and Complementary Medicine

Address: 30 Station Approach, West Byfleet, Surrey KT14 6NF; *Tel*: 09323 49123/6.

Activity: *JACM*, for practitioners of all forms of healing, is published monthly by Argus Publishing Services, sponsors of the annual Alternative Practitioners' Exhibition in London in April.

Kesteven Natural Health Trust

Address: Church Farm, Great Hale, Sleaford, Lincs. *Tel*: 0529 60536.

Activity: Natural therapies promotion group; health and education centre.

Education: 1-year certificate course in holistic medicine; 2-year diploma course in holistic medicine; 1-day self-help courses.

Publication: Newsletter.

Size: Under 100 members.

Leamington Spa Health Foundation

Address: 21 Mason Road, Lillington, Leamington Spa, Warks. CV32 7QE; *Tel*: 0926 44279.

Activity: Natural therapies support group—information centre.

Education: Occasional talks.

Publications: Occasional leaflets.

Size: Under 20 members.

International Health Research Network

Address: 11 Woodbury Avenue, Havant, Hants PO9 1RH.

Activity: Promotion of research and gathering information on natural medicine.

Martindale Trust Ltd

Address: Moorlands, 24 South Road, Newton Abbot, Devon TQ12 1HQ; *Tel*: 06266 5493.

Activity: Natural therapies promotion group; information and consultative service.

Education: Offers scholarships to students of approved teaching colleges and organizations.

National College of Holistic Medicine

Address: 26 Sea Road, Boscombe, Bournemouth, Dorset BH5 1DF; *Tel*: 0202 36354.

Activity: Teaches courses in holistic medicine: an introductory course in nutrition, followed by a Diploma in Holistic Medicine course including nutrition and preventive medicine, and an advanced-level course leading to membership of the National Guild of Holistic Practitioners.

Size: 60 students.

Natural Health Foundation

Address: 159 George Street, London W1H 5LB; *Tel*: 01-723 7256.

Activity: Organizes public events, promotes education, disseminates information, and generally supports natural medicine and self-help.

Natural Health Network

Address: 51 Rodney Road, Cheltenham, Glos. GL50 7HX; *Tel*: 0242 25437.

Activity: Natural therapies support group; health centres.

Education: Seminars; short courses (several evenings or weekend).

Publication: Informational leaflets.

Associated with: Represents 12 natural health centres throughout the UK.

Size: Under 100 members (including all 12 health centres).

New Approaches to Cancer

Address: C/o The Seekers' Trust, Addington Park, Maidstone, Kent ME19 5BL; *Tel*: 0732 848336.

Activity: Holistic and complementary approaches to cancer: national focus for holistic groups throughout the UK, providing education courses for practitioners and providing patient referral organization.

Portland Centre

Address: 16 Preston Street, Brighton, Sussex; *Tel*: 0273 27464.

Activity: General health promotion group; health centre; bookshop.

Education: Lectures; seminars; workshops.

Size: Under 20 members.

Research Council for Complementary Medicine

Address: Suite 1, 19a Cavendish Square, London W1M 9AD; *Tel*: 01-493 6930.

Activity: A committee set up to direct and promote research, channel support, publish findings and represent complementary medicine to medical, lay, and patients' organizations and charities. Publishes newsletter, and the journal *Complementary Medical Research*. Has established a National Information Access Centre on Complementary Medicine.

The Scientific and Medical Network

Address: Lake House, Ockley, near Dorking, Surrey RH5 5NS; *Tel*: 0306 711268.

Activity: Publishes a newsletter. Encourages research.

Education: Occasional workshops, conferences, seminars.

Size: Over 400 members.

Shrewsbury Natural Health Centre

Address: 33/34 Abbey Foregate, Shrewsbury SY2 6BL.

Activity: Holistic medicine and health centre, book room, information and educational centre; cancer self-help; seminars and weekend courses.

Size: 60 members.

Society for Environmental Therapy

Address: 31 Sarah Street, Darwen, Lancs. BB3 3ET; *Tel*: 0254 775867.

Activity: Anti-environmental pollution and general health promotion group; research service, specializes in treating and preventing allergies.

Education: Conferences.

Size: Under 100 members.

Society of Students of Holistic Health

Address: 160 Upper Fant Road, Maidstone, Kent ME16 8DG.

Activity: Integration of different therapies; interaction between different disciplines; organizing workshops and conferences to promote holistic concepts.

Size: Approx. 300 members.

Scientific Information Centre

Address: The library, British School of Osteopathy, 1–4 Suffolk Street, London SW1Y 4HG; *Tel*: 01-930 9254.

Activity: A national information and documentation centre on complementary medicine, linked to the British Library, the Centre for Complementary Health Studies at Exeter University, and the Research Council for Complementary Medicine.

Tyringham Naturopathic Clinic

Address: Newport Pagnell, Buckinghamshire MK16 9ER; *Tel*: 0908 610450.

Activity: Naturopathy—residential health centre.

Associated with: Tyringham Foundation Ltd.

Size: Under 100 members.

The Vegan Society Ltd

Address: 33–35 George Street, Oxford OX1 2AY; *Tel*: 0865 722166.

Activity: Cookery courses, medical/nutrition lectures, nutritional advice in Vegan nutrition.

Size: 4000 members.

Vegetarian Society

Address: Parkdale, Dunham Road, Altrincham, Cheshire WA14 4QG; *Tel*:

061 928 0793. Or 53 Marloes Road, Kensington, London W8; *Tel*: 01-937 1714.

Activities: Courses in vegetarian cooking and nutrition. Publish magazine *The Vegetarian*, also *The International Vegetarian Handbook* and various leaflets.

Size: 10,000 members in 1986.

Warden Court

Address: Presteigne, Powys LD8 2DD, Wales; *Tel*: 05 444 205.

Activity: Natural therapies—commercial organization and health centre.

Education: Monthly seminars or weekend workshops.

Size: Under 20 members.

Wessex Healthy Living Foundation

Address: 72 Bellevue Road, Southbourne, Bournemouth BH6 3DX; *Tel*: 0202 422087.

Activity: Natural therapies support group; information centre; lectures and short courses; clinic (with nominal fees); vegetarian cookery lessons.

Publications: Newsletter.

Size: 24 voluntary practitioners. Over 2,000 members.

Wholefood School of Nutrition

Address: 12 Coton Lane, Erdington, Birmingham B23 6TP; *Tel*: 021 382 4393.

Activity: Nutrition—educational centre; general health promotion group.

Education: Local courses in wholefood cooking; intensive learning and teacher training weekends.

Publication: Magazine.

Size: Under 20 members.

Wholistic Research Co

Address: Bright Haven, Robin's Lane, Lolworth, Cambridge CB3 8HH; *Tel*: 0954 81074.

Activity: Information, instruction, equipment and products for natural birth control, environmental pollution, iridology, magnetic therapy, and natural health.

Wrekin Trust

Address: Marbury House, St Owen Street, Hereford HR1 2PR; *Tel*: 0432 266551.

Activity: An educational charity concerned with the spiritual nature of man and the universe. Has pioneered courses and conferences on the holistic world view and now offers, in addition, a curriculum for spiritual training; residential and non-residential weekend courses, day events and summer schools.

Publications: Newsletter, course brochures, cassettes. Book sales.

Yoga Biomedical Trust

Address: PO Box 140, Cambridge CB1 1PU; *Tel*: 0223 65771.

Activity: To promote and advance for the public benefit the study and practice of and research into the therapeutic effects of yoga as a means of improving the mental, physical and spiritual health of the community and to publish the useful results of any such research. There is no official membership, except for the Yoga Teacher Service, through which the Trust recommends people to yoga teachers throughout the UK.

Publications: *Yoga Biomedical Bulletin, Yoga for a Healthy Old Age*, and bibliographies.

Bibliography

Complementary and holistic
medicine—general

Ardell, D.B. (1977). *High level wellness*. Rodale Press, Emmaus, Pennsylvania.

Dossey, L. (1982). *Space, time and medicine*. Routledge & Kegan Paul, London. (A seminal philosophy of medicine, bringing it up to date with the new discoveries in physics)

Fraser, J.L. (1981). *The medicine men: A guide to natural medicine*. London, Thames TV/Methuen.

Guirdham, A. (1957). *A theory of disease*. Neville Spearman, London. (A classical pioneering philosophical discourse)

Hastings, A.C. (eds) (1981). *Health for the whole person*. Westview Press, Boulder, Colorado. (Highly recommended)

Hill, A. (ed.) (1979). *A visual encyclopedia of unconventional medicine*. New English Library, London.

Inglis, B. (1984). *Fringe Medicine*. Faber and Faber, London.

——, B. (1978). *Natural medicine*. Collins, London. (Highly recommended)

——, B. and West, R. (1983). *The alternative health guide*. Michael Joseph, London. (Good popular guide)

Kaptchuck, T. and Croucher, M. (1985). *The healing arts*. BBC Publications, London.

Kaslov, L. (1978). *Wholistic dimensions in healing*. Doubleday, New York. (A classical work)

Kenyon, J. (1986). *21st Century medicine: A layman's guide to the medicine of the future*. Thorsons, Wellingborough.

Leibrich, J., Hickling, J. and Pitt, G. (1987). *In search of well-being. Exploratory research into complementary therapies*. Health Services Research and Development Unit, Department of Health, Wellington, New Zealand.

LeShan, L. (1984). *Holistic health: How to understand and use the revolution in medicine*. Turnstone, Wellingborough.

Lewith, G.T. (ed.) (1985). *Alternative therapies. A guide to complementary medicine for the health professional*. Heinemann, London.

Pelletier, K.R. (1979). *Holistic medicine; from stress to optimum health*. Delta, N.Y.

Reason, P. and Rowan, J. (eds) (1981). *Human inquiry: A sourcebook of new paradigm research*. Wiley, Chichester.

Richman, J. (1987). *Medicine and Health*. Longman, London.

Salmon, J.W. (ed.) (1985). *Alternative medicines: Popular and policy perspectives*. Tavistock, London and New York. (First sociological text)

Sobel, D. (1979). *Ways of health: Holistic approaches in ancient and contemporary medicine*. Viking, New York.

Stanway, A. (1982). *Alternative medicine. A guide to natural therapies*. Penguin, Harmondsworth, Middlesex.

Walker, B. (1978). *Encyclopaedia of metaphysical medicine*. Routledge and Kegan Paul, London.

Wallis, R. and Morley, P. (eds) (1976). *Marginal medicine*. Peter Owen, London.

Weil, A. (1983). *Health and healing: Understanding conventional and alternative medicine*. Houghton Mifflin, Los Angeles. (Highly recommended)

Werbach, M.R. (1986). *Third Line Medicine*. Routledge, London.

West, R. and Trevelyan, J.E. (1985). *Alternative medicine: A bibliography of books in English*. Mansell, London.

Critiques of conventional medicine

Carlson, R.J. (1975). *The end of medicine*. Wiley-Interscience, New York. (Pioneering work)

Carter, C.O. and Peel, J. (1969). *Equalities and inequalities in health*. Academic Press, New York.

Draper, P. *et al.*, (1978). *The NHS in its next 30 years*. The Unit for the Study of Health Policy; Guy's Hospital Medical School, London.

Dubos, Rene (1968). *Man, medicine and environment*. Praeger, New York.

Fulder, S. (1987). *How to survive medical treatment*. Century-Hutchinson, London.

Gould, D. (1985). *The Black and White Medicine Show*. Hamish Hamilton, London.

Howe, G.M. (1977). *Man, environment and disease in Britain*. Pelican Books, Harmondsworth, Middlesex. (Invaluable statistical and historical review)

Illich, I. (1977). *Medical nemesis: The expropriation of health*. Bantam, New York. (Highly recommended)

Inglis, B. (1981). *Diseases of civilisation*. Hodder and Stoughton, London.

McKeown, T. (1979). *The role of medicine: Dream, mirage or nemesis*. Rock Carling Memorial Lecture, Blackwell's, Oxford.

Medawar, C. (1984). *The Wrong Kind of Medicine*. Hodder & Stoughton and the Comsumers Association, London.

Mellville, A. and Johnson, C. (1982). *Cured to death, the effect of prescription drugs*. Secker and Warburg, London.

Office of Population Census and Surveys (1974).*Morbidity statistics from general practice: Second national study 1970–71*. HMSO, London.

Richards, D. (1982). *The topic of cancer. When the killing has to stop*. Pergamon Press, Oxford and New York. (A strong case, by a scientist, against radical treatment of cancer)

Royal Commission on the NHS (1979). *Report Cmnd. 7615*. HMSO, London.

Weitz, M. (1980). *Health shock: How to avoid ineffective and hazardous medical treatment*. Prentice-Hall, Englewood Cliffs, N.J. David and Charles, London.

History

Brock, A.J. (1921). *Greek medicine*. Dent and Sons, New York.

Grossinger, R. (1980). *Planet medicine*. Shambhala, Colorado.

Inglis, B. (1979b). *A history of medicine*. Fontana/Collins, London.

Institute of History of Medicine and Medical Research. Department of Philosophy of Medicine and Science (1973). *Theories and philosophies of medicine: with particular reference to Greco-Arab medicine; Ayurveda and traditional Chinese medicine*. (2nd edn) New Delhi.

Traditional

Bannerman, R.H., Burton, J., and Wen-Chieh, C. (1983). *Traditional Medicine and Health Care Coverage*. WHO, Geneva.

CIBA Foundation (1977). *Health and disease in tribal societies*. CIBA Symposium No. 49. Elsevier, Excerpta Medica, Amsterdam.

Croizier, R.C. (1968). *Traditional medicine in modern China; Science, nationalism, and the tensions of cultural change*. Harvard University Press, Cambridge, Mass.

Foster, G.M. (1984). *Medical Anthropology*. Wiley, New York.

Furst, B.G. (1974). *Traditional medicine and indigenous practitioners*. American, Public Health Association, International Health Programs, Washington D.C.

Harrison, I.E. and Cosminsky, S. (1976). *Traditional medicine: Implications for ethno-medicine, ethnopharmacology, maternal and child health, mental health, and public health; an annotated bibliography of Africa, Latin America and the Caribbean*. Garland, New York.

—— and Dunlop, David W. (eds) (1974). *Traditional healers, use and non-use in health care delivery*. Michigan University Press, East Lansing, Michigan.

Helman, C. (1985). *Culture, Health and Illness*. Wright, Bristol.

Hillier, S.M. and Jewell, J.A. (1984). *Health care and traditional medicine in China*. Routledge and Kegan Paul, London.

Hunan (Province) Revolutionary Health Committee. *A barefoot doctor's manual*. Routledge and Kegan Paul, London.

Kleimann *et al.* (ed.) (1975). *Medicine in Chinese cultures: Comparative studies of health care in Chinese and other societies—Conference sponsored by John E. Fogarty Centre (NIH)*. US Government Printing Office, DHEW Pub. No. (NIH) 95–653, Washington D.C.

Landy, D. (ed.) (1977). *Culture, disease and healing: Studies in medical anthropology*. Macmillan, New York.

Maclean, U. (1971). *Magical medicine; A Nigerian case-study*. Penguin, Harmondsworth, Middlesex.

Self-help (see also Naturopathy)

Benjamin, H. (1983). *Everybody's guide to nature cure*. Thorsons, Wellingborough.

Billings, L. (1982). *The Billings method: Controlling fertility without drugs or devices*. Penguin, Harmondsworth, Middlesex.

Bricklin, M. *The practical encyclopedia of natural healing*. Rodale Press, Emmaus, Pennsylvania.

Brook, D. (1984). *Naturebirth: you, your body and your baby*. Penguin, Harmondsworth, Middlesex.

Clark, L.A. (1983). *Get well naturally*. Arco, New York. (Classical pioneering book)

Cott, A. (1981). *Fasting: the ultimate diet*. Bantam, New York.

Drake, K. and Drake, J. (1984). *Natural birth control*. Thorsons, Wellingborough.

Forbes, A. (1976). *Try being healthy*. Health Science Press, Holsworthy. (Highly recommended)

Fulder, S. (1983). *An end to ageing?*. Thorsons, Wellingborough.

Gann, R. (1986). *The health information handbook*. Gower, London.

Haas, E.M. (1983). *Staying healthy with the seasons*. Celestial Arts Berkeley, California.

Halvorsen, B. (1987). *The natural dentist*. Century Arrow, London.

Inglis, B. and West, R. (1983). *The alternative health guide*. Michael Joseph, London.

Kübler-Ross, E. (1975). *Death: The final stage of growth*. Prentice-Hall, Englewood Cliffs, N.J.

Llewellyn-Jones, D. (1980). *Every body, a nutritional guide to life*. Oxford University Press, Oxford.

Mayes, A. (1985). *Dictionary of nutritional health*. Thorsons, Wellingborough.

Null, G. (1984). *The complete guide to health and nutrition*. Arlington, London.

O'Neill, B. and Phillips, R. (1985). *Biorhythms: how to live with your life cycles*. Signet, New York.

Acupuncture

Austin, M. (1982). *Acupuncture therapy*. Turnstone Books, Wellingborough, Northants.

Campbell, A. (1987). *Acupuncture: the modern scientific approach*. Faber and Faber, London.

Chan, P. (1974). *Finger acupuncture*. Price, Stern and Sloan, Los Angeles, California.

Chen, James, Y.P., *Acupuncture Anesthesia in the People's Republic of China, 1973*. Bethesda, Maryland, National Institutes of Health, DHEW publication (1975).

College of Traditional Chinese Medicine, Peking, *An Outline of Chinese Acupuncture*. Peking, Foreign Language Press (1975).

Hill, S. and Playfair, G. (1979). *The cycles of heaven*. Pan, London.

Jenerick, H.P. (ed.) (1973). *Proceedings of the National Institute of Health Acupuncture Research Conference*. Bethesda, Maryland. Department of Health, Education and Welfare (NIH), Publication No. 74–165 (1973). (Standard text)

Kao, F.F. (1979). *Recent advances in acupuncture research*. Institute for Advanced Research in Asian Science and Medicine, Garden City, New York.

Kapchuk, T. (1984). *The web that has no weaver*. Hutchinson, London. (Highly recommended)

Kenyon, J.N. (1985). *Modern techniques of acupuncture: practical guide to electroacupuncture*. Thorsons, Wellingborough.

Lawson-Wood, D. and Lawson-Wood, J. (1976). *Five elements of acupuncture and Chinese massage*. Health Science Press, Holsworthy.

Lewith, G.T. (1982). *Acupuncture: Its place in Western medical science*. Thorsons, Wellingborough. (Recommended)

—— and Lewith, R.N. (1986). *Modern Chinese acupuncture*. Thorsons, Wellingborough.

Macdonald, A. (1984). *Acupuncture from ancient art to modern medicine*. Unwin, London.

Mann, F. (1982). *The treatment of disease by acupuncture. Part 1: Function of acupuncture points. Part 2: Treatment of disease*. (4th edn). Heinemann Medical Books, London.

Needham, J. and Gwei-Djen, L. (1980). *Celestial lancets: A history and rationale of acupuncture and moxa*. Cambridge University Press. (Highly recommended)

O'Connor, J. and Bensky, D. (eds) (1981). *Acupuncture: A comprehensive text*. Shanghai College of Traditional Medicine. Eastland Press, Chicago. (The best complete work available)

Pálos, S. (1982). *The Chinese art of healing*. Bantam, New York.

People's Medical Publishing House (1979). *National symposium of acupuncture, moxibustion and acupuncture anaesthesia*. World Books, Peking.

Pokert, M. *The theoretical foundation of Chinese medicine: Systems of correspondence*. MIT Press, Cambridge, Mass. (Theoretical text)

Tan, L.T., Tan, M., and Veith, I. (1975). *Acupuncture therapy, current Chinese practice*. Routledge and Kegan Paul, London.

Veith, I. (transl.) (1966). *The Yellow Emperor's classic of internal medicine (The Nei Ching)*. University of California Press.

Woollerton, H. and MacLean, C.J. (1983). *Acupuncture energy in health and disease*. Thorsons, Wellingborough.

Worsley, J.R. (1973). *Is acupuncture for you?* Harper and Row, New York.

Alexander and Feldenkrais Techniques

Alexander, F.M. (1971). (ed. E. Maisel) *The resurrection of the body*. Dell, New York. (The classic book by the originator of the technique)

Alexander, F.M. (1985). *The use of the self*. Gollancz, London.

Barlow, W. (1982). *The Alexander principle*. Gollancz, London. (A comprehensive description of the technique)

Feldenkrais, M. (1972). *Awareness through movement: Health exercises for personal growth*. Harper and Row, New York. (The main book by the originator of the Feldenkrais technique)

Fenton, J. (1973). *Practical movement control* (original title: *The choice of habit*). Macdonald and Evans, London.

Jones, F.P. (1976). *Body awareness in action: A study of the Alexander Technique*. Schocken, New York. (Excellent section on research)

Maisel, E. (1969). *The resurrection of the body*. University Books, New York.

Anthroposophical medicine

Bott, V. (1985). *Anthroposophical medicine*. Thorsons, Wellingborough.

Bott, V. (1986). *Anthroposophical guide to family medicine*. Thorsons, Wellingborough.

Buhler, W. (1979). *Living with your body*. Rudolf Steiner Press, London.

Hauschke, M. (1979). *Rhythmical massage*. Rudolf Steiner Press, London.

Leroi, A. (1973). *The cell, the human organism and cancer*. New Knowledge Books, East Grinstead.

Lievegoed, B. (1982). *Phases—crisis and development in the individual*. Rudolf Steiner Press, London.

Pelikan, W. (1978). *Healing plants*. Rudolf Steiner Press, London.

Steiner, R. (1948). *Spiritual science and medicine*. Rudolf Steiner Press, London.

—— (1979*a*). *The philosophy of freedom*. Rudolf Steiner Press, London.

—— (1979*b*). *Occult science—an outline*. Rudolf Steiner Press, London.

Chiropractic (see also Osteopathy)

Beurger, A.A. and Tobis, J.S. (eds) (1977). *Approaches to the validation of a manipulative therapy*. Charles Thomas, Springfield, Illinois.

Brennan, M.J. (ed.) (1981). *The resource guide to chiropractic: a bibliography of chiropractic and related areas*. American Chiropractors' Association, Washington D.C.

Cyriax, J. (1971). *Treatment by manipulation, massage and injection*. Williams and Williams, Baltimore, Maryland.

Dintenfuss, J. (1975). *Chiropractic: A modern way to health*. Pyramid, New York.

Fisk, J.W. (1977). *A practical guide to the management of the painful neck and back*. Charles C. Thomas, Springfield, Illinois. (A good presentation of possibilities, by an open-minded doctor, on medical manipulation and chiropractic)

International Chiropractic Association (1979). *Modern developments in the principles and practice of chiropractic*. Appleton-Century-Crofts, New York.

Kunert, W. (1963). *The vertebral column, autonomic nervous system and internal organs*. Enke, Stuttgart.

Maitland, G.B. (1964). *Vertebral manipulation*. Butterworth, London. (A classical medical text on manipulation—*not* chiropractic)

National Institute of Neurological Communicable Disorders and Stroke (1975). *The research status of spinal manipulative therapy*. Department of Health, Education and Welfare: NIH, Washington D.C.

Report of the Commission of Inquiry (1979). *Chiropractic in New Zealand*, New Zealand Government Printer. Wellington.

Scofield, A.G. (1982). *Chiropractic: The science of specific spinal adjustment*. Thorsons, Wellingborough.

Valentine, T. and Valentine, C. (1985). *Applied kinesiology: Muscle response in diagnosis, therapy, and preventive medicine*. Thorsons, Wellingborough.

White, A.A. (1983). *Your aching back*. Bantam, New York.

Creative and sensory therapies

Alvin, J. (1985). *Music therapy*. Hutchinson, London.

Alvin, J. (1976). *Music therapy for the handicapped child*. Oxford University Press.

Birren, F. (1950). *Colour psychology and colour therapy: A factual study of the influence of colour on human life*. McGraw-Hill, New York.

Clark, L.A. (1975). *Ancient art of colour therapy*. Devin-Adair, Old Greenwich, Connecticut.

Feldman, E.B. (1970). *Becoming human through art*. Prentice-Hall, Englewood Cliffs, N.J.

Fring-Keyes, M. (1976). *The inward journey: Art as therapy for you*. Celestial Arts, Millbrae, California.

Halpern, S. and Savary, S. (1985). *Sound health: music and sounds that make us whole*. Harper & Row, New York.

Jennings, S. (1977). *Creative therapy*. Pitman, London.

McLaughlin, T. (1970). *Music and communication*. Faber and Faber, London.

Michel, D. (1985). *Music therapy: an introduction*. Charles C. Thomas, Springville, Illinois.

Ott, J.N. (1984). *Health and light: The effects of natural and artificial light on man and other living things*. Devin-Adair, Old Greenwich, Connecticut.

Stebbing, L. (1975). *Music therapy—A new anthology*. Knowledge Books, Horsham.

Ethnic medicine

Dash, B. (1974). *Ayurvedic treatment for common diseases*. Delhi Diary, Delhi.

Dasher, J.F. (1978). *Everybody's guide to Ayurvedic medicine*. D.B. Taraporevala, Bombay.

Fazal, U. and Razzack, H. M.A. (eds) (1976). *A handbook of common remedies in Unani system of medicine*. Central Council for Research in Indian Medicine and Homeopathy, New Delhi.

Jaggi, O.P. (1973*a*). *Indian system of medicine*. Ram, Delhi.

—— (1973*b*). *Yogic and Tantric medicine*. Ram, Delhi.

Khan, M.S. (1985). *Islamic medicine*. Routledge and Kegan Paul, London.

Thakhur, C. (1974). *Introduction to Ayurveda*. ASI Publishers, New York.

Udupa, K.N. (ed.) (1970). *Advances in research in Indian medicine*. Banaras Hindu University, Varanasi.

Healing

Bloomfield, B. (1984). *The mystique of healing*. Skilton and Shaw, Edinburgh.

Easthope, G. (1987). *Healers and alternative medicine: a sociological examination*. Gower, Aldershot.

Edmunds, Henry Tudor (ed.) (1976). *Some unrecognized factors in medicine*. Theosophical Publishing House, Wheaton, Illinois.

Edwards, H. (n.d.). *A guide to the understanding and practice of spiritual healing*. The Harry Edwards Spiritual Healing Sanctuary Trust, Guildford.

Eliade, M. (1964). *Shamanism: Archaic technique of ecstasy*. Princeton University Press. (Highly recommended)

Gennaro, L., Guzzon, F., and Marsigli, P. (1986). *Kirlian photography*. East West Publications, London.

Halifax, J. (1982). *Shaman, the wounded healer*. Thames and Hudson, London.

Karagulla, S. (1967). *Breakthrough to Creativity*. De Vorss Press, Marina del Ray, California. (A pioneering book)

Krippner, S. and Villoldo, A. (1976). *Realms of healing*. Celestial Arts, Millbrae, California.

Le Shan, L. (1985). *From Newton to ESP*. Viking, New York.

MacManaway, B. (1983). *Healing*. Thorsons, Wellingborough.

Meek, G.W. (1977). *Healers and the healing process*. Quest Books, Wheaton, Illinois.

Morris, J.D. Morris, R.L., and Roth, W.G. (eds) (1976). *Research in parapsychology 1975*. Scarecrow Press, Methuen, N.J.

Moss, T. (1979). *The body electric*. Granada, St Albans. (The best account of research into Kirlian photography)

Playfair, G.L. (1987). *Medicine, mind and magic*. Aquarian Press, Wellingborough.

Puharich, G. (1977). *Beyond telepathy*. Granada, St Albans.

Regush, N.M. (ed.) (1974). *The human aura*. Berkeley Medallion, New York.

Sargant, W.W. (1973). *The mind possessed: A physiology of possession, mysticism and faith healing*. Heinemann, London.

Valentine, T. (1973). *Psychic surgery*. Pocket Books, New York.

Young, A. (1983). *Spiritual healing: Miracle or mirage?* De Vorss Press, Marina del Ray, California.

Wolman, B.B. (1977). *Handbook of parapsychology.* Van Nostrand Rheinhold, New York.

Herbalism

Blackwood, J. and Fulder, S. (1986). *Garlic: Nature's original remedy*. Javelin Books, Poole, Dorset.

Chopra, Ram Nath (1958). *Indigenous drugs of India*. Dhur, Calcutta.

Culpeper, N. (1979). *Culpeper's complete herbal*. Foulsham, Slough, Middlesex.

—— (Potterton, D. Ed.) (1983). *Culpeper's colour herbal*. Foulsham, Slough, Middlesex.

De Bairacli-Levy, J. (1982). *The illustrated herbal handbook*. Faber and Faber, London.

De Vries, J. (1985). *Traditional home and herbal remedies*. Mainstream, London.

Dincin B.D. (1979). *Herbal medicine: The natural way to get well and stay well*. The Herb Society/Hutchinson, London. (Recommended)

Fluck, H. (1976). *Medicinal plants*. Foulsham, Slough, Middlesex.

Fulder, S. (1982). *The Tao of medicine: Ginseng, Oriental remedies and the pharmacology of harmony*. Destiny Books, Rochester, Vermont.

Grieve, M. (1982). *A modern herbal*. Jonathan Cape, London; Peregrine, Harmondsworth, Middlesex.

Griggs, B. (1981). *Green pharmacy: A history of herbal medicine*. Jill Norman, London. (Highly recommended)

Griggs, B. (1982). *The home herbal*. Jill Norman, London.

Hoffman, D. (1986). *Holistic herbal way to successful stress control*. Thorsons, Wellingborough.

Hutchins, A.R. (1982). *Indian herbology of North America*. Merce, Ontario.

Kloss, J. (1984). *Back to Eden*. Woodbridge Press, Santa Barbara, California.

Krieg, M.B. (1965). *Green medicine*. Harrap, London and Toronto.

Launert, E. (1981). *Edible and medicinal plants of Britain and Northern Europe*. Hamlyn, London.

Lewis, W.H. and Elvin-Lewis, P.F. (1977). *Medical botany: Plants affecting man's health*. Wiley, New York.

Li, Chen-p'ien (1975). *Chinese herbal medicine*. National Institutes of Health, DHEW publication. NIH, Bethesda, Maryland.

Mességué, M. (1979). *Health secrets of plants and herbs*. Collins, London.

Mills, S. (1986). *The dictionary of modern herbalism: The complete guide to herbs and herbal therapy*. Thorsons, Wellingborough.

Price, S. (1976). *Practical aromatherapy*. Thorsons, Wellingborough.

Rose, J. (1976). *Jeanne Rose's herbal body book*. Grosset and Dunlop, New York.

Steiner, R.P. (1986). *Folk medicine, the art and the science*. American Chemical Society, Washington D.C.

Stuart, M. (ed.) (1979). *The encyclopaedia of herbs and herbalism*. Orbis, London.

Swain, T. (ed.) (1972). *Plants in the development of modern medicine*. (Papers presented at a symposium) Harvard University Press, Cambridge, Mass.

Tierra, M. (1980). *The way of herbs*. Unity Press, Santa Cruz, California. (Highly recommended)

Tisserand, R.B. (1985). *The art of aromatherapy*. C.W. Daniel, Saffron Walden, Destiny Books, Rochester, Vermont.

Vogel, V.J. (1982). *American Indian medicine*. University of Oklahoma Press, Norman.

Wagner, H. and Wolff, P. (1977). *New natural products and plant drugs with pharmacological, biological and therapeutic activity*. Springer-Verlag, Heidelberg.

Weiner, M.A. (1984). *The people's herbal*. Putnam, New York.

Wren, R.W. (1979). *Potters new cyclopaedia of botanical drugs and preparations*. Health Science Press, Holsworthy.

Wyatt, C. (1978). *Chinese herbal medicine*. Wildwood House, London.

Homeopathy

Babbington Smith, C. (1986). *Champion of homeopathy, the life of Margery Blackie*. John Murray, London.

Blackie, M.G. (1984). *The patient, not the cure: The challenge of homeopathy*. Unwin, London. (An acclaimed personal book by one of the leading UK homeopaths)

—— (1986). *Classical homeopathy*. Beaconsfield Library, Beaconsfield.

Boyd, H. (1981). *Introduction to homeopathic medicine*. Beaconsfield Library, Beaconsfield, Bucks.

Campbell, A. (1984). *The two faces of homeopathy*. Hale, London.

Coulter, H.L. (1981). *Homeopathic science and modern medicine*. North Atlantic Books, Berkeley, California.

Resh, G. and Gutman, V. (1987). *The scientific foundations of homeopathy*. Bartel and Bartel, Berg Am Starnberger See, West Germany.

Sharma, C.H. (1975). *A manual of homeopathy and natural medicine*. Turnstone, Wellingborough.

Shepherd, D. (1979). *The magic of minimum dose*. Health Science Press, Holsworthy.

—— (1982). *Homeopathy for the first aider*. Health Science Press, Holsworthy.

Smith, T. (1982). *Homeopathic medicine*. Thorsons, Wellingborough.

—— (1984). *Homeopathic constitutional medicine*. Thorsons, Wellingborough.

—— (1986). *The principles, art and .practice of homeopathy*. Insight Publications, Worthing, Sussex.

Stephenson, J.H. (1976). *A doctor's guide to helping yourself with homeopathic remedies*. Parker Publishing Company, New York.

Vithoulkas, G. (1986). *The science of homeopathy*. Thorsons, Wellingborough. (An intelligent guide to homeopathy)

—— (1981). *Homeopathy—medicine of the new man*. Arco Press, New York. (Perhaps the best short introduction available)

Weeks, Nora (1979). *Medical discoveries of Edward Bach, physician*. Keats Publishers, New Canaan, Connecticut.

Wheeler, C.E. and Kenyon, J.D. (1980). *Introduction to the principles and practice of homeopathy*. C.W. Daniel, Saffron Walden.

Whitmore, E. (1981). *Psyche and substance*. North Atlantic Books, Richmond, California. (Highly recommended to those interested in the metaphysics of homeopathy)

Hypnosis

Ambrose, G. and Newbold, G. (1980). *A handbook of medical hypnosis*. Ballière Tindall, Eastbourne.

Barber, T.X., Spanos, N.P., and Chaves, J.F. (1986). *Hypnosis, imagination and human potentialities*. Pergamon Press, Oxford and New York.

Black, S. (1969). *Mind and Body*. London, W. Kimber.

Cheek, D. and Le Cron, L. (1986). *Clinical hypnotherapy*. Grune and Stratton, New York. (The presentation of the author's results on hypnosis in surgery, with the unconscious, and with ideometer methods)

Erickson, M. and Rossi, E. (1980). *Hypnotherapy: An exploratory casebook*. Irvington Publishers, New York.

Hartland, J. (1971). *Medical and dental hypnosis*. Ballière and Tindall, London. (The classic book for medical professionals)

Hilgard, E.R. and Hilgard, J.R. (1984). *Hypnosis in the relief of pain*. William Kaufmann, Los Altos, California.

Rogers, C. (1973). *Client centred therapy*. McGraw-Hill, New York.

Shone, R. (1985). *Autohypnosis: A step by step guide to self-hypnosis*. Thorsons, Wellingborough.

Shreeve, C. and Shreeve, D. (1984). *Healing power of hypnotism*. Thorsons, Wellingborough.

Udolf, K. (1986). *Handbook of hypnosis for professionals*. van Nostrand Rheinhold, New York.

Waxman, D. (1981). *Hypnosis: A guide for patients and practitioners*. Allen and Unwin, London. (Recommended)

Manual therapies

Bahr, F. (1982). *The acupressure health book*. Unwin, London.

Bergson, A. and Tuchak, V. (1974). *Zone therapy*. Pinnacle, New York.

Bayly, D. (1982). *Reflexology today*. Thorsons, Wellingborough.

Birdwhistell, R.L. (1970). *Kinesics and context: Essays on body motion communication*. University of Pennsylvania Press. (Pioneering work on applied kinesiology and muscle balancing)

Blate, M. (1982). *The natural healers acupressure handbook: G-J fingertip technique*. Routledge and Kegan Paul, London. (Recommended)

—— (1982). *How to heal yourself using hand acupuncture*. Routledge and Kegan Paul, London.

Downing, G. (1972). *The massage book*. Random House, New York. (Perhaps the best all-round book on massage)

—— (1974). *Massage and meditation*. Random House, New York.

Hessel, S. (1978). *The articulate body*. St Martin's, New York.

Hofer, J. (1976). *Total massage*. Grosset and Dunlap, New York.

Johnson, D. (1977). *The protean body*. Harper and Row, New York. (Deep massage and structural integration)

Kaye, A. and Matchan, D.C. (1985). *Reflexology: Techniques of foot massage for health and fitness*. Thorsons, Wellingborough.

Kunz, K. and Kunz, B. (1985). *The complete guide to foot reflexology*. Thorsons, Wellingborough.

Marquardt, H. (1983). *Reflex zone therapy of the feet*. Thorsons, Wellingborough.

Montagu, A. (1972). *Touching: The human significance of skin*. Harper and Row, New York.

Namikoshi, T. (1972). *Shiatzu: Japanese finger-pressure therapy*. Japan Publications, San Francisco.

—— (1977). *Shiatzu therapy, theory and practice*. Wehmann Brothers, New Jersey.

Ohashi, W. (1978). *Do-it-yourself Shiatsu: How to perform the ancient Japanese art of 'acupuncture without needles'*. Unwin, London.

Rolf, I. (1977). *Rolfing—The integration of human structures*. Dennis Landmann, Santa Monica, California.

Stone, R. (1978). *Health building*. Parameter Press, Orange County, California. (On polarity therapy)

Thie, J. and Marks, M. (1979). *Touch for health*. De Vorss Press, Santa Monica, California.

Mind–Body therapies

Achterberg, J. (1985). *Imagery in healing—shamanism and modern medicine.* Shambhala, Boston.

Achterberg, J., Simonton, C., and Simonton, S. (1976). *Stress, psychological factors, and cancer.* New Medicine Press, Fort Worth.

Assagioli, R. (1971). *Psychosynthesis.* Hobbs, Dorman, New York. (Classic book on Assagioli's visualization and meditative psychotherapies)

Benson, H. (1976). *The relaxation response.* Morrow, New York. (The classic book on the psychophysiological effects of relaxation)

Bloomfield, H.H. *et al.* (1975). *TM: Discovering inner energy and overcoming stress.* Delacorte, New York. (A summary of psychophysiological effects of transcendental meditation)

Brena, S.F. (1973). *Yoga and medicine.* Penguin, New York.

Brown, B. (1978). *Stress and the art of biofeedback.* Canfield, London.

—— (1984). *New mind, new body. Biofeedback: new direction for the mind.* Irvington, New York.

Cade, C.M. and Coxhead, N. (1987). *The awakened mind—Biofeedback and the development of higher states of awareness.* Element, Shaftesbury, Dorset. (Leading UK biofeedback researchers)

Carroll, D. (1984). *Biofeedback in practice.* Longmans, Harlow.

Dychtwald, K. (1977). *Bodymind.* Random House, New York. (Excellent summary of theory, methods and results of body awareness techniques of all kinds)

Elbert, T. (ed.) (1984). *Self-regulation of the brain and behaviour.* Springer-Verlag, Berlin, New York.

Everly, G.S. and Rosenfeld, R. (1981). *The nature and treatment of the stress response.* Plenum, New York.

Friedman, M. and Rosenman, R. (1974). *Type A behaviour and your heart.* Fawcett, New York.

Garfield, S., Bergin, A.E. (1986). *Psychotherapy and behaviour change.* John Wiley, Chichester.

Gratchel, R.J. (1979). *Clinical application of biofeedback: Appraisal and status.* Pergamon Press, Oxford and New York.

Garde, R.K. (1970). *Principles and practice of yoga therapy.* Tarnhelm, Lakemont.

Glasser, R. (1976). *The body is the hero.* Random House, New York.

(Classic book on the possibilities gained through body awareness)

Green, E. and Green, A. (1977). *Beyond biofeedback*. Delacorte, New York.

Grunderson, E. and Rahe, R. (eds) (1974). *Life, stress and illness*. (Proceedings of a NATO-sponsored conference on stress and disease) Charles C. Thomas, Springfield, Illinois.

Huxley, Aldous L. (1974). *Art of seeing*. Montanu Books, Seattle. (Aldous Huxley's account of the return of his sight using the Bates method)

James, G., Dennis, J. and Bresler, D. (eds) (1981). *Mind, body and health: Towards an integral medicine*. National Institute of Mental Health, Rockville, Maryland. (Summaries by many top authorities and practitioners of holistic methods of health care)

Krakowski, A.J. and Chase, P. (1983). *Psychosomatic medicine, theoretical, clinical and transcultural aspects*. Plenum, New York.

Lamb, W. and Watson, E. (1982). *Body code. The meaning in movement*. Routledge and Kegan Paul, London. (A new summary of knowledge of the body as an expression of the mind)

Lewis, H.R. and Lewis, M. (1972). *Psychosomatics*. Viking, New York.

Lowen, A. (1978). *Bioenergetics*. Penguin, London.

Luthe, W. (1976). *Creative mobilisation technique*. Grune and Stratton, New York. (Manual of autogenic therapy)

Meares, A. (1983). *Relief without drugs*. Fontana, London.

Motofsky, D.I. (1976). *Behaviour control and the modification of physiological activity*. Prentice-Hall, Englewood Cliffs, N.J. (Summary of research)

Oyle, I. (1975). *The healing mind*. Celestial Arts, Millbrae, California.

Pelletier, K. (1977). *Mind as healer, mind as slayer: A holistic approach to preventing stress disorders*. Delacorte, New York. (Highly recommended)

Rosa, C. (1976). *You and autogenic training*. Dutton, New York.

Rowan, J. (1980). *Ordinary ecstasy*. Routledge and Kegan Paul, London. (Well-known summary of alternative psychotherapeutic techniques)

Selye, Hans (1976). *The stress of life*. McGraw-Hill, New York. (Personal account of biochemical and physiological discoveries by the man who 'discovered' the stress response)

Simonton, O.C., Matthews-Simonton, S., and Creighton, J. (1978). *Getting well again*. Tarcher Books, Los Angeles. (The book covers the use of visualization and meditation in overcoming cancer)

Tanner, O. (1977). *Stress*. Time-Life International, The Netherlands.

Tohei, K. (1978). *The book of Ki: Coordinating mind and body in daily life*. Japan Publications, San Francisco.

Naturopathy and nutrition therapy
(see also self-help)

Adams, R. and Murray, F. (1985). *Body, mind and B vitamins*. Larchmont, New York.

Bland, J. (ed.) (1986). *Yearbook of nutritional medicine*. Keats Publishing, New Canaan, Connecticut.

Brandt, J. (1971). *The grape cure*. Benedict Lust, Simi Valley, California.

Budd, M.L. (1981). *Low blood sugar*. Thorsons, Wellingborough.

Cheraskin, E. and Ringsdorf, W. (1980). *Psychodietetics: Food as the key to emotional health*. Stein and Day, New York.

—— Ringsdorf, W., and Clark, J.W. (1977). *Diet and disease*. Keats Publishing, New Canaan, Connecticut. (Recommended)

Colgan, M. (1982). *Your personal vitamin profile*. Blond and Briggs, London.

Cott, A. (1981). *Fasting: the ultimate diet*. Bantam, New York.

Davies, S. and Stewart, A. (1987). *Nutritional medicine*. Pan, London.

Davis, A. (1983). *Let's get well*. Unwin, London.

Dubos, R. (1968). *So human an animal*. Scribners, New York.

Forbes, A. (1984). *The Bristol Diet*. Century Hutchinson, London.

Garrison, R. and Somer, E. (1985). *Nutrition desk reference*. Keats Publishing, New Canaan, Connecticut.

Gerson, M. (1977). *Cancer therapy: a result of 50 cases*. Totality Books, Delmar, California.

Horrobin, D. (ed.) (1982). *Clinical uses of essential fatty acids*. Eden Press, Montreal.

Hunter, B.T. (1972). *Consumer beware!*. Simon and Schuster, New York.

International vegetarian health food handbook (1986). Daniel, Saffron Walden.

Jarvis, D. (1983). *Folk medicine: A doctor's guide to good health*. Pan, London.

Kirschmann, J.D. (1979). *Nutrition almanac*. McGraw-Hill, New York.

Kohnlechner K. (1979). *Handbuch der Naturheilkunde*. (2 Vols). Wilhelm Heyne Verlag, Munich. (The comprehensive reference book of Heilpraktiker).

Krause, M.V. and Hauscher, M.A. (1977). *Food, nutrition and diet therapy*. W.B. Saunders, Philadelphia.

Kushi, M., Esko, E. and van Canwenberghe, M. (eds.) (1983). *The macrobiotic approach to major illnesses*. East West Foundation, Boston.

Kriege, T. (1969). *The fundamental basis of iridiagnosis*. Fowler, London.

Law, T. (1980). *You are how you eat*. Turnstone, Wellingborough.

Lindlahr, V.H. (1983). *Natural therapeutics*. (2 Vols). C.W. Daniel, Saffron Walden. (The classical work)

Mayes, A. (1985). *Dictionary of nutritional health*. Thorsons, Wellingborough.

Mackarness, R. (1976). *Not all in the mind*. Pan, London.

—— (1980). *Chemical victims*. Pan, London.

Mervyn, L. (1986). *Dictionary of minerals*. Thorsons, Wellingborough.

Newman-Turner, R. (1984). *Naturopathy*. Thorsons, Wellingborough. (Recommended)

Null, G. (1984). *The complete guide to health and nutrition*. Arlington, London.

Passwater, R. (1982). *Supernutrition for healthy hearts*. Thorsons, Wellingborough.

Pauling, L. (1986). *How to live longer and feel better*. W.H. Freeman, New York.

Pfeiffer, C.C. (1975). *Mental and elemental nutrients: A physician's guide to nutrition and health care*. Keats Publishing, New Canaan, Connecticut.

Pizzorno, J. and Murray, M. (1985). *A textbook of natural medicine*. John Bastyr College Publications, Seattle.

Royal College of Physicians. (1981). *Medical aspects of dietary fibre*. Pitman medical, London.

Soyka, S. and Edmonds, A. (1978). *The ion effect*. Dutton, New York.

Stone, I. (1979). *Healing factor: Vitamin C against disease*. Grosset and Dunlap, New York.

Williams, R.J. (1977). *A physicians' handbook of nutritional science*. Pergamon, Oxford.

Williams, R.J. (1979). *Biochemical individuality*. Wiley, New York.

Williams, R. (1981). *Nutrition against disease*. Bantam, New York. (Highly recommended)

Wilson, F.A. (1980). *Food fit for humans*. C.W. Daniel, Saffron Walden.

Osteopathy (see also Chiropractic)

Chaitow, L. (1982). *Osteopathy: Head-to-toe health through manipulation*. Thorson, Wellingborough.

—— (1987). *Soft tissue manipulation*. Thorsons, Wellingborough.

Hoag, J.M., Cole, W.V., and Bradford, S.G. (1980). *Osteopathic Medicine*. McGraw Hill, New York.

Korr, I.M. (1978). *The neurobiologic mechanisms in manipulative therapy*. Plenum, New York.

Lettvin, M. (1979). *The back book: Healing the hurt in your lower back*. Fontana, London.

Still, A.T. (1910). *Osteopathy—Research and practice*. (Privately published, A.T. Still, Missouri)

Stoddard, A. (1983). *Manual of osteopathic technique*. Hutchinson, London.

Upledger, J. and Vredevoord, J. (1983). *Craniosacral therapy*. Eastland Press, Chicago.

Radionics and psionic medicine

Baerlin, E. and Dower, H.L.G. (1980). *Healing with radionics*. Thorsons, Wellingborough.

Burr, H.S. (1973). *The fields of life*. Ballantine, New York.

Reyner, J.H., Laurence, G., and Upton, C. (1980). *Psionic medicine*. Routledge and Kegan Paul, London. (Highly recommended)

Russell, E. (1973). *Report on radionics*. Neville Spearman, London.

Tansley, D.V. (1980). *Dimensions of radionics*. Health Science Press, Holsworthy.

—— (1982). *Radionics: Science or magic?* Daniel, Saffron Walden, Essex.

Westlake, A.T. (1973). *The pattern of health: A search for a greater understanding of the life force in health and disease*. Shambhala, Colorado.

Index

Abrams, Dr. Albert 260-1
abdominal disorders 110, 122
acidity 181
Aconite 266
Acropolis 80
acupuncture 3, 5, 13, 14, 27-8, 31,
   42-4, 46, 54-6, 59, 67, 74,
   79-80, 90, 108-10, 119-33, 216,
   221
   anaesthesia 19, 119
   analgesia 206
   in Australia 34, 100-4
   in back problems 48
   British Association of 59
   British College of 54, 59
   in China 107-11
   College of Traditional 54
   diagnosis in 6, 7, 46, 56, 122-6
   diet and 122, 126
   ear 7, 129
   and EEC 96-8
   in Finland 96
   in France 91, 129
   and Government 18, 64-5, 74,
      79-80, 109
   with herbalism 185
   in kidney function 9
   meridians and points 6, 7, 23, 108,
      122-4, 127-9, 216-17
   and moxibustion 107, 125-6
   NHS clinics 67
   needles in 13, 119, 125-6, 216
   problems suitable for treatment
      by 33-4, 127-9
   in pregnancy 126
   and professional associations 59-61
   pulse reading in 6, 56, 123-5
   with radionics 267
   registration of 61, 74, 101-2
   research in 20, 23, 127-9
   Society of International 91
   success rate of 128

techniques of 122-6
in Third World 110
training in 50-6, 112
in USA 88
in USSR 98, 99
in West Germany 89
and WHO 110, 127
addictions 127, 129
Advertising Standards Authority 75-6
Aesculapius 12-13
Africa 104-6, 201
agriculture 239, 267
alchoholism 236, 250
Alexander, F.M. 135, 137
Alexander Technique 5, 6, 50, 135-7
All-China Association of Traditional
   Chinese Medicine 109
allergic conditions 32-3, 179, 197, 203,
   206-8, 217, 236, 242, 245, 267
Alma-Ata, USSR 105
Aloe Vera 180, 183
alteratives 179
American Holistic Medical
   Association 8
American Naturopathic
   Association 223
amnesia 207
anaesthesia 19, 99, 119, 128-9, 207-8,
   213, 217
analgesia 19, 129, 207
Angelica 182
angina 127, 196, 228
Anglo-European College of
   Chiropractic 52, 57, 157
animal treatment 166-7, 185, 268
Anorexia nervosa 124, 127
Anthroposophical Medical
   Association 149
anthroposophical medicine 5, 89,
   139-50, 155
   diagnosis in 14
   four principles of 141

399

TERESA MCLEAN

METAL JAM

By the time Teresa McLean was twenty-one, she'd been asked to leave her school but had gone to Oxford and come out with a good degree as well as a cricket Blue.

She'd done an array of student jobs, taught, travelled to India and worked with Mother Teresa. She'd always been a try-anything enthusiast, both thoughtful and energetic.

Then came diabetes.

That was over twelve years ago. *Metal Jam* is the story, honest and unflinching, painful but often funny, of those years.

'Excellently written . . . I laughed aloud on several occasions, empathised with some of the less severe incidents and was horrified by others'

Balance

'Thorough and lucid . . . a notable feat of balance'
The Sunday Times

'I couldn't put it down. Packed with information, it is also lively, shocking and extremely funny. An eye-opener of a book, entirely lacking in self-pity'
Mary Craig, author of *Blessings*

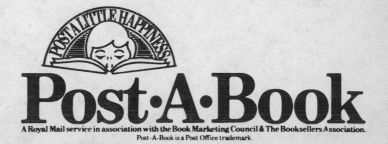

POST A LITTLE HAPPINESS

Post·A·Book

A Royal Mail service in association with the Book Marketing Council & The Booksellers Association.
Post-A-Book is a Post Office trademark.

ANDREW TYLER

STREET DRUGS

Prescribed, trafficked or stolen, drugs are swallowed, smoked, sniffed and injected at all levels of society. Patterns of use and abuse change and change again. Yet accurate information and level-headed advice are hard to come by.

Instead we are bombarded by a succession of panic headlines as scare follows scare. Even medical opinion reverses: yesterday's wonder prescription is today's killer. Fact and fiction are muddled. The law and government policies either limp along behind reality or become sidetracked by moral crusades. History is ignored and lessons never learned.

STREET DRUGS is a much-needed guide to the whole range of drugs – legal and illegal – in use today. Effects and side-effects, trade names and street names, history and geography, methods and fashions, benefits and dangers, are all clearly described.

STREET DRUGS is for drug workers, drug users, teachers, parents, for everyone who needs or wants to know about drugs and drug taking in the Eighties.

HODDER AND STOUGHTON PAPERBACKS

LAURIE TAYLOR AND BOB MULLAN

UNINVITED GUESTS

— *CALVIN (40): "I don't think I've ever once seen an Arab in Dallas. I know America has got its own oil industry but they must have to collaborate with the Arabs from time to time. I don't think I've ever seen an Arab negotiating."*

Previous studies of Britain's viewing and listening habits have been dry sociological surveys. In UNINVITED GUESTS it's the audiences themselves – rather than the academics – who give their views on the programmes which are such an integral part of our popular culture. Their comments – perceptive, knowledgeable and often very funny – form the basis of this highly entertaining account of the *real* effects of television and radio on us all.

'A book full of pleasure and insights: at once an original look at television and a portrait of Britain today . . . valuable and entertaining'

Melvyn Bragg in Punch

'Wholly original, immensely readable and often very funny'

Christopher Dunkley of the Financial Times

HODDER AND STOUGHTON PAPERBACKS

VICTORIA PRINCIPAL

THE DIET PRINCIPAL

Life is a rush. That's true for Victoria Principal and it's true for most women today. There just isn't time for hours spent working out in the gym, for the endless preparation of special foods, for long-winded shopping expeditions.

You really can't plan your life round your diet. Your diet – and Victoria Principal's diet – has to fit in with your life.

So here is how she manages it: not one but *three* complete and easy-to-follow diets, each with its own specific objective and each worked out by Victoria Principal from her own experience (incredibly, she was once 40 pounds overweight).

THE BIKINI DIET: a speedy and safe seven-day plan to help you lose those extra pounds fast.

THE 30-DAY DIET: a more sustained plan to take-off rather more unwanted pounds and to revitalise your body through maximum nutrition.

THE DIET FOR LIFE: a long-term plan to *keep* those pounds off, to maintain your fittest weight and to lead the way to a lifetime of good health.

Three diets with two things in common – They work and they're delicious.

Eating on the run, fitting in with the family or entertaining; *The Diet Principal* makes healthy eating glamorous and practical.

HODDER AND STOUGHTON PAPERBACKS

ELIZABETH WARD

TIMBO: A STRUGGLE FOR SURVIVAL

Many people in Britain today carry a kidney donor card, yet few probably have any idea how, where or why the practice originated. TIMBO, A STRUGGLE FOR SURVIVAL is the personal story that lies behind these cards.

In September 1966, Elizabeth Ward suddenly discovered that her 13-year-old son Timbo had developed a severe kidney problem. It was a discovery that changed the lives not only of the Ward family but of thousands of kidney sufferers throughout Britain, and led to the founding of the British Kidney Patient Association in 1975.

But for Elizabeth Ward, the constant deterioration of Timbo's health was the most painful way to learn about any disease. Together they fought against hospitals, failed transplants, a lack of public awareness, and the disease itself. This book is the story of that struggle.

'Fascinating reading on both human and ethical grounds'
Good Housekeeping

'A story that tugs the heart'
Church Times

'A harrowing and heroic story . . . an inspiring example'
Emlyn Williams

HODDER AND STOUGHTON PAPERBACKS

JOHN LEWIS

A DOCTOR'S OCCUPATION

In 1939 Dr John Lewis was building up a successful general practice in Jersey.

In 1940, as the Germans were poised to invade the Channel Islands, he managed to get his pregnant wife safely across to England. He then returned to Jersey to look after his patients.

In 1945 the German garrison surrendered to the British. Five years of occupation were at an end.

This is the story of Dr Lewis's experiences during those years: a first-hand account of life in the only British territory to be controlled by Nazi Germany during World War II.

HODDER AND STOUGHTON PAPERBACKS

MORE TITLES AVAILABLE FROM
HODDER AND STOUGHTON PAPERBACKS